Immunology
and Evolution of
Infectious Disease

Immunology and Evolution of Infectious Disease

STEVEN A. FRANK

Princeton University Press
Princeton and Oxford

Library of Congress Cataloging-in-Publication Data

Frank, Steven A., 1957–
Immunology and Evolution of Infectious Disease /
Steven A. Frank. p.   cm.
Includes bibliographic references and index.
ISBN 0-691-09594-9 (cloth : alk. paper)
ISBN 0-691-09595-7 (pbk. : alk. paper)
1. Immunogenetics. 2. Host-parasite relationships—
Genetic aspects. 3. Microorganisms—Evolution.
4. Antigens. 5. Molecular evolution.
6. Parasite antigens—Variation. I. Title.
[DNLM: 1. Communicable Diseases—immunology.
2. Evolution, Molecular. 3. Genetics, Population.
4. Immunity—genetics. WC 100 F828i 2002]
QR184 .F73 2002
616.9′0479—dc21   2002018384

British Library Cataloging-in-Publication Data is available

Typeset by the author with TEX
Composed in Lucida Bright

Printed on acid-free paper. ∞

www.pupress.princeton.edu

Printed in the United States of America

10 9 8 7 6 5 4 3 2

10 9 8 7 6 5 4 3 2
(Pbk.)

Contents

PART V: STUDYING EVOLUTION

Acknowledgments

My wife, Robin Bush, read earlier drafts and helped in every way. Camille Barr provided comments on the entire manuscript. My department, led by Chair Al Bennett, gave me the freedom to read and write over nearly two years. The National Science Foundation and the National Institutes of Health funded my research. My web pages at http://stevefrank.org/ provide information and updates for this book.

Immunology and Evolution of Infectious Disease

1   Introduction

Multidisciplinary has become the watchword of modern biology. Surely, the argument goes, a biologist interested in the biochemical pathways by which genetic variants cause disease would also want to understand the population processes that determine the distribution of genetic variants. And how can one expect to understand the interacting parts of complex immune responses without knowing something of the historical and adaptive processes that built the immune system?

Working in the other direction, evolutionary biologists have often treated amino acid substitutions within a parasite lineage as simply statistical marks to be counted and analyzed by the latest mathematical techniques. More interesting work certainly follows when hypotheses about evolutionary change consider the different selective pressures caused by antibody memory, variation among hosts in MHC genotype, and the epidemiological contrasts between rapidly and slowly spreading infectious diseases.

Synthesis between the details of molecular biology and the lives of organisms in populations will proceed slowly. It is now hard enough to keep up in one's own field, and more difficult to follow the foreign concepts and language of other subjects. The typical approach to synthesis uses an academic discipline to focus a biological subject. I use the biological problem of parasite variation to tie together many different approaches and levels of analysis.

Why should parasite variation be the touchstone for the integration of disciplines in modern biology? On the practical side, infectious disease remains a major cause of morbidity and mortality. Consequently, great research effort has been devoted to parasites and to host immune responses that fight parasites. This has led to rapid progress in understanding the biology of parasites, including the molecular details about how parasites invade hosts and escape host immune defenses. Vaccines have followed, sometimes with spectacular success.

But many parasites escape host defense by varying their *antigenic* molecules recognized by host immunity. Put another way, rapid evolution of antigenic molecules all too often prevents control of parasite populations. The challenge has been to link molecular understanding of parasite molecules to their evolutionary change and to the antigenic variation in populations of parasites.

On the academic side, the growth of information about antigenic variation provides a special opportunity. For example, one can find in the literature details about how single amino acid changes in parasite molecules allow escape from antibody binding, and how that escape promotes the spread of variant parasites. Evolutionary studies no longer depend on abstractions—one can pinpoint the physical basis for success or failure and the consequences for change in populations.

Molecular understanding of host-parasite recognition leads to a comparative question about the forces that shape variability. Why do some viruses escape host immunity by varying so rapidly over a few years, whereas other viruses hardly change their antigens? The answer leads to the processes that shape genetic variability and evolutionary change. The causes of variability and change provide the basis for understanding why simple vaccines work well against some viruses, whereas complex vaccine strategies achieve only limited success against other viruses.

I did not start out by seeking a topic for multidisciplinary synthesis. Rather, I have long been interested in how the molecular basis of recognition between attackers and defenders sets the temporal and spatial scale of the battle. Attack and defense occur between insects and the plants they eat, between fungi and the crop plants they destroy, between viruses and the bacteria they kill, between different chromosomes competing for transmission through gametes, and between vertebrate hosts and their parasites. The battle often comes down to the rates at which attacker and defender molecules bind or evade each other. The biochemical details of binding and recognition set the rules of engagement that shape the pacing, scale, and pattern of diversity and the nature of evolutionary change.

Of the many cases of attack and defense across all of biology, the major parasites of humans and their domestic animals provide the most information ranging from the molecular to the population levels. New advances in the conceptual understanding of attack and defense will likely rise from the facts and the puzzles of this subject. I begin by putting the diverse, multidisciplinary facts into a coherent whole. From that foundation, I describe new puzzles and define the key problems for the future study of parasite variation and escape from host recognition.

I start at the most basic level, the nature of binding and recognition between host and parasite molecules. I summarize the many different ways in which parasites generate new variants in order to escape molecular recognition.

Next, I build up the individual molecular interactions into the dynamics of a single infection within a host. The parasites spread in the host, triggering immune attack against dominant antigens. The battle within the host develops through changes in population numbers—the numbers of parasites with particular antigens and the numbers of immune cells that specifically bind to particular antigens.

I then discuss how the successes and failures of different parasite antigens within each host determine the rise and fall of parasite variants over space and time. The distribution of parasite variants sets the immune memory profiles of different hosts, which in turn shape the landscape in which parasite variants succeed or fail. These coevolutionary processes determine the natural selection of antigenic variants and the course of evolution in the parasite population.

Finally, I consider different ways to study the evolution of antigenic variation. Experimental evolution of parasites under controlled conditions provides one way to study the relations between molecular recognition, the dynamics of infections within hosts, and the evolutionary changes in parasite antigens. Sampling of parasites from evolving populations provides another way to test ideas about what shapes the distribution of parasite variants.

My primary goal is to synthesize across different levels of analysis. How do the molecular details of recognition and specificity shape the changing patterns of variants in populations? How does the epidemiological spread of parasites between hosts shape the kinds and amounts of molecular variation in parasite antigens?

I compare different types of parasites because comparative biology provides insight into evolutionary process. For example, parasites that spread rapidly and widely in host populations create a higher density of immune memory in their hosts than do parasites that spread slowly and sporadically. Host species that quickly replace their populations with offspring decay their population-wide memory of antigens faster than do host species that reproduce more slowly. How do these epidemiological and demographic processes influence molecular variation of parasite antigens?

I end each chapter with a set of problems for future research. These problems emphasize the great opportunities of modern biology. At the molecular level, new technologies provide structural data on the three-dimensional shape of host antibody molecules bound to parasite antigens. At the population level, genomic sequencing methods provide detailed data on the variations in parasite antigens. One can now map the nucleotide variations of antigens and their associated amino acid substitutions with regard to the three-dimensional location of antibody binding. Thus, the spread of nucleotide variations in populations can be directly associated with the changes in molecular binding that allow escape from antibody recognition.

No other subject provides such opportunity for integrating the recent progress in structural and molecular analysis with the conceptual and methodological advances in population dynamics and evolutionary biology. My problems for future research at the end of each chapter emphasize the new kinds of questions that one can ask by integrating different levels of biological analysis.

Part I of the book gives general background. Chapter 2 summarizes the main features of vertebrate immunity. I present enough about the key cells and molecules so that one can understand how immune recognition shapes the diversity of parasites.

Chapter 3 describes various benefits that antigenic variation provides to parasites. These benefits explain why parasites vary in certain ways. For example, antigenic variation can help to escape host immunity during a single infection, extending the time a parasite can live within a particular host. Or antigenic variation may avoid the immunological memory of hosts, allowing the variant to spread in a population that previously encountered a different variant of that parasite. Different benefits favor different patterns of antigenic variation.

Part II introduces molecular processes. Chapter 4 describes the attributes of host and parasite molecules that contribute to immune recognition. The nature of recognition depends on specificity, the degree to which the immune system distinguishes between different antigens. Sometimes two different antigens bind to the same immune receptors, perhaps with different binding strength. This cross-reactivity protects hosts against certain antigenic variants, and sets the molecular distance by which antigenic types must vary to escape recognition. Cross-reactivity may also interfere with immune recognition when immune receptors bind a variant sufficiently to prevent a new response but not strongly enough to clear the variant.

Chapter 5 summarizes the different ways in which parasites generate antigenic variants. Many parasites generate variants by the standard process of rare mutations during replication. Baseline mutation rates vary greatly, from about 10^{-5} per nucleotide per generation for the small genomes of some RNA viruses to about 10^{-11} for larger genomes. Although mutations occur rarely at any particular site during replication, large populations generate significant numbers of mutations in each generation. Some parasites focus hypermutation directly on antigenic loci. Other parasites store within each genome many genetic variants for an antigenic molecule. These parasites express only one genetic variant at a time and use specialized molecular mechanisms to switch gene expression between the variants.

Part III focuses on the dynamics of a single infection within a particular host. Chapter 6 emphasizes the host side, describing how the immune response develops strongly against only a few of the many different antigens that occur in each parasite. This immunodominance arises from interactions between the populations of immune cells with different recognition specificities and the population of parasites within the host. Immunodominance determines which parasite antigens face strong pressure from natural selection and therefore which antigens are likely to vary over space and time. To understand immunodominance, I step through the dynamic processes that regulate an immune response and determine which recognition specificities become amplified.

Chapter 7 considers the ways in which parasites escape recognition during an infection and the consequences for antigenic diversity within hosts. The chapter begins with the role of escape by mutation in persistent infections by HIV and hepatitis C virus. I then discuss how other parasites extend infection by switching gene expression between variants stored within each genome. This switching leads to interesting population dynamics within the host. The different variants rise and fall in abundance according to the rate of switching between variants, the time lag in the expansion of parasite lineages expressing a particular variant, and the time lag in the host immune response to each variant.

Part IV examines variability in hosts and parasites across entire populations. Chapter 8 considers genetic differences among hosts in immune response. Hosts differ widely in their major histocompatibility complex (MHC) alleles, which cause different hosts to recognize and focus their immune responses on different parasite antigens. This host variability can strongly affect the relative success of antigenic variants as they attempt to spread from host to host. Hosts also differ in minor ways in other genetic components of specific recognition. Finally, host polymorphisms occur in the regulation of the immune response. These quantitative differences in the timing and intensity of immune reactions provide an interesting model system for studying the genetics of regulatory control.

Chapter 9 describes differences among hosts in their molecular memory of antigens. Each host typically retains the ability to respond quickly to antigens that it encountered in prior infections. This memory protects the host against reinfection by the same antigens, but not against antigenic variants that escape recognition. Each host has a particular memory profile based on past infections. The distribution of memory profiles in the host population determines the ability of particular antigenic variants to spread between hosts. Hosts retain different kinds of immunological memory (antibody versus T cell), which affect different kinds of parasites in distinct ways.

Chapter 10 reviews the genetic structure of parasite populations. The genetic structure of nonantigenic loci provides information about the spatial distribution of genetic variability, the mixing of parasite lineages by transmission between hosts, and the mixing of genomes by sexual processes. The genetic structure of antigenic loci can additionally be affected by the distribution of host immunological memory, because parasites must avoid the antigen sets stored in immunological memory. Host selection on antigenic sets could potentially structure the parasite population into distinct antigenic strains. Finally, each host forms a separate island that divides the parasite population from other islands (hosts). This island structuring of parasite populations can limit the exchange of parasite genes by sexual processes, causing a highly inbred structure. Island structuring also means that each host receives a small and stochastically variable sample of the parasite population. Stochastic fluctuations may play an important role in the spatial distribution of antigenic variation.

Part V considers different methods to study the evolutionary processes that shape antigenic variation. Chapter 11 contrasts two different ways to classify parasite variants sampled from populations. Immunological assays compare the binding of parasite isolates to different immune molecules. The reactions of each isolate with each immune specificity form a matrix from which one can classify antigenic variants according to the degree to which they share recognition by immunity. Alternatively, one can classify isolates phylogenetically, that is, by time since divergence from a common ancestor. Concordant immunological and phylogenetic classifications frequently arise because immunological distance often increases with time since a common ancestor, reflecting the natural tendency for similarity by common descent. Discordant patterns of immunological and phylogenetic classifications indicate some evolutionary pressure on antigens that distorts immunological similarity. I show how various concordant and discordant relations point to particular hypotheses about the natural selection of antigenic properties in influenza and HIV.

Chapter 12 introduces experimental evolution, a controlled method to test hypotheses about the natural selection of antigenic diversity. This chapter focuses on foot-and-mouth disease virus. This well-studied virus illustrates how one can measure multiple selective forces on particular amino acids. Selective forces on amino acids in viral surface molecules include altered binding to host-cell receptors and changed binding to host antibodies. The selective forces imposed by antibodies and by attachment to host-cell receptors can be varied in experimental evolution studies to test their effects on amino acid change in the parasite. The amino acid substitutions can also be mapped onto three-dimensional structural models of the virus to analyze how particular changes alter binding properties.

Chapter 13 continues with experimental evolution of influenza A viruses. Experimental evolution has shown how altering the host species favors specific amino acid changes in the influenza surface protein that binds to host cells. Experimental manipulation of host-cell receptors and antibody pressure can be combined with structural data to understand selection on the viral surface amino acids. These mechanistic analyses of selection can be combined with observations on evolutionary change in natural populations to gain a better understanding of how selection shapes the observed patterns of antigenic variation.

Chapter 14 discusses experimental evolution of antigenic escape from host T cells. The host T cells can potentially bind to any short peptide of an intracellular parasite, whereas antibodies typically bind only to the surface molecules of parasites. T cell binding to parasite peptides depends on a sequence of steps by which hosts cut up parasite proteins and present the resulting peptides on the surfaces of host cells. Parasite escape from T cell recognition can occur at any of the processing steps, including the digestion of proteins, the transport of peptides, the binding of peptides by the highly specific host MHC molecules, and the binding of peptide-MHC complexes to receptors on the T cells. One or two amino acid substitutions in a parasite protein can often abrogate binding to MHC molecules or to the T cell receptors. Experimental evolution has helped us to understand escape from T cells because many of the steps can be controlled, such as the MHC alleles carried by the host and the specificities of the T cell receptors. Parasite proteins may be shaped by opposing pressures on physiological performance and escape from recognition.

Chapter 15 turns to samples of nucleotide sequences from natural populations. A phylogenetic classification of sequences provides a historical reconstruction of evolutionary relatedness and descent. Against the backdrop of ancestry, one can measure how natural selection has changed particular attributes of parasite antigens. For example, one can study whether selection caused particular amino acids to change rapidly or slowly. The rates of change for particular amino acids can be compared with the three-dimensional structural location of the amino acid site, the effects on immunological recognition, and the consequences for binding to host cells. The changes in natural populations can also be compared with patterns of change in experimental evolution, in which one controls particular selective forces. Past evolutionary change in population samples may be used to predict which amino acid variants in antigens are likely to spread in the future.

The last chapter recaps some interesting problems for future research that highlight the potential to study parasites across multiple levels of analysis.

PART I

BACKGROUND

2 Vertebrate Immunity

"The CTLs destroy host cells when their TCRs bind matching MHC-peptide complexes." This sort of jargon-filled sentence dominates discussions of the immune response to parasites. I had initially intended this book to avoid such jargon, so that any reasonably trained biologist could read any chapter without getting caught up in technical terms. I failed—the quoted sentence comes from a later section in this chapter.

The vertebrate immune system has many specialized cells and molecules that interact in particular ways. One has to talk about those cells and molecules, which means that they must be named. I could have tried a simpler or more logically organized naming system, but then I would have created a private language that does not match the rest of the literature. Thus, I use the standard technical terms.

In this chapter, I introduce the major features of immunity shared by vertebrates. I present enough about the key cells and molecules so that one can understand how immune recognition shapes the diversity of parasites. I have not attempted a complete introduction to immunology, because many excellent ones already exist. I recommend starting with Sompayrac's (1999) *How the Immune System Works*, which is a short, wonderfully written primer. One should keep a good textbook by one's side—I particularly like Janeway et al. (1999). Mims's texts also provide good background because they describe immunology in relation to parasite biology (Mims et al. 1998, 2001).

The first section of this chapter describes nonspecific components of immunity. Nonspecific recognition depends on generic signals of parasites such as common polysaccharides in bacterial cell walls. These signals trigger various killing mechanisms, including the complement system, which punches holes in the membranes of invading cells, and the phagocytes, which engulf invaders.

The second section introduces specific immunity, the recognition of small regions on particular parasite molecules. Specific recognition occurs when molecules of the host immune system bind to a molecular shape on the parasite that is not shared by other parasites. Sometimes all parasites of the same species share the specificity, and recognition differentiates between different kinds of parasites. Other times, different parasite genotypes vary in molecular shape, so that the host molecules that bind specifically to one parasite molecule do not bind another parasite molecule that differs by as little as one amino acid. A parasite molecule that stimulates specific recognition is called an *antigen*. The small region of the parasite molecule recognized by the host is called an *epitope*. Antigenic variation occurs when a specific immune response against one antigenic molecule fails to recognize a variant antigenic molecule.

The third section presents the B cells, which secrete antibodies. Antibodies are globular proteins that fight infection by binding to small regions (epitopes) on the surface molecules of parasites. Different antibodies bind to different epitopes. An individual can make billions of different antibodies, each with different binding specificity. Diverse antibodies provide recognition and defense against different kinds of parasites, and against particular parasites that vary genetically in the structure of their surface molecules. Antibodies bind to surface molecules and help to clear parasites outside of host cells.

The fourth section focuses on specific recognition by the T cells. Host cells continually break up intracellular proteins into small peptides. The hosts' major histocompatibility complex (MHC) molecules bind short peptides in the cell. The cell then transports the bound peptide-MHC pair to the cell surface for presentation to roving T cells. Each T cell has receptors that can bind only to particular peptide-MHC combinations presented on the surface of cells. Different T cell clones produce different receptors. When a T cell binds to a peptide-MHC complex on the cell surface and also receives stimulatory signals suggesting parasite invasion, the T cell can trigger the death of the infected cell. T cells bind to parasite peptides digested in infected cells and presented on the infected cell's surface, helping to clear intracellular infections.

The final section summarizes the roles of antibodies and T cells in specific immunity.

2.1 Nonspecific Immunity

Nonspecific immunity recognizes parasites by generic signs that indicate the parasite is an invader rather than a part of the host. The nonspecific complement system consists of different proteins that work together to punch holes in the surfaces of cells. Host cells have several surface molecules that shut off complement attack, causing complement to be directed only against invading cells. Common structural carbohydrates found on the surfaces of many parasites trigger complement attack, whereas the host cells' carbohydrate molecules do not trigger complement.

Phagocytic cells such as macrophages and neutrophils engulf invading parasite cells. Various signals indicate to the phagocytes that nearby cells are invaders. For example, certain lipopolysaccharides commonly occur in the outer walls of gram-negative bacteria such as *E. coli*. Mannose, which occurs in the cell walls of many invaders, also stimulates phagocytes. In addition, phagocytes respond to signs of tissue damage and inflammation.

Nonspecific defense by itself may not entirely clear an infection, and in some cases parasites can avoid nonspecific defense. For example, the protective capsules of staphylococci and the surface polysaccharide side chains of salmonellae protect those bacteria from attachment by nonspecific killing molecules (Mims et al. 1993, p. 12.2).

2.2 Specific Immunity: Antigens and Epitopes

Nonspecific immunity recognizes common, repetitive structural features that distinguish parasites from the host's cells. By contrast, specific immunity recognizes small regions of particular parasite molecules. Specific recognition may depend on just five or ten amino acids of a parasite protein. Such specificity means that different parasite species often differ at recognition sites. Indeed, different parasite genotypes may vary such that a host can recognize particular sites on one genotype but not on another.

This book is about parasite variation in regard to specific immunity, so it is important to get the jargon right. Specific host immunity recognizes and binds to an *epitope,* which is a small molecular site within a larger parasite molecule. An *antigen* is a parasite molecule that stimulates a specific immune response because it contains one or more epitopes. For example, if one injects a large foreign protein into a host, the host recognizes thousands of different epitopes on the surface of the protein antigen.

Antigenic variation occurs when a specific immune response against one antigenic molecule fails to recognize a variant antigenic molecule. The antigenic variants differ at one or more epitopes, the sites recognized by specific immunity.

2.3 B Cells and Antibodies

B cells mature in the bone marrow (bursa in birds). They then develop into lymphocytes, immune cells that circulate in the blood and lymph systems. B cells express globular proteins (immunoglobulins) on their cell surfaces. These immunoglobulins form the B cell receptors (BCRs). B cells also secrete those same immunoglobulins, which circulate as antibodies. In other words, antibodies are simply secreted BCRs. I will often use the word *antibody* for *B cell immunoglobulin,* but it is important to remember that the same immunoglobulins can be either BCRs or antibodies. Immunoglobulin is usually abbreviated as Ig.

The B cells generate alternative antibody specificities by specially controlled recombination and mutation processes (fig. 2.1). The host maintains a huge diversity of antibody specificities, each specificity in low abundance. Novel parasite epitopes often bind to at least one rare antibody specificity. Binding stimulates the B cells to divide, forming an expanded clonal lineage that increases production of the matching antibody.

Each antibody molecule has two kinds of amino acid chains, the heavy chains and the light chains (fig. 2.1). A heavy chain has three regions that affect recognition, variable (V), diversity (D), and joining (J). A light chain has only the V and J regions. In humans, there are approximately one hundred different V genes, twelve D genes, and four J genes (Janeway 1993).

Each progenitor of a B cell clone undergoes a special type of DNA recombination that brings together a V-D-J combination to form a heavy chain coding region. There are $100 \times 12 \times 4 = 4,800$ V-D-J combinations. A separate recombination event creates a V-J combination for the light chain, of which there are $100 \times 4 = 400$ combinations. The independent formation of heavy and light chains creates the potential for $4,800 \times 400 = 1,920,000$ different antibodies. In addition, randomly chosen DNA bases are added between the segments that are brought together by recombination, greatly increasing the total number of antibody types.

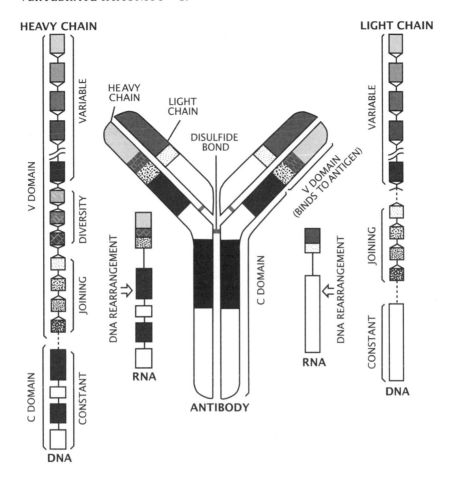

Figure 2.1   The coding and assembly of antibody molecules. Randomly chosen alternatives of the variable (V), diversity (D), and joining (J) regions from different DNA modules combine to form an RNA transcript, which is then translated into a protein chain.   Two heavy and two light chains are assembled into an antibody molecule.   The constant region is sometimes referred to as the Fc fragment, and the variable region as the Fab fragment. Redrawn from Janeway (1993), with permission from Roberto Osti.

Recombination creates a large number of different antibodies.   Initially, each of these antibodies is rare.   Upon infection a few of these rare types may match a parasite epitope, stimulating amplification of the B cell clones.   The matching B cells increase their mutation rate, creating many slightly different antibodies that vary in their affinity to the

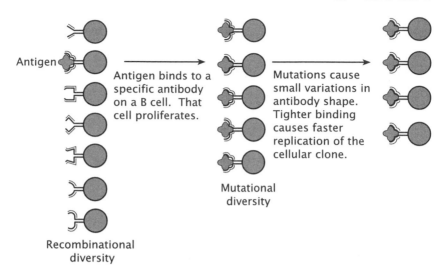

Antigen

Antigen binds to a specific antibody on a B cell. That cell proliferates.

Mutations cause small variations in antibody shape. Tighter binding causes faster replication of the cellular clone.

Mutational diversity

Recombinational diversity

Figure 2.2 Clonal selection of B cells to produce antibodies that match an epi-tope of an invading antigen. Recombinational mechanisms produce a wide va-riety of different antibody molecules (fig. 2.1). All B cells of a particular clone are derived from a single ancestral cell that underwent recombination. Mem-bers of a clone express only a single antibody type. Cells are stimulated to divide rapidly when an epitope matches the antibody receptor. This creates a large population of B cells that can bind the epitope. These cells undergo in-creased mutation in their antibody gene during cell division, producing a set of antibodies that vary slightly in their binding properties. Stronger binding causes more rapid cellular reproduction. This affinity maturation enhances the antibody-epitope fit. Modified from Golub and Green (1991).

invader (fig. 2.2). Those mutant cells that bind more tightly are stimu-lated to divide more rapidly. This evolutionary fine-tuning of the B cell population is called *affinity maturation.*

Naive B cells produce IgM immunoglobulins before stimulation and affinity maturation. After affinity maturation, B cells produce various types of immunoglobulins by changing the constant region (fig. 2.1). The most common are IgG in the circulatory system and IgA on mucosal surfaces.

On first encounter with a novel parasite, the rare, matching antibodies cannot control infection. While the host increases production of match-ing antibodies, the infection spreads. Eventually the host may produce sufficient antibody to clear parasites that carry the matching epitope. If the parasites, in turn, vary the matched epitope, the host must expand new antibody types to clear the variant parasites.

Once the host expands an antibody specificity against a matching epitope, it maintains a memory of that epitope. Upon later exposure to the same epitope, the host can quickly produce large numbers of matching antibodies. This memory allows the host to clear subsequent reinfection without noticeable symptoms.

Antibodies typically bind to surface epitopes of parasites. Thus, antibodies aid clearance of parasites circulating in the blood or otherwise exposed to direct attack. Once an intracellular parasite enters a host cell, the host must use other defenses such as T cells.

2.4 T Cells and MHC

Host cells continually break up intracellular proteins into small peptides. The host's major histocompatibility complex (MHC) molecules bind these short peptides within the cell. The cell then transports the bound peptide-MHC pair to the cell surface for presentation to roving T cells. T cells are lymphocytes that mature in the thymus.

T cell receptors (TCRs) vary in binding specificity. Each T cell receptor can bind only to particular peptide-MHC combinations presented on the surface of cells. Different T cell clones produce different TCRs. The TCR variability is generated by a process similar to the recombinational mechanisms that produce antibody diversity in B cells. However, T cells do not go through affinity maturation, so once the recombination process sets the TCR for a T cell lineage, the TCR does not change much for that lineage.

A parasite peptide is called an epitope when it binds to MHC and a TCR. In this case, an antigen is the protein from the which the epitope is digested.

There are two different kinds of MHC molecules and two main classes of T cells. Most cells of the body express the MHC class I molecules, presenting class I peptide-MHC complexes on their surface. The class I molecules bind a subset of T cells that have the cellular determinant protein CD8 on their surface, the CD8$^+$ T cells. When the CD8$^+$ T cells are stimulated by various signals of attack, they become armed with killing function and are known as cytotoxic T lymphocytes (CTLs). The CTLs destroy host cells when their TCRs bind matching peptide-MHC complexes. The CTLs play a central role in clearing intracellular infections.

Specialized antigen-presenting cells (APCs) take up external proteins including parasite proteins, digest those proteins into short peptides, and present the peptides bound to MHC class II molecules. T cells with the cellular determinant protein CD4 on their surface, the CD4$^+$ T cells, can bind to class II peptide-MHC complexes presented on the surfaces of APCs if they have matching TCRs. The CD4$^+$ cells are often called *helper T cells* because they frequently provide a helping signal needed to stimulate an antibody or CTL response.

Upon first exposure to a parasite, some of the parasite epitopes presented by MHC will match rare TCR specificities. TCR binding along with other stimulatory signals trigger rapid division of T cell clones with matching TCR specificities. The first infection by a parasite may spread widely in the host before matching T cells can be amplified. After amplification, eventual clearance of parasites with matching epitopes may end the infection or may favor the rise of variant epitopes, which must also be recognized and cleared. Once the host expands a TCR specificity against a matching epitope, it often maintains a memory of that epitope. Upon later exposure to the same epitope, the host produces large numbers of matching T cells more quickly than on first exposure.

T cells can recognize only those epitopes that bind to MHC for presentation. MHC class I binding specificity depends on short peptides of about 8–10 amino acids; class II binds to a sequence of about 13–17 amino acids (Janeway et al. 1999). The highly polymorphic MHC alleles vary between host individuals, causing each individual to have a particular spectrum of presentation efficiencies for different peptides. Thus, the strength of a host's response to a particular epitope depends on its MHC genotype.

2.5 Summary

I have greatly simplified the immune response. For example, different kinds of "helper" T cells regulate B cell stimulation, antibody affinity maturation, deployment and maintenance of CTLs, and other immune responses. Among antibodies, specialized types stimulate different inflammatory responses or killing mechanisms.

In spite of this complexity, antibodies do play a key role in clearing parasites located outside of cells, and MHC presentation to specific T cell receptors plays a key role in defense against parasites located within cells. B and T cell recognition is highly specific to particular epitopes, which are often small sets of amino acids. Parasites can escape that specific recognition by varying only one or two amino acids in an epitope. This recognition and escape provides the basis for antigenic variation.

3   Benefits of Antigenic Variation

In this chapter, I describe the benefits that antigenic variation provides to parasites. These benefits help to explain why parasites vary in certain ways.

The first section examines how antigenic variants can extend the time a parasite maintains an infection within a host. The initial parasite type stimulates an immune response against its dominant antigens. If the parasite changes those antigens to new variants, it escapes immunity and continues a vigorous infection until the host generates a new response against the variants. Some parasites generate novel antigens by random mutations during replication. Other parasites store in their genomes alternative genes encoding variants of dominant antigens. Such parasites occasionally switch expression between the archived variants, allowing escape from specific immunity.

The second section presents how antigenic variants can reinfect hosts with immune memory. Host immune memory recognizes and mounts a rapid response against previously encountered antigens. Antigenic variants that differ from a host's previous infections escape that host's memory response. The distribution of immune memory profiles between hosts determines the success of each parasite variant.

The third section suggests that particular antigenic variants can attack some host genotypes but not others. For example, hosts vary in their MHC genotype, which determines the T cell epitopes each host can recognize. An epitope often can be recognized by one rare MHC allele but not by others. Each antigenic variant has its own distribution of host genotypes on which it does best at avoiding MHC recognition. Hosts also vary in the cellular receptors used for attachment by parasite surface antigens. Variation in surface antigens may allow parasites to attach with variable success to cellular receptors of different host genotypes.

The fourth section proposes that variable surface antigens sometimes enhance parasite fitness by allowing colonization of different host tissues. For example, certain antigenic variants of the blood-borne spirochete *Borrelia turicatae* sequester in the brain, protected from immune pressure. Antigenic variants of *Plasmodium falciparum* affect cytoad-herence to capillary endothelia, which influences the tendency of the parasite to be hidden from sites of powerful immune activity. Sequestered variants may prolong infection or provide a source for reestablishing infection after the majority of parasites have been cleared from other body compartments. Many antigenic variants of *B. turicatae* and *P. falciparum* arise during a single infection because both species change surface antigens by switching gene expression between loci in a genomic archive of variants. Those surface variants stimulate strong antibody responses, suggesting that both immune escape and variable tissue tropism can provide important benefits for antigenic variation.

The fifth section describes how some antigenic variants interfere with the immune response to other variants. For example, a host may first encounter a particular antigenic type and then later become infected by a cross-reacting variant. The second infection sometimes stimulates a host memory response to the first variant rather than a new, specific response to the second variant. The memory response to the first variant may not clear the second variant effectively. Thus, hosts' memory profiles can benefit certain cross-reacting variants. In other cases, one variant may interfere with a host's ability to respond to another variant. This antagonism may cause the interacting variants to occur together because one or both variants enjoy the protection created by the presence of the other variant.

The final section outlines promising topics of study for future research.

3.1 Extend Length of Infection

Many parasites follow a simple pattern of infection and clearance. The measles virus, for example, multiplies and develops a large population in the host upon first infection (Griffin 2001). As the initial parasitemia builds, the host develops a specific immune response that eventually clears the infection. That same host rapidly clears later measles reinfections by specific immunity against the measles virus. Immunity that protects against reinfection develops from special memory components of the immune system. The immune system attacks conserved epitopes of the measles virus that do not vary significantly between viruses. Thus, measles does not escape immunity by changing its dominant antigens.

Other parasites begin their infection cycle in the same way—a large initial parasitemia followed by reduction when the host mounts a specific immune response against a dominant epitope. But some parasites can alter their dominant epitope. Antigenic variants escape recognition by the first wave of specific host defense against the initial antigenic type, extending the length of infection.

Trypanosoma brucei changes its dominant antigenic surface glycoprotein at a rate of 10^{-3} to 10^{-2} per cell division (Turner 1997). The trypanosome changes to another surface coat by altering expression between different genes already present in the genome. Infections lead to successive waves of parasitemia and clearance as novel antigenic types spread and are then checked by specific immunity.

Some viruses, such as HIV, escape immune attack by mutating their dominant epitopes (McMichael and Phillips 1997). Mutational changes to new, successful epitopes may be rare in each replication of the virus. But the very large population size of viruses within a host means that mutations, rare in each replication, often occur at least once in the host in each parasite generation.

For parasites that produce antigenic variants within hosts, the infection continues until the host controls all variants, raises an immune response against a nonvarying epitope, or clears the parasite by nonspecific defenses.

Antigenic variation can extend the total time before clearance (Moxon et al. 1994; Deitsch et al. 1997; Fussenegger 1997). Extended infection benefits the parasite by increasing the chances for transmission to new hosts.

3.2 Infect Hosts with Prior Exposure

Hosts often maintain memory against antigens from prior infections. Host memory of particular antigens blocks reinfection by parasites carrying those antigens. Parasites can escape host memory by varying their antigens.

Cross-reaction between antigenic variants occurs when a host can use its specific recognition from exposure to a prior variant to fight against a later, slightly different variant. Cross-reactive protection may provide only partial defense, allowing infection but clearing the parasite more rapidly than in naive hosts.

In the simplest case, each antigenic type acts like a separate parasite that does not cross-react with other variants. The distribution of antigenic variants will be influenced by the rate at which new variants arise and spread and the rate at which old variants are lost from the population. As host individuals age, they become infected by and recover from different antigenic variants. Thus, the host population can be classified by resistance profiles based on the past infection and recovery of each individual (Andreasen et al. 1997).

Two extreme cases define the range of outcomes. On the one hand, each variant may occasionally spread epidemically through the host population. This leaves a large fraction of the hosts resistant upon recovery, driving that particular variant down in frequency because it has few hosts it can infect. The variant can spread again only after many resistant hosts die and are replaced by young hosts without prior exposure to that antigen. In this case, three factors set the temporal pacing for each antigenic variant: host age structure, the rapidity with which variants can spread and be cleared, and the waiting time until a potentially successful variant arises.

Variants may, on the other hand, be maintained endemically in the host population. This requires a balance between the rate at which infections lead to host death or recovery and the rate at which new susceptible hosts enter the population. The parasite population maintains as many variants as arise and do not cross-react, subject to "birth-death" processes governing the stochastic origin of new variants and the loss of existing variants.

These extreme cases set highly simplified end points. In reality, variants may differ in their ability to transmit between hosts and to grow within hosts. Nonspecific immunity or partial resistance to nonvarying or secondary epitopes also complicate the dynamics. Nonetheless, the epidemiology of the parasite, the host age structure and resistance profiles, and the processes that generate new variants drive many aspects of the dynamics.

Cross-reactivity between variants adds another dimension (Andreasen et al. 1997; Lin et al. 1999). The resistance profiles of individual hosts can still be described by history of exposure. However, a new variant's ability to infect a particular host depends on the impedance to the variant caused by the host's exposure profile and the cross-reactivity between antigens.

3.3 Infect Hosts with Genetically Variable Resistance

Host genotype can influence susceptibility to different parasite variants. For example, MHC genotype determines the host's efficiency in presenting particular epitopes to T cells. From the parasite's point of view, a particular antigenic variant may be able to attack some host genotypes but not others.

Hill (1998) pointed out that hepatitis B virus provides a good model for studying the interaction between MHC and parasite epitopes. Preliminary reports found associations between MHC genotype and whether infections were cleared or became persistent (van Hattum et al. 1987; Almarri and Batchelor 1994; Thursz et al. 1995; Hohler et al. 1997). The hepatitis B virus genome is very small (about 3,000 base pairs, or bp), which should allow direct study of how variation in viral epitopes interacts with the host's MHC genotype.

Host genotype can also affect the structure of the cellular receptors to which parasites attach. For example, the human CCR5 gene encodes a coreceptor required for HIV-1 to enter macrophages. A 32bp deletion of this gene occurs at a frequency of 0.1 in European populations. This deletion prevents the virus from entering macrophages (Martinson et al. 1997; O'Brien and Dean 1997; Smith et al. 1997).

It is not clear whether minor variants of cellular receptors occur sufficiently frequently to favor widespread matching variation of parasite surface antigens. Several cases of this sort may eventually be found, but in vertebrate hosts genetic variation of cellular receptors may be a relatively minor cause of parasite diversity.

3.4 Vary Attachment Characters

Parasite surface antigens often play a role in attachment and entry into host cells or attachment to particular types of host tissue. Varying these attachment characters allows attack of different cell types or adhesion to various tissues. Such variability can provide the parasite with additional resources or protection from host defenses.

Several species of the spirochete genus *Borrelia* cause relapsing fever (Barbour and Hayes 1986; Barbour 1987, 1993). Relapses occur because the parasite switches expression between different genetic copies of the major surface antigen. The host develops fever and then clears the initial parasitemia, but suffers a few rounds of relapse as the antigenic variants rise and fall. A subset of antigenic variants of these blood-borne bacteria have a tendency to accumulate in the brain, where they can avoid the host's immune response (Cadavid et al. 2001). Those bacteria in the brain may cause later relapses after the host has cleared the pathogens from the blood. The differing tissue tropisms of the antigenic variants may combine to increase the total parasitemia.

Protozoan parasites of the genus *Plasmodium* cause malaria in a variety of vertebrate hosts. Several *Plasmodium* species switch antigenic type (Brannan et al. 1994). Switching has been studied most extensively in *P. falciparum* (Reeder and Brown 1996). Programmed mechanisms of gene expression choose a single gene from among many archival genetic copies for the *P. falciparum* erythrocyte membrane protein 1 (PfEMP1) (Chen et al. 1998). As its name implies, the parasite expresses this antigen on the surface of infected erythrocytes. PfEMP1 induces an antibody response, which likely plays a role in the host's ability to control infection (Reeder and Brown 1996).

PfEMP1 influences cytoadherence of infected erythrocytes to capillary endothelia (Reeder and Brown 1996). This adherence may help the parasite to avoid clearance in the spleen. Thus, antigenic variants can influence the course of infection by escaping specific recognition and by hiding from host defenses (Reeder and Brown 1996). Full understanding of the forces that have shaped the archival repertoire, switching process, and course of infection requires study of both specific immune recognition and cytoadherence properties of the different antigenic variants.

The bacteria that cause gonorrhea and a type of meningitis have antigenically varying surface molecules. The variable Opa proteins form a family that influences the colony opacity (Malorny et al. 1998). *Neisseria gonorrhoeae* has eleven to twelve *opa* loci in its genome, and *N. meningitidis* has three to four *opa* loci. Any particular bacterial cell typically expresses only one or two of the *opa* loci; cellular lineages change expression in the *opa* loci (Stern et al. 1986). Both conserved and hypervariable regions occur among the loci. The bacteria expose the hypervariable regions on the cell surface (Malorny et al. 1998; Virji et al. 1999). The exposed regions contain domains that affect binding to host cells and to antibody epitopes.

The different antigenic variants within the Opa of proteins family affect tropism for particular classes of host cells (Gray-Owen et al. 1997;

Virji et al. 1999). For *N. gonorrhoeae*, some Opa proteins have an affinity for the host cell surface protein CD66e found on the squamous epithelium of the uterine portio. Other Opa variants bind more effectively to CD66a found on the epithelium of the cervix, uterus, and colon tissues. Thus, the CD66-specific Opa variants may mediate the colonization of different tissues encountered during gonococcal infection (Gray-Owen et al. 1997).

HIV provides the final example for this section. This virus links its surface protein gp120 to two host-cell receptors before it enters the cell (O'Brien and Dean 1997). One host-cell receptor, CD4, appears to be required by most HIV variants (but see Saha et al. 2001). The second host-cell receptor can be CCR5 or CXCR4. Macrophages express CCR5. A host that lacks functional CCR5 proteins apparently can avoid infection by HIV, suggesting that the initial invasion requires infection of macrophages. HIV isolates with tropism for CCR5 can be found throughout the infection; this HIV variant is probably the transmissive form that infects new hosts.

As an infection proceeds within a host, HIV variants with tropism for CXCR4 emerge (O'Brien and Dean 1997). This host-cell receptor occurs on the surface of the $CD4^+$ (helper) T lymphocytes. The emergence of viral variants with tropism for CXCR4 coincides with a drop in $CD4^+$ T cells and onset of the immunosuppression that characterizes AIDS.

These examples show that variable surface antigens may sometimes occur because they provide alternative cell or tissue tropisms rather than, or in addition to, escape from immune recognition.

3.5 Antigenic Interference

Prior exposure of the host to particular epitopes sometimes reduces the host's ability to raise an immune response against slightly altered parasite variants. This interference was first observed in influenza (Fazekas de St. Groth and Webster 1966a, 1966b). In this case, if a host first encounters a variant, *x*, then a later cross-reacting variant, *y*, restimulates an antibody response against *x* rather than stimulating a specific response against *y*. This phenomenon is called *original antigenic sin* because the host tends to restimulate antibodies against the first antigen encountered. A similar pattern has been observed for the cytotoxic T cell response of mice against lymphocytic choriomeningitis virus (Klenerman and Zinkernagel 1998).

In some cases, antibodies from a first infection appear to enhance the success of infection by later, cross-reacting strains (see references in Ferguson et al. 1999). The mechanisms are not clear for many of these cases, but the potential consequences are important. If cross-reactive strains interfere with each other's success, then populations of parasites tend to become organized into nonoverlapping antigenic variants that define strains (Gupta et al. 1998). By contrast, if similar epitopes enhance each other's success, then well-defined strain clustering is less likely (Ferguson et al. 1999).

Simultaneous infection by two related epitopes sometimes interferes with binding by cytotoxic T cells. This interference, called *altered peptide ligand antagonism,* has been observed in HIV, hepatitis B virus, and *Plasmodium falciparum* (Bertoletti et al. 1994; Klenerman et al. 1994; Gilbert et al. 1998). In *P. falciparum,* the MHC molecule HLA-B35 binds two common epitopes of the circumsporozoite protein, cp26 and cp29, but does not bind two other epitopes, cp27 and cp28 (Gilbert et al. 1998). In hosts with HLA-B35, simultaneous infection with cp26 and cp29 appears to limit T cell responsiveness. In natural infections, hosts harbored both cp26 and cp29 variants more often than expected if epitopes were distributed randomly between hosts. Gilbert et al. (1998) suggest that the excess cp26-cp29 infections may have occurred because these two epitopes act synergistically to interfere with T cell response.

3.6 Problems for Future Research

1. Measures of parasite fitness. The first section of this chapter described how antigenic variation potentially extends the length of infection within a single host. Longer infections probably increase the transmission of the parasites to new hosts, increasing the fitness of the parasites. Other attributes of infection dynamics may also contribute to transmission and fitness. For example, the density of parasites in the host may affect the numbers of parasites transmitted by vectors. If so, then a good measure of fitness may be the number of parasites in the host summed over the total length of infection. It would be interesting to study experimentally the relations between infection length, parasite abundance, and transmission success. These relations between parasite characters and fitness strongly influence how selection shapes antigenic variation within hosts.

2. Interference between antigens in archival libraries of variants. Reports of original antigenic sin and altered peptide ligand antagonism have come from observations of antigenic variants generated by mutation. It would be interesting to learn whether parasites with archival variants also induce these phenomena. One might, for example, find that some variants induce a memory response that interferes with the host's ability to generate a specific response to other variants. Thus, the antigenic repertoire in archival libraries may be shaped both by the tendency to avoid cross-reaction and by the degree to which variants can interfere with the immune response to other variants.

PART II

MOLECULAR PROCESSES

4 Specificity and Cross-Reactivity

In this chapter, I describe the attributes of host and parasite molecules that determine immune recognition. Two terms frequently arise in discussions of recognition. Specificity measures the degree to which the immune system differentiates between different antigens. Cross-reactivity measures the extent to which different antigens appear similar to the immune system. The molecular determinants of specificity and cross-reactivity define the nature of antigenic variation and the selective processes that shape the distribution of variants in populations.

The first section discusses antibody recognition. The surfaces of parasite molecules contain many overlapping antibody-binding sites (epitopes). An antibody bound to an epitope covers about 15 amino acids on the surface of a parasite molecule. However, only about 5 of the parasite's amino acids contribute to the binding energy. A change in any of those 5 key amino acids can greatly reduce the strength of antibody binding.

The second section focuses on the paratope, the part of the antibody molecule that binds to an epitope. Antibodies have a variable region of about 50 amino acids that contains many overlapping paratopes. Each paratope has about 15 amino acids, of which about 5 contribute most of the binding energy for epitopes. Paratopes and epitopes define complementary regions of shape and charge rather than particular amino acid compositions. A single paratope can bind to unrelated epitopes, and a single epitope can bind to unrelated paratopes.

The third section introduces the different stages in the maturation of antibody specificity. Naive B cells make IgM antibodies that typically bind with low affinity to epitopes. A particular epitope stimulates division of B cells with relatively higher-affinity IgM antibodies for the epitope. As the stimulated B cell clones divide rapidly, they also mutate their antibody-binding regions at a high rate. Mutant lineages that bind with higher affinity to the target antigen divide more rapidly and outcompete weaker-binding lineages. This mutation and selection produces high-affinity antibodies, typically of type IgA or IgG.

The fourth section describes "natural" antibodies, a class of naive IgM antibodies. Each natural antibody can bind with low affinity to many different epitopes. Natural antibodies from different B cell lineages form a diverse set that binds with low affinity to almost any antigen. One in vitro study of HIV suggested that these background antibodies bind to the viruses with such low affinity that they do not interfere with infection. By contrast, in vivo inoculations with several different pathogens showed that the initial binding by natural antibodies lowered the concentrations of pathogens early in infection by one or two orders of magnitude.

The fifth section contrasts affinity and specificity. Poor binding conditions cause low-affinity binding to be highly specific because detectable bonds form only between the strongest complementary partners. By contrast, favorable binding conditions cause low-affinity binding to develop a relatively broad set of complementary partners, causing relatively low specificity. The appropriate measure of affinity varies with the particular immune process. Early stimulation of B cells appears to depend on the equilibrium binding affinity for antigens. By contrast, competition between B cell clones for producing affinity-matured antibodies appears to depend on the dynamic rates of association between B cell receptors and antigens.

The sixth section compares the cross-reactivity of an in vivo, polyclonal immune response with the cross-reactivity of a purified, monoclonal antibody. Polyclonal immune responses raise antibodies against many epitopes on the surface of an antigen. Cross-reactivity declines linearly with the number of amino acid substitutions between variant antigens because each exposed amino acid contributes only a small amount to the total binding between all antibodies and all epitopes. By contrast, a monoclonal antibody usually binds to a single epitope on the antigen surface. Cross-reactivity declines rapidly and nonlinearly with the number of amino acid substitutions in the target epitope because a small number of amino acids control most of the binding energy.

The seventh section discusses the specificity and cross-reactivity of T cell responses. Four steps determine the interaction between parasite proteins and T cells: the cellular digestion of parasite proteins, the transport of the resulting peptides to the endoplasmic reticulum, the binding of peptides to MHC molecules, and the binding of peptide-MHC complexes to the T cell receptor (TCR). Mason (1999) estimates that each

TCR cross-reacts with $\sim 10^5$ different peptides. If a TCR reacts with a specific peptide, then the probability that it will react with a second, randomly chosen peptide is only $\sim 10^{-4}$. Thus, the TCR can be thought of as highly cross-reactive or highly specific depending on the point of view.

The eighth section lists the ways in which hosts vary genetically in their responses to antigens. MHC alleles are highly polymorphic. The germline genes that contribute to the T cell receptor have some polymorphisms that influence recognition, but the germline B cell receptor genes do not carry any known polymorphisms.

The final section takes up promising lines of study for future research.

4.1 Antigens and Antibody Epitopes

An antigenic molecule stimulates an immune response. Each specific subset of an antigenic molecule recognized by an antibody or a T cell receptor defines an epitope. Each antigen typically has many epitopes. For example, insulin, a dimeric protein with 51 amino acids, has on its surface at least 115 antibody epitopes (Schroer et al. 1983). Nearly the entire surface of an antigen presents many overlapping domains that antibodies can discriminate as distinct epitopes (Benjamin et al. 1984).

Epitopes have approximately 15 amino acids when defined by spatial contact of antibody and epitope during binding (Benjamin and Perdue 1996). Almost all naturally occurring antibody epitopes studied so far are composed of amino acids that are discontinuous in the primary sequence but brought together in space by the folding of the protein.

The relative binding of a native and a mutant antigen to a purified (monoclonal) antibody defines one common measure of cross-reactivity. The native antigen is first used to raise the monoclonal antibody. $C50_{mut}$ is the concentration of the mutant antigen required to cause 50% inhibition of the reaction between the native antigen and the antibody. Similarly, $C50_{nat}$ is the concentration of the native antigen required to cause 50% inhibition of the reaction between the native antigen and the antibody (self-inhibition). Then the relative equilibrium binding constant for the variant antigen, $C50_{nat}/C50_{mut}$, measures cross-reactivity (Benjamin and Perdue 1996).

Site-directed mutagenesis has been used to create epitopes that vary by only a single amino acid. This allows measurement of relative binding caused by an amino acid substitution. Studies differ considerably in the methods used to identify the amino acid sites defining an epitope, the choice of sites to mutate, the amino acids used for substitution, and the calculation of changes in equilibrium binding constants or the free-energy of binding. Benjamin and Perdue (1996) discuss these general issues and summarize analyses of epitopes on four proteins.

Five tentative conclusions about amino acid substitutions suffice for this review. First, approximately 5 of the 15 amino acids in each epitope strongly influence binding. Certain substitutions at each of these strong sites can reduce the relative binding constant by two or three orders of magnitude. These strong sites may contribute about one-half of the total free-energy of the reaction (Dougan et al. 1998).

Second, the other 10 or so amino acids in contact with the antibody may each influence the binding constant by up to one order of magnitude. Some sites may have no detectable effect.

Third, the consequences of mutation at a particular site depend, not surprisingly, on the original amino acid and the amino acid used for substitution.

Fourth, theoretical predictions about the free-energy consequences of substitutions based on physical structure and charge can sometimes be highly misleading. This problem often occurs when the binding location between the antibody and a particular amino acid is highly accessible to solvent, a factor that theoretical calculations have had difficulty incorporating accurately.

Fifth, antibodies raised against a particular epitope might not bind optimally to that epitope—the antibodies sometimes bind more strongly to mutated epitopes. In addition, antibodies with low affinity for an antigen can have higher affinity for related antigens (van Regenmortel 1998).

4.2 Antibody Paratopes

An antibody contains a variety of binding sites. Each antibody binding site defines a paratope, composed of the particular amino acids of that antibody that physically bind to a specific epitope. Approximately 50 variable amino acids make up the potential binding area of an antibody (van Regenmortel 1998). Typically, only about 15 of these 50 amino acids physically contact a particular epitope. These 15 or so contact residues define the structural paratope. Only 5 or so of these amino acids dominate in terms of binding energy. However, in both epitope and paratope, substitutions both in and away from the binding site can change the spatial conformation of the binding region and affect the binding reaction (Wedemayer et al. 1997; van Regenmortel et al. 1998; Lavoie et al. 1999).

The antibody's 50 or so variable amino acids in its binding region define many overlapping groups of 15 amino acids. Thus, an antibody has a large number of potential paratopes. A paratope does not define a single complementary epitope; rather it presents certain molecular characteristics that bind antigenic sites with varying affinity. This leads to four aspects of antibody-antigen specificity.

First, an antibody can have two completely independent binding sites (paratopes) for unrelated epitopes (Richards et al. 1975). Bhattacharjee and Glaudemans (1978) showed that two purified mouse antibodies (M384 and M870) each bind methyl α D-galactopyranoside and phosphorylcholine at two different sites in the antigen-binding region of the antibody.

Second, an antibody presumably has many overlapping paratopes that can potentially bind to a variety of related or unrelated epitopes. I did not, however, find any studies that defined for a particular antibody the paratope map relative to a set of variable epitopes. The potential distribution of paratopes may change as a B cell clone matures in response to challenge by a matching antigen—I take this up in the next section (4.3), on *Antibody Affinity Maturation*.

Third, a single paratope can bind two unrelated epitopes (mimotopes, Pinilla et al. 1999; Gras-Masse et al. 1999). Kramer et al. (1997) scanned a library of synthetically generated peptides for competition in binding to a monoclonal (purified) antibody. X-ray diffraction of three competing peptides showed that they all bound to the same site on the antibody (Keitel et al. 1997).

Fourth, a particular epitope can be recognized by two different paratopes with no sequence similarity. For example, Lescar et al. (1995) used x-ray diffraction to study the physical contact between guinea fowl lysozyme and two different antibodies. The two antibodies contact the same 12 amino acids of the antigen. However, the antibodies have different paratopes with no identical amino acids in the region that binds the antigen. The two antibodies also have different patterns of cross-reactivity with other antigens.

Experimental studies of specificity frequently compare pairwise affinities between an epitope and various paratopes or between a paratope and various epitopes. In these pairwise measures, one first raises antibody to a monomorphic (nonvarying) antigenic molecule and then isolates a single epitope-paratope binding—in other words, one raises a monoclonal antibody that binds to a single antigenic site. Variations in affinity are then measured for different epitopes holding the paratope constant or for different paratopes holding the epitope constant.

Alternatively, one can challenge a host with a polymorphic population of antigens. One controlled approach varies the antigens only in a small region that defines a few epitopes (Gras-Masse et al. 1999). If exact replicas of each epitope occur rarely, then antibodies will be selected according to their binding affinity for the aggregate set of varying epitopes (mixotopes) to which they match. This method may be a good approach for finding antibodies with high cross-reactivity to antigenic variants of a particular epitope.

4.3 Antibody Affinity Maturation

The host's naive B cells make antibodies of the immunoglobulin M class (IgM). An antibody is a secreted form of a receptor that occurs on the surfaces of B cells. Each B cell clone makes IgM with different binding characteristics—that is, the variable binding regions of the IgMs differ. The host has a large repertoire of naive B cells that produce a diverse array of IgM specificities.

An antigen on first exposure to a host will often bind rather weakly to several of the naive IgM. Those B cell clones with relatively high-affinity IgM for the antigen divide rapidly and come to dominate the antibody response to the antigen.

The dividing B cell clones undergo affinity maturation for particular epitopes. During this process, elevated mutation rates occur in the DNA that encodes the antibody binding region. This hypermutation in dividing B cell lineages creates a diversity of binding affinities. Those B cells with relatively higher binding affinities are stimulated to divide more rapidly than B cells with lower affinities. This process of mutation and selection creates high-affinity antibodies for the antigen.

The B cells that win the competition and produce affinity matured antibodies switch from producing IgM to immunoglobulin G (IgG). This class switch occurs by a change in the nonvariable region of the antibody that is distinct from the variable binding region.

Wedemayer et al. (1997) studied the changes in the variable antibody binding region during affinity maturation to a particular epitope. The matured antibody had an affinity for the epitope 30,000 times higher than the original, naive antibody. This increased affinity resulted from nine amino acid substitutions during affinity maturation. Wedemayer et al. (1997) found that the naive antibody significantly changed its shape during binding with the epitope. By contrast, the mature antibody had a well-defined binding region that provided a lock-and-key fit to the epitope. Wedemayer et al. (1997) speculated that naive antibodies may have more flexible binding regions in order to recognize a wide diversity of antigens, whereas matured antibodies may develop relatively rigid and highly specific binding sites.

Wedemayer et al.'s (1997) study suggests that naive IgM may bind a broader array of antigens at lower affinity, whereas matured IgG may bind a narrower array of antigens at higher affinity. Most analyses of epitope binding focus on IgG antibodies that have been refined by affinity maturation. Recently, attention has turned to the binding characteristics and different types within the IgM class, including the natural antibodies.

4.4 Natural Antibodies—Low-Affinity Binding to Diverse Antigens

Some purified antibodies bind to a wide array of self- and nonself-antigens. These polyreactive antibodies are sometimes referred to as natural or background antibodies because they occur at low abundance independently of antigen stimulation (Avrameas 1991). Natural antibodies are typically of the IgM class and have few mutations relative to the germline genotype, suggesting that natural antibodies usually have not gone through hypermutation and affinity maturation to particular antigens (Harindranath et al. 1993).

Chen et al. (1998) sampled the antibody repertoire of adult and new-born humans. They tested B cells for ability to bind insulin and β-galactosidase. Among adults, 21% of B cells bound insulin, 28% bound β-galactosidase, and 11% bound both antigens. Among newborns, 49% bound insulin, 54% bound β-galactosidase, and 33% bound both antigens. They concluded that low-affinity background reactivity commonly occurs in antibodies. Not surprisingly, newborns have a higher percentage of polyreactive antibodies than adults because adults have been exposed to many challenges and have a higher percentage of specific IgG antibodies.

Llorente et al. (1999) studied the natural antibody repertoire against the gp120 antigen of HIV-1. Among uninfected human blood donors, gp120 bound 2–5% of peripheral B cells. Llorente et al. (1999) analyzed in more detail the full repertoire of a single uninfected donor. None of the IgG isolates bound gp120, whereas 86% of the IgM clones bound the HIV-1 antigen. The IgM binding affinities were low, about an order of magnitude lower than a specific IgG antibody for gp120 that has been through the affinity maturation process. The low-affinity IgM antibodies did not inhibit in vitro infection by HIV-1. The authors suggested that these polyreactive antibodies do not provide protection against infection in vivo.

Ochsenbein et al. (1999) tested the role of natural antibodies in immunity against infection. They compared the ability of antibody-free and antibody-competent mice to resist infection against various viruses and the bacterium *Listerium monocytogenes*. In early infection kinetics, the pathogens were detected in concentrations one to two orders of magnitude lower in antibody-competent mice. Natural IgM but not IgG were found against most of the pathogens tested. By contrast with Llorente et al.'s (1999) conclusions, Ochsenbein et al. (1999) suggest that natural antibodies can help to contain infection during the early stages of invasion.

4.5 Affinity versus Specificity

The consequences of antigenic variation depend on how the host's immune system recognizes and reacts to variants. For example, if host immunity reacts in the same way to two parasite genotypes, then the host immune response does not exert differential effects of natural selection on those variants.

The ability of host immunity to discriminate between antigenic variants can be measured in different ways. For the sake of discussion, I focus on antibody-antigen binding. The same issues apply to any binding reaction.

An antibody's equilibrium affinity for different antigens can be compared by the relative inhibition tests described above in section 4.1, *Antigens and Antibody Epitopes.* Measures of relative inhibition can be easily translated into the free-energy difference in binding between an antibody and two different antigens (Benjamin and Perdue 1996).

Dynamic rather than equilibrium aspects of affinity drive certain processes in host immunity. For example, B cells compete for antigen to stimulate clonal expansion and enhanced expression of the associated antibodies. Several authors have argued that different processes influence the selection and maturation of antibodies during different phases of the immune response (reviewed by Lavoie et al. 1999; Rao 1999).

Rao (1999) summarizes the argument as follows. The early stimulation of B cells in response to initial exposure to an antigen depends on relative equilibrium binding affinities of the B cell receptors and associated antibodies. Those B cells that receive a threshold level of stimulation increase secretion of antibodies. Typically, a variety of B cells receive threshold stimulation. Thus, the early immune response tends to produce diverse antibodies that recognize various epitopes.

By contrast, dynamic association rates of reaction rather than equilibrium binding constants may determine the next phase of antibody response. Rao's (1999) lab compared antibodies that had developed in response to two related antigens. These antibodies were isolated from the later stages of the immune response and had therefore been through affinity maturation. They found no detectable difference in the equilibrium binding affinities of an antibody to the antigen to which it was raised versus the other antigenic variant. By contrast, the on-rates of antigen binding did differ.

Apparently, those B cell receptors with higher rates of antigen acquisition outcompete B cell receptors with lower rates of acquisition. This makes sense because affinity maturation occurs when the B cell clones are highly prone to apoptosis (suicide) unless they receive positive stimulation. Thus, the selection process during affinity maturation tends to optimize antigen acquisition rates rather than equilibrium binding constants.

Other studies have also analyzed the maturation of antibody binding properties during the course of an immune response (reviewed by Lavoie et al. 1999). Those studies also found differences in how the affinity constants and rates of association and dissociation changed over time. The appropriate type of affinity and measure of immune recognition depend on the dynamic processes of the immune response. I take this up in more detail in chapter 6.

Specificity defines another dimension of immune recognition. Specificity is the degree to which an immune response discriminates between antigenic variants. A simple approach measures the relative binding affinities of purified antibodies or T cell receptors for different antigens. Discrimination depends on the range of parasite variants bound, on the binding affinity, and on the stringency of the conditions under which one conducts the assay.

Figure 4.1 shows that relatively low-affinity binding can often provide greater specificity when measured at intermediate stringency. This occurs because low-affinity receptors bind fewer kinds of antigens as conditions limit the assay's sensitivity for low-affinity binding. Thus, the relative specificity of different antibodies or T cells depends on both affinity and conditions of measurement.

4.6 Cross-Reaction of Polyclonal Antibodies to Divergent Antigens

I have discussed the cross-reactivity of a particular antibody to antigenic variants and the extent to which a particular antigenic variant reacts with different antibodies. These issues focus on the affinity and specificity of particular binding reactions when one perturbs either the antibody or the antigen. For example, affinity decreases in a highly non-linear way with amino acid substitutions in either the antibody or the antigen. Substitutions in just a few key amino acids can reduce the equilibrium binding constants by several orders of magnitude.

Those studies of affinity and specificity were typically conducted with purified (monoclonal) antibodies of a single type. By contrast, the immune response to an antigen often raises many different antibodies to

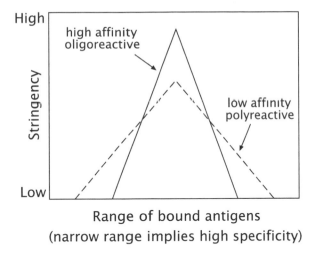

Range of bound antigens
(narrow range implies high specificity)

Figure 4.1 Affinity versus specificity of host immunity. The two triangles show the range of antigens bound by a particular antibody or T cell. A narrow range implies high discrimination between parasite antigens and high specificity. Detection of binding depends on the stringency of conditions used in the assay. For example, if only very strong binding can be detected in the assay (high stringency), then typically the antibody or T cell will appear to bind a narrower range of antigens and will therefore have higher specificity. Reducing the concentration of antibodies or T cells also increases the stringency because fewer host-parasite complexes form. In the example shown, the relation between affinity and specificity changes with stringency. Low stringency raises the relative specificity of the high-affinity antibody or T cell, medium stringency causes higher relative specificity for the low-affinity antibody or T cell, and high stringency drops the low-affinity reaction below the detection threshold.

the various exposed epitopes on the antigen. The initial polyclonal response may narrow over time as the various B cell clones receive positive or negative signals for expansion and the development of memory. I consider those dynamics in a later section. Here, I am concerned with the nature of cross-reactivity of the polyclonal immune response to a whole antigen as compared with the cross-reactivity of a monoclonal antibody to the antigen.

Benjamin et al. (1984) emphasized that the strength of cross-reactivity between antigens decreases linearly with the number of amino acid substitutions when measured by the polyclonal sera of the full immune response (see update in Prager 1993). The linear relationship explains

80% or more of the total variation in cross-reactivity between phylogenetically diverged variants of proteins such as myoglobin. Other major
studies have focused on lysozyme c and cytochrome c.

The linear relationship between polyclonal cross-reactivity and amino
acid substitutions arises because the surface of a protein antigen appears to present a nearly continuous and overlapping set of epitopes.
Each exposed amino acid probably contributes only a small amount to
the total binding between all antibodies and all epitopes.

4.7 T Cell Epitopes

Antibodies bind directly to free pathogens in the blood, lymph, or
mucosal surfaces. Antibodies cannot get at intracellular pathogens. To
fight intracellular infections, the host uses cell-mediated defenses spear-
headed by the cytotoxic T lymphocytes (CTL), also referred to as CD8$^+$ T
cells. The entire pathway leading to a CTL response against a pathogen
has several components that act as regulatory checks and balances. But
the bottom line often amounts to CTLs killing host cells that contain
specific epitopes of intracellular pathogens.

I start with a brief outline of specific recognition and then expand
on the key issues. First, host cells cut up the proteins of an intracellular pathogen. Second, transporter of antigen presentation (TAP) moves
peptides from the cytosol to the endoplasmic reticulum. Third, some
of these cut-up peptides bind to the host cell's major histocompatibility
complex (MHC) class I molecules. Fourth, peptide-MHC complexes move
to the cell surface, exposing the bound peptide to the outside. Fifth, the
T cell receptors (TCR) on free T cells can bind to certain peptide-MHC
combinations. Sixth, if the TCRs of some CTLs bind pathogen peptide-
MHC complexes on the surface of a cell, and some supporting signals
prevail, then the CTLs kill the host cell.

Several variations on T cell immunity occur. But this scenario captures the essential features of specific recognition: cutting pathogen
peptides, transporting peptides to the endoplasmic reticulum, binding
of pathogen peptides to class I MHC, presentation on cell surfaces, and
binding of specific TCRs to the peptide-MHC complex (Deng et al. 1997;
Davis et al. 1998; Germain and Štefanová 1999).

The last part of this section addresses the relation between specificity
and cross-reactivity for the TCR. On the one hand, each TCR probably

cross-reacts widely with different epitopes. On the other hand, T cell responses appear to be highly specific—variant epitopes often avoid the T cell response generated against the initial challenge. The resolution may follow from numerical considerations. Each TCR reacts with many different epitopes, perhaps as many as 10^5 different peptides. However, if a TCR reacts with one epitope, then the probability that it reacts with another, randomly chosen epitope may be as low as 10^{-4} because of the large number of possible epitopes. In terms of the total number of epitopes bound, TCRs appear widely cross-reactive, but in terms of the frequency of epitopes bound, TCRs appear highly specific.

INTRACELLULAR PEPTIDE PROCESSING AND TRANSPORT

MHC class I molecules typically bind peptides with 8–10 amino acids. Any short peptide within any pathogen protein is a candidate for MHC binding. Peptides have polarity, with carboxyl (C-terminal) and amino (N-terminal) ends. Many processes cut proteins into shorter peptides, but the proteasomes seem to be particularly important for generating peptides of the right length for MHC presentation (Rock and Goldberg 1999; York et al. 1999). Proteasome digestion creates a nonrandom population of peptides relative to the potential set defined by the amino acid sequence of whole proteins. Digestion appears to be particularly specific for the C-terminal cut, less so for the N-terminal cut (Niedermann et al. 1999).

The MHC class I molecules have biases for certain amino acids at the C-terminal site of peptides (Rammensee et al. 1995). Niedermann et al. (1999) have shown a correlation between the preferred C-terminal cuts of proteasome digestion and the favored C-terminal amino acids bound by MHC class I molecules. Thus, the proteasomes appear to be preferentially generating peptides that can be presented by MHC.

A peptide that binds MHC with relatively high affinity may not be generated in sufficient quantity to be a dominant epitope for immune recognition. In vitro studies of proteasome digestion provide the easiest way to quantify peptide generation. Although in vivo results may differ, the preliminary data from in vitro studies provide interesting hints. For example, mice were immunized with chicken ovalbumin, and the CTL response was studied by in vitro reactions with peptides presented by the class I MHC molecule K^b. The peptide $Ova_{257}SIINFEKL_{264}$ dominated the CTL response (Chen et al. 1994; Niedermann et al. 1995), where the capital letters define the peptide sequence based on the single-letter amino acid code and the subscripts give the location of the peptide within the primary sequence of the protein. A secondary, weaker response to $Ova_{55}KVVRFDKL_{62}$ can be generated under some conditions.

Dick et al. (1994) found that proteasome digestion of full-length ovalbumin proteins yielded $Ova_{257}SIINFEKL_{264}$ but not $Ova_{55}KVVRFDKL_{62}$. Niedermann et al. (1995, 1996) studied in detail the proteasome digestion patterns of synthetic peptides with 22 or 44 amino acids containing the two potential epitopes. They found major cleavage sites at the two ends of the dominant $Ova_{257}SIINFEKL_{264}$ epitope and relatively little cleavage within the epitope. By contrast, a dominant cleavage site occurred between amino acids 58 and 59 of $Ova_{55}KVVRFDKL_{62}$, yielding only traces of the intact epitope. Several other studies reviewed by Niedermann et al. (1999) support the hypothesis that proteasomal digestion frequently reduces the number of copies of potential epitopes sufficiently to prevent a strong CTL response.

It may eventually be possible to predict the probabilities of proteasomal cleavage sites (Niedermann et al. 1999). However, many factors influence the concentration of different peptides available for MHC binding. For example, sequences flanking antigenic peptides influence cleavage (Yewdell and Bennink 1999). Interferon-γ changes the distribution of proteases affecting antigenic peptide production, perhaps enhancing peptides with MHC binding motifs (York et al. 1999). TAP transports different peptides at different rates from the cytosol to the endoplasmic reticulum, where MHC class I binding of peptides occurs (Yewdell and Bennink 1999).

I have focused on the MHC class I molecules, which are present in many cell types. By contrast, MHC class II molecules operate in specialized antigen-presenting cells. Those cells take in antigen from the outside environment, process the proteins into peptides, bind peptides to MHC class II molecules, and present the peptide-MHC complexes on the cell surface. These peptide–class II complexes bind to a subset of $CD4^+$ T cells with specific, matching T cell receptors. The $CD4^+$ cells are often called *helper T cells* because they provide stimulation to CTLs or to B cells and antibody production.

Different cellular locations and proteases occur in the MHC class I and class II pathways. Nakagawa and Rudensky (1999) and Villadangos et al. (1999) review the proteases involved in class II peptide processing. Kropshofer et al. (1999) review transport and loading of peptides onto class II molecules.

INTRACELLULAR PRODUCTION AND EXOGENOUS UPTAKE OF ANTIGENS

The timing and quantity of production for different antigens in infected cells has received relatively little attention (Schubert et al. 2000), but certainly affects the influx of peptides available for MHC binding. In addition, exogenous antigens may be taken up by antigen-presenting cells and carried to lymphoid tissue for presentation to T cells (Schumacher 1999; Sigal et al. 1999). Intracellular production and exogenous uptake of antigens most likely influence the distribution of epitopes presented to T cells.

PEPTIDE-MHC BINDING

The class I MHC molecules bind peptides of 8-10 amino acids. For peptides with 9 amino acids (nonamers), the 20 different amino acids that can occur at each site combine to make $20^9 = 512 \times 10^9$ different peptide sequences. The human genome has three loci with class I molecules that present to CTLs. These loci are highly polymorphic; thus, each diploid individual typically carries six different class I alleles for CTL presentation. Clearly, if the molecules encoded by these six alleles are to bind and present a reasonable fraction of parasite peptides, then each molecule must bind to a large diversity of peptides.

Class I binding is indeed highly degenerate with regard to peptide sequence. Yewdell and Bennink (1999) estimate that each molecule binds approximately 1/200 of the possible peptide sequences, or on the order of roughly 10^7 different nonamers. An individual with six different alleles binds approximately 6/200 = 3% of candidate peptides. Here, binding means with sufficient affinity to stimulate a CTL response.

The specificity of MHC binding influences which parasite epitopes dominate an immune response. Current understanding of MHC binding is rather crude. Prediction of which parasite sequences would bind strongly to MHC molecules might help in vaccine design and in understanding the different patterns in immune response between different individuals. Given this widespread interest, the field is moving rapidly.

The three human class I loci that present to CTLs have 614 currently known alleles (http://www.anthonynolan.com/HIG/index.html). Many of the MHC molecules have been characterized by a specific binding motif—the amino acid sequence pattern to which they typically bind (Marsh et al. 2000).

Buus (1999) reviews the different methods to estimate binding motif and alternative techniques for prediction of binding. Details vary for the different alleles, but often an MHC class I molecule has two anchor positions near the ends of the peptide among the 9 or so amino acids of the peptide. Each anchor position has a favored amino acid or sometimes a limited set of alternatives. However, prediction based on anchor positions is only moderately successful; about 30% of peptides carrying the predicted motif actually bind, and sequences lacking anchor residues can bind. More complex statistical approaches have improved prediction above 70%.

Class II molecules also bind a region of about 10 amino acids. However, by contrast to class I molecules, the class II molecules have open-ended binding grooves, allowing class II molecules to bind peptides of varying lengths in which differing numbers of amino acids hang out of each end of the groove (Marsh et al. 2000). These varying peptide lengths have made it difficult to establish binding motifs; thus relatively less is known about class II binding.

Class II molecules appear to be less specific (more degenerate) in their binding compared with class I molecules (Marsh et al. 2000). A few detailed studies of class II binding have been developed (e.g., Latek and Unanue 1999). It may be that class II's relatively less specific binding has to do with its role in stimulating helper T cells that regulate the immune response rather than in directly killing parasites, but there is little evidence for this at present.

The class I and class II molecules bind only to peptides. Recent work has shown that the CD1 MHC system presents lipids and glycolipids to T cells, providing an opportunity for T cell response to nonprotein antigens (Porcelli and Modlin 1999; Prigozy et al. 2001). No doubt this system plays some role in immunity, but its relative importance is not clear at present.

T Cell Receptor Binding to Peptide-MHC Complexes

The immune system can generate highly specific memory responses against particular antigens. For example, first infection by a measles virus typically leads to symptomatic infection and eventual clearance. Second infection rapidly induces specific antibody and T cell responses based on a pool of memory cells from prior infection. This type of observed memory response naturally led to the belief that TCR recognition is highly specific for particular epitopes. However, recent work demonstrated that the TCR binds in a highly degenerate way, each TCR binding on the order of 10^4–10^7 different epitopes (Mason 1999). In addition, limited data suggest that a single peptide stimulates several different T cell clones (Maryanski et al. 1997; Mason 1999). However, different studies and different methods have given variable estimates for the number of clones stimulated by a single peptide (Yewdell and Bennink 1999).

How can the TCR binding be so degenerate, yet the immune response be so specific? Most of the details are not understood at present, but some reasonable hypotheses are beginning to take shape.

I first review relevant aspects of T cell binding. The TCR on CTLs (CD8$^+$ T cells) binds to peptide-MHC class I complexes presented on the surface of most cell types. The TCR on the helper (CD4$^+$) T cells binds to peptide-MHC class II complexes presented on the surface of specialized antigen-presenting cells. Binding and signal strength are quantitative factors, but again I use *binding* qualitatively to mean sufficient signal strength to stimulate a T cell response against an epitope.

Now consider some magnitudes with regard to the problem of recognition (Mason 1999). Define T as the number of T cell clones with different TCRs in the naive T cell repertoire, $T(p)$ as the number of T cell clones that respond to the same peptide, N as the number of possible peptides to be recognized, and $P(t)$ as the number of different peptide-MHC complexes recognized by a particular TCR. Thus,

$$T(p) \times N = P(t) \times T, \tag{4.1}$$

because both sides describe the total number of recognition specificities over all T cell clones. Immune response probably depends more on the frequencies of T cell clones that respond to particular peptides, $F(p) = T(p)/T$, rather than total numbers of clones in the body, so it is also useful to write

$$F(p) = P(t)/N, \qquad (4.2)$$

which shows that the frequency of T cell clones responding to a particular peptide equals the frequency of presented peptides stimulating a particular T cell clone. If we assume that, in the naive T cell repertoire, each clone with a unique TCR has about the same number of cells, then $F(p)$ is also the frequency of individual T cells that respond to a particular peptide. Equation (4.2) can be rewritten to emphasize cross-reactivity of the TCR as

$$P(t) = F(p) \times N, \qquad (4.3)$$

which is the probability that if a T cell receptor binds one epitope, then it also binds to a second, randomly chosen epitope.

The number of possible specificities, N, for peptides with n amino acids, is $20^n \times S$, where S is the fraction of peptides that can be presented by MHC alleles. Considering nonamers with $n = 9$, and setting $S \approx 10^{-2}$ as discussed above for MHC binding, we have $N \approx 20^9 \times 10^{-2} = 5 \times 10^9$.

The lower bound for $F(p)$, the frequency of T cell clones that respond to a peptide, occurs when every T cell is unique and each peptide stimulates only a single T cell. Mice have about 10^8 T cells, so the minimum value of $F(p)$ is 10^{-8}, and thus, from equation (4.3), the minimum value for the number of peptides bound by a TCR is $P(t) \approx 50$. This is certainly a gross underestimate, because each TCR clone has more than one cell on average, and each peptide likely stimulates more than one clone. Nonetheless, this extreme case shows that the magnitude of the recognition problem demands some degeneracy in TCR binding in mice.

Mason (1999) suggests that a more realistic description follows if one accepts the experimental estimate by Butz and Bevan (1998) that, in the naive repertoire, three different viral epitopes each stimulated a frequency $F(p) \approx 10^{-4}$ of mouse CTL cells. In a mouse with 10^7–10^8 naive CTLs, this gives an estimate of 10^3–10^4 CTLs potentially responding to each epitope. Using $F(p) = 10^{-4}$ in equation (4.3) gives the number of peptides bound by a single TCR as $P(t) \approx 5 \times 10^5$, a value that is in line with other estimates obtained by various methods (Mason 1999).

The estimated frequency $F(p) \approx 10^{-4}$ based on Butz and Bevan (1998) refers to the frequency of individual T cells responding to a peptide. It was not clear from that study how many different T cell clones were involved. It is challenging to estimate the number of different clones from the naive repertoire that respond to a particular peptide, although recent technical breakthroughs may soon provide more data (Yewdell and Bennink 1999). Among the better studies available, Maryanski et al. (1996) estimated that an epitope from the human class I molecule HLA-CW3 stimulated fifteen to thirty different T cell clones in a mouse. The response in this case may have been limited because the human MHC molecule is similar to mouse MHC molecules, causing the tested peptide to be seen as similar to a self-peptide of the mouse. In another study by the same research group, the clonal diversity of CTLs responding to a *Plasmodium berghei* peptide was much higher than against HLA-CW3, but the methods did not permit a comparable estimate for the number of clones (Jaulin et al. 1992).

Humans have about 10^{11} T cells compared with about 10^8 T cells in mice. If the frequency, $F(p)$, of T cells responding to a peptide is about the same in humans as in mice, then, from equation (4.3), the cross-reactivity of each TCR receptor, $P(t)$, is about the same in humans as in mice. The value estimated above is each TCR binding $P(t) \approx 5 \times 10^5$ different peptides.

How can such high cross-reactivity be reconciled with observed specificity? First, the probability of any particular T cell cross-reacting with two different epitopes remains low. If a T cell reacts with one epitope, the probability that it reacts with a second, randomly chosen epitope is $P(t)/N \approx 10^{-4}$.

Second, the observed specificity has to do with the number of different T cell clones that actually expand in response to an epitope. The number of expanding clones is certainly lower than the potential set of clones that bind sufficiently strongly to stimulate a response (Yewdell and Bennink 1999). Competition between clones for the epitope and for other stimulatory signals limits clonal expansion. I return to this topic in chapter 6. Here I simply note that the broad and highly cross-reactive repertoire of the naive T cells may be important for fighting primary exposure, much as the natural antibodies provide background protection against first infection. The secondary or memory response may be much narrower because it is limited to those binding clones that received additional stimulatory signals during primary infection.

SUMMARY OF T CELL EPITOPES

Yewdell and Bennink (1999) calculate an overall probability of 1/2,000 for a peptide of a foreign antigen to stimulate a dominant CTL response. By their calculation only ~1/5 of potential epitopes survive proteolytic digestion and transport to the endoplasmic reticulum for loading onto MHC molecules; of these, only ~1/200 bind MHC molecules above the threshold affinity required for immunogenicity; finally, limitations in the TCR repertoire for binding peptide-MHC complexes cause ~1/2 of presented peptides to stimulate a response. This is only a very rough approximation based on the limited data available.

MHC presentation and TCR binding are just the first steps in a T cell response. Typically, several TCRs may receive sufficient stimulation, but only a subset continue to develop strong clonal expansion. I discuss the factors that influence which clones do and do not expand in chapter 6.

4.8 Every Host Differs

The epitopes that stimulate an immune response depend on an interaction between the host and parasite. Different hosts vary in several attributes of immune recognition; thus the dominant epitopes will change from one host to the next even for an unvarying parasite.

The MHC class I and II molecules are the most strikingly polymorphic of all human loci. The three main class I loci for presenting peptides, designated A, B, and C, currently have 175, 349, and 90 alleles described, respectively. The class II molecules have separate designations for individual components of each molecule. The highly polymorphic components tend to be in the β_1 chains that contact bound peptides (Marsh et al. 2000). The β_1 chains for the DR, DQ, and DP class II molecules currently have 246, 44, and 86 alleles described, respectively. The IMGT/HLA on-line database lists recent allelic counts, as described in Robinson et al. (2000).

The MHC molecules shape the TCR repertoire. As T cells mature in the thymus, they bind to MHC molecules presenting self-antigens. Those TCRs that bind too strongly cause the associated T cells to die. Those TCRs that bind too weakly fail to provide sufficiently strong reinforcing signals, again causing the associated T cells to die. Fewer than 1% of T cells pass these checks to survive (Marsh et al. 2000). Thus, the naive

TCR repertoire is strongly influenced by the particular MHC alleles of each individual. The individual naive repertoires lead to different TCR clones being stimulated in different individuals when challenged by the same epitope (Maryanski et al. 1996, 1999). Because helper T cells influence antibody response and other aspects of immune regulation, the variable TCR repertoire may have additional consequences beyond CTL variability.

Proteolysis of antigens and transport of peptides determine the peptides available for MHC binding. Strong challenge by a particular parasite could lead to selection favoring or disfavoring specific patterns of proteolysis. However, I am not aware of any evidence for proteasome polymorphism. The peptide transporter, TAP, is polymorphic: the two subunits TAP1 and TAP2 have six and four sequences listed in the IMGT/HLA database (Robinson et al. 2000). So far, no functional differences among alleles have been found (Marsh et al. 2000).

Somatic mutation and recombination between various germline loci generate the DNA that encodes the TCR (Janeway et al. 1999). These generative mechanisms allow each individual to produce a huge variety of TCR binding specificities. The intensity of direct selection on germline polymorphisms may be rather weak because the somatic mechanisms of variation and selection shield the germline from the selective processes imposed by diverse antigens. However, the germline alleles do set the initial conditions on which somatic processes build, so it is certainly possible that germline polymorphisms influence individual tendencies to react to particular antigens.

The limited data available show some germline polymorphisms for the TCR (e.g., Reyburn et al. 1993; Hauser 1995; Moffatt et al. 1997; Moody et al. 1998; Sim et al. 1998; see also http://imgt.cines.fr). One interesting study found an interaction between a human germline polymorphism in a subunit of the TCR (VA8.1) and an MHC class II polymorphism (HLA-DRB1) (Moffatt et al. 1997). The authors analyzed two variants of the VA8.1 allele and the six most common HLA-DRB1 alleles. Individuals with enhanced allergic response to a dust mite antigen tended to have one of the two VA8.1 variants combined with the HLA-DRB1*1501 allele.

Moffatt et al. (1997) measured allergic response by the titer of IgE antibodies, which are known to be directly involved in stimulating allergic symptoms (Janeway et al. 1999). Most likely, the TCR and MHC class II polymorphisms influence IgE via helper T cells, because TCR binding to antigens presented by MHC class II stimulate helper T cells, and such T cell response is typically required for antibody stimulation. Thus, specific recognition by the TCR and MHC can affect specific recognition by antibodies.

The B cell receptor (BCR) is generated by a process of somatic recombination and mutation similar to the process that generates TCRs. Antibodies are secreted forms of the BCR. I did not find any comparable reports of germline variation in the alleles that make up the components of the BCR. Hauser (1995) suggested that somatic hypermutation (affinity maturation) of the BCR protects the germline from direct selection. The TCR has limited somatic mutation after the initial genetic recombinations, perhaps exposing germline TCRs to more intense selective pressures than BCRs. However, the difference may simply reflect less study of the BCR germline genes.

Finally, a complex network of quantitative or threshold signals regulates many aspects of the immune response. Quantitative aspects of immune regulation probably also vary among individuals. Those variable regulatory controls may influence different hosts' specific responses to antigens, because response often depends on a cascade of quantitative signals triggered by an antigen. Thus, it seems likely that variable patterns of specific recognition between individuals will be influenced by quantitative variability in regulatory control.

4.9 Problems for Future Research

1. Recognition by naive versus affinity-matured antibodies. Wedemayer et al.'s (1997) study suggests that naive IgM and affinity-matured IgA/IgG antibodies differ in the nature of the antibody-epitope bond. IgM antibodies may have rather flexible binding regions that significantly change shape when attaching to an epitope. By contrast, the affinity-matured antibodies seem to have relatively rigid, well-defined binding regions that provide a highly specific lock-and-key fit to the epitope. I suspect that an epitope must change more drastically to escape from flexible IgM binding than from the more rigid IgA/IgG binding. Thus, naive and affinity-matured antibodies may impose different selective pressures on the molecular changes between antigenic variants.

Affinity-matured antibodies in a memory response probably play the dominant role in blocking repeat infection by most pathogens (Janeway et al. 1999; Plotkin and Orenstein 1999). But some parasites may be more strongly limited by naive antibodies. For example, IgM antibodies seem to play the dominant role in fighting a sequence of different antigenic variants of the spirochete *Borrelia hermsii* (Barbour and Bundoc 2001). This parasite switches its antigenic surface molecules during a single infection. The parasite achieves this by occasionally copying into a single expression site different genes for antigenic variants stored within the genome. In this case, the major selective pressure differentiating antigenic variants most likely concerns cross-reaction with previously expressed variants during the same infection cycle.

In a parasite that rapidly switches antigenic variants, a particular epitope may need relatively more changes in amino acid composition to escape cross-reaction with naive IgM antibodies. By contrast, other pathogens may require relatively fewer amino acid changes to escape affinity-matured IgA/IgG antibodies.

It would be valuable to have more data on the degree to which IgM or affinity-matured antibodies dominate against different parasites. The IgM response may dominate only against parasites that present to the host a rapid sequence of antigenic variants. In those cases, escape from IgM rather than affinity-matured antibodies may determine the molecular changes needed for antigenic variants to escape cross-reactivity.

2. Binding stringency affects the affinity-specificity relationship. Figure 4.1 shows how specificity and cross-reactivity change with interactions between binding affinity and binding stringency. The degree of cross-reactivity determines how much molecular change parasites require to escape immune pressure directed against related antigens. Thus, the combined effects of binding affinity and stringency influence cross-reactivity, which in turn shapes molecular aspects of antigenic variation.

Controlled experiments in vitro could apply monoclonal antibodies with different affinities to cultured parasites under different binding stringencies. The type of molecular change required to escape immune pressure should vary in response to interactions between stringency and affinity.

3. Equilibrium versus kinetic aspects of affinity. Different stages of the immune response probably depend on different aspects of binding affinity to antigens. For example, clearance of antigens by antibodies may depend on the equilibrium affinity of antibody-epitope bonds, whereas the relative stimulation of different B cell lineages may depend on kinetic rates of association with antigens. Different kinetic consequences probably follow from different molecular attributes of binding between immune effectors and antigens. Complete understanding of antigenic variation requires one to trace the chain: types of molecular variation → aspects of binding kinetics → control of the immune response.

5   Generative Mechanisms

In this chapter, I summarize the different ways in which parasites generate antigenic variants. The amount of new variation and the kinds of new variants influence antigenic polymorphism and the pace of evolutionary change (Moxon et al. 1994; Deitsch et al. 1997; Fussenegger 1997).

The first section describes baseline mutation rates and special hypermutation processes that raise rates above the baseline. Microbial mutation rates per nucleotide decline with increasing genome size, causing a nearly constant mutation rate per genome per generation of about 0.003. Genome-wide hypermutation can raise the mutation rate at all sites within the genome. Such mutator phenotypes probably have altered replication enzymes. Low frequencies of mutator phenotypes have been observed in stable populations of *Escherichia coli*, whereas fluctuating populations appear to maintain higher frequencies of mutators. In some cases, hypermutation may be targeted to certain genes by DNA repeats and other DNA sequence motifs that promote local replication errors.

The second section presents three common mechanisms that parasites use to change gene expression between antigenically variable copies of a gene, potentially allowing escape from immune recognition. Replication errors of short nucleotide repeats can alter regulatory sequences or disrupt translation of coding sequences. Gene conversion can copy variant genes from different genomic locations into a single expression site. Invertible pieces of DNA occasionally change the direction of nucleotide sequences, altering the expression of nearby genes. Different *Plasmodium* species have different families of antigenically variable surface molecules. The mechanisms by which *Plasmodium* species switch expression between antigenic variants are not fully understood.

The third section focuses on parasites that store antigenic variants within each genome. Some parasite genomes have dozens or hundreds of variants but express only one archival copy at a time. Intragenomic recombination between archived copies may create new variants. Studies of the spirochete *Borrelia hermsii* and the protozoan *Trypanosoma brucei* provide evidence of recombination between archival copies.

The fourth section lists different mechanisms that can mix genetic material between lineages of parasites to create new antigenic variants. Segregation brings together in one individual different chromosomes from distinct lineages. Intergenomic recombination mixes genetic sequences from different lineages. Horizontal transfer moves pieces of DNA from one individual into another by processes such as bacterial uptake of naked DNA from the environment.

The final section outlines promising topics of study for future research.

5.1 Mutation and Hypermutation

There are many different ways to measure mutation rates and many different processes that influence mutations (Drake et al. 1998). I focus in this section on errors in nucleotide replication that change the antigenic properties of the encoded molecule.

BASELINE MUTATION RATES

RNA virus populations typically have high frequencies of mutants and often evolve rapidly (Holland 1992; Knipe and Howley 2001). However, few studies have provided direct estimates of mutation rates. The limited data suggest relatively high mutation rates on the order of 10^{-4}–10^{-5} per base per replication (Holland 1992; Coffin 1996; Preston and Dougherty 1996; Drake et al. 1998; Drake and Holland 1999).

Drake et al. (1998) summarized mutation rates for various microbes with DNA chromosomes (table 5.1). The table shows an amazingly consistent value of approximately 0.003 mutations per genome per generation. This value holds over genomes that vary in total size by four orders of magnitude; consequently the per base mutation rates also vary over four orders of magnitude.

GENOME-WIDE HYPERMUTATION

None of the microbes in table 5.1 face intense, constant selective pressure on antigens imposed by vertebrate immunity—it is unlikely that *E. coli* depends on antigenic variation to avoid clearance from its hosts. It would be interesting to know if pathogens under very intense selection by host immunity have higher baseline mutation rates than related microbes under less intense immune pressure.

Table 5.1 Mutation rates per replication in various microbes

Organism	G	μ_b	μ_g
Bacteriophage M13	6.4×10^3	7.2×10^{-7}	0.0046
Bacteriophage λ	4.9×10^4	7.7×10^{-8}	0.0038
Bacteriophages T2 & T4	1.7×10^5	2.4×10^{-8}	0.0040
Escherichia coli	4.6×10^6	5.4×10^{-10}	0.0025
Saccharomyces cerevisiae	1.2×10^7	2.2×10^{-10}	0.0027
Neurospora crassa	4.2×10^7	7.2×10^{-11}	0.0030
Mean			0.0034

Values are from Drake et al. (1998). All microbes listed here have DNA chromosomes. G is the total number of bases in the genome, μ_b is the mutation rate per base per replication, and μ_g is the mutation rate per genome per replication.

High genome-wide mutation rates arise in bacteria by spontaneous mutator mutations, in which the mutator alleles raise the error rate during replication (Drake et al. 1998). The mutator alleles probably are various DNA replication and repair enzymes. Ten or more genes of *E. coli* can develop mutator mutations. Assuming that each gene has about 1,000 bases, then the overall mutation rate of mutator loci is $10 \times 1,000 \times 5 \times 10^{-10} \approx 10^{-6}$–$10^{-5}$, based on the per base mutation rate in table 5.1. Some mutations will be nearly neutral; others will cause extremely high mutation rates and will never increase in frequency.

Typical *E. coli* cultures accumulate mutator mutants at a frequency of less than 10^{-5} (Mao et al. 1997), probably because most mutations are deleterious and therefore selection does not favor increased mutation rates. However, mutators can be strongly favored when the competitive conditions and the selective environment provide opportunities for the mutators to generate more beneficial mutations than the nonmutators (Chao and Cox 1983; Mao et al. 1997). In this case, mutators increase because they are linked with a higher frequency of beneficial mutations.

Although mutators are typically rare in freshly grown laboratory cultures, hospital isolates of *E. coli* and *Salmonella enterica* sometimes have mutator frequencies above 10^{-2} (Jyssum 1960; Gross and Siegel 1981; LeClerc et al. 1996). Extensive serial passage in the laboratory can also lead to high frequencies of mutators (Sniegowski et al. 1997). Thus, it appears that rapid change of hosts or culture conditions can increase the frequency of mutators 1,000-fold relative to stable environmental conditions. As Drake et al. (1998) point out, theory suggests that mutators can speed adaptation in asexual microbes (Leigh 1970; Moxon et al.

1994; Taddei et al. 1997). It would be interesting to compare naturally occurring frequencies of mutators in stable and rapidly changing selective environments.

DNA damage induces the SOS response of *E. coli* (Walker 1984). This response causes higher mutation rates even in the undamaged parts of the genome. Radman (1999) argues that this stress-induced mutagenesis is an adaptation to generate variability in the face of challenging environments. But it is not clear whether the special replication enzymes induced by SOS serve primarily to replicate DNA under difficult conditions, albeit with high mutation, or whether certain aspects of SOS are particularly designed to raise mutation above the minimum level that could be achieved efficiently during emergency. In any case, it is interesting to consider whether some microbes facultatively induce increased genome-wide mutation when challenged by host immunity.

LOCALIZED HYPERMUTATION

Targeting mutations to key loci would be more efficient than raising the genome-wide mutation rate. Various mechanisms can increase the mutation rate over short runs of nucleotides (Fussenegger 1997; Ripley 1999). For example, *Streptococcus pyogenes* coats its surface with a variable M protein, of which eighty antigenically distinct variants are known (Lancefield 1962; Fischetti 1991). The amino acid sequence of the M6 serotype revealed repeats in three regions of the protein (Hollingshead et al. 1986, 1987). Region 1 has five repeats of 42 bp, each repeat containing two nearly identical 21 bp repeats; region 2 has five 75 bp repeats; and region 3 has two repeats of about 81 bp. In regions 1 and 2, the two outermost repeats vary slightly in sequence from the three identical repeats in the interior.

Sequence analysis of variant M proteins suggests that mutations occur by generating both gains and losses of the duplications. These mutations probably arise by intragenic recombination between the DNA repeats, but may be created by slippage during replication. Slippage mutations over repeated DNA lead to gain or loss in the number of repeats and occur at frequencies much higher than typical replication errors (Charlesworth et al. 1994). The repeats of the M protein are multiples of 3 bases; thus changes in repeat number do not cause frameshift mutations. Some of the repeats vary slightly in base composition, so recombinations can alter sequence composition as well as total length.

Fussenegger (1997) reviews several other cases of bacterial cell-wall proteins that have repeated sequences, most of which occur in multiples of 3 bp. Repeats are often associated with binding domains for other proteins or polysaccharides (Wren 1991), so perhaps the ability to generate variable-length domains provides an advantage in attachment to host tissues or in escape from host immunity.

Other mutational mechanisms besides repeats may increase local mutation rates (Ripley 1999). For example, when double-stranded DNA splits to be replicated, the complementary bases on a single strand may bind to each other to form "hairpin" structures. Such hairpins may increase errors in replication. Caporale (1999) suggests that certain genomic regions, such as antigenic sites, may have DNA base compositions that promote higher mutation rates.

Apart from the well-known case of repeats and replication slippage, no evidence at present associates antigenic sites with higher replication errors. But this would certainly be an interesting problem to study further. One could, for example, focus on associations between mutation rate and nucleotide sequence. Comparison would be particularly interesting between epitopes that evolve rapidly and conserved regions of antigenic molecules that evolve slowly. Such comparison may help to identify aspects of nucleotide composition that promote higher error rates in replication.

5.2 Stochastic Switching between Archival Copies

Many pathogens change critical surface molecules by switching expression between alternative genes. Three types of switch mechanisms commonly occur: replication errors that turn expression on or off, gene conversion into fixed expression sites, and invertible promoters that change the direction of transcription.

REGULATORY SWITCHES BY REPLICATION ERRORS OF SHORT REPEATS

Short, repeated nucleotide sequences often lead to high error rates during replication. Repeats have recurring units typically with 1–5 bases per unit. Short, repeated DNA sequences probably lead to replication errors by slipped-strand mispairing (Meyer 1987; Levinson and Gutman

1987; Charlesworth et al. 1994). Errors apparently arise when a DNA polymerase either skips forward a repeat unit, causing a deletion of one unit, or slips back one unit, producing a one-unit insertion.

Gene expression can be turned on or off by insertions or deletions. Inserted or deleted repeats within the coding sequence cause frameshift mutations that prevent translation and production of a full protein. For example, the eleven opacity genes of *Neisseria meningitidis* influence binding to host cells and tissue tropism. These genes each have between eight and twenty-eight CTCTT repeats, which can disrupt or restore the proper translational frame as the number of repeats changes (Stern et al. 1986; Stern and Meyer 1987). The limited repertoire of eleven genes and the crude on-off switching suggest that variable expression has more to do with altering cell tropism than with escape from host immunity (Fussenegger 1997).

On-off switches can also be created by short repeats in transcriptional control regions. *Bordetella pertussis* controls expression of two distinct fimbriae by transcriptional switching (Willems et al. 1990). Fimbriae are bacterial surface fibers that attach to host tissues. Particular cells produce both, only one, or neither of the fimbrial types. Sequences of about 15 C nucleotides in the transcriptional promoters of each of the two genes influence expression. The actual length of the poly-C sequence varies, probably by slipped-strand mispairing during replication. The length affects transcription of the attached gene. Thus, by the stochastic process of replication errors, the individual loci are turned on and off. Again, this sort of switching may have more to do with tissue tropism than with escape from immune recognition.

Gene Conversion

Some pathogens store many variant genes for a surface antigen, but express only one of the copies at any time. For example, there may be a single active expression site at which transcription occurs. Occasionally, one of the variant loci copies itself to the expression site by gene conversion—a type of intragenomic recombination that converts the target without altering the donor sequence. The genome preserves the archival library without change, but alters the expressed allele.

The spirochete *Borrelia hermsii* has approximately thirty alternative loci that encode an abundant surface lipoprotein (Barbour 1993). There is a single active expression site when the spirochete is in mammalian hosts (Barbour et al. 1991). The expression site is changed by gene conversion to one of the variant archival copies at a rate of about 10^{-4}–10^{-3} per cell division (Stoenner et al. 1982; Barbour and Stoenner 1985). A small number of antigenic variants dominate the initial parasitemia of this blood-borne pathogen. The host then clears these initial variants with antibodies. Some of the bacteria from this first parasitemia will have changed antigenic type. Those switches provide new variants that cause a second parasitemia, which is eventually recognized by the host and cleared. The cycle repeats several times, causing relapsing fever.

The protozoan *Trypanosoma brucei* has hundreds of alternative loci that encode the dominant surface glycoprotein (Barry 1997; Pays and Nolan 1998). Typically, each cell expresses only one of the alternative loci. Switches in expression occur at a rate of up to 10^{-2} per cell division (Turner 1997). The switch mechanism is similar to that in *Borrelia hermsii*—gene conversion of archival copies into a transcriptionally active expression site. *T. brucei* has approximately twenty alternative transcription sites, of which only one is usually active. Thus, this parasite can also change expression by switching between transcription sites. It is not fully understood how different transcription sites are regulated.

INVERTIBLE SEQUENCES

E. coli stores two alternative fimbriae genes adjacent to each other on its chromosome (Abraham et al. 1985). A promoter region between the two genes controls transcription. The promoter triggers transcription in only one direction, thus expressing only one of the two variants. Occasionally, the promoter flips orientation, activating the alternative gene. The ends of the promoter have inverted repeats, which play a role in the recombination event that mediates the sequence inversion. *Salmonella* uses a similar mechanism to control flagellum expression (Silverman et al. 1979).

Moraxella species use a different method to vary pilin expression (Marrs et al. 1988; Rozsa and Marrs 1991). The variable part of the pilin gene has alternate cassettes stored in adjacent locations. Inverted repeats flank the pair of alternate cassettes, causing the whole complex occasionally to flip orientation. The gene starts with an initial constant region and continues into one of the cassettes within the invertible complex. When the complex flips, the alternate variable cassette completes the gene. Several bacteriophage use a similar inversion system to switch genes encoding their tail fibers, which determine host range (Kamp et al. 1978; Iida et al. 1982; van de Putte et al. 1984).

Fussenegger (1997) reviews other invertible-sequence mechanisms. These low-diversity switches provide only a limited advantage against immunity because, even if the switch rates were low, an infection would soon contain all variants at appreciable abundance. Thus, these switch mechanisms may serve mainly to generate alternative attachment variants.

OTHER ARCHIVAL SWITCH MECHANISMS

Plasmodium species are a diverse and polyphyletic group of protozoans that cause malarial symptoms in vertebrate hosts. Antigenic variation appears to be common and to be caused by diverse mechanisms. I briefly summarize three examples.

Infection and reproduction in host erythrocytes determine the build-up of parasite numbers within the host (Mims et al. 1998). *P. falciparum* expresses the *var* gene within erythrocytes. The gene product, PfEMP1, moves to the surface of the host cell, where it influences cellular adhesion and recognition by host immunity (Deitsch and Wellems 1996). The *var* genes are highly diverse antigenically (Su et al. 1995). Each parasite exports only one *var* type to the erythrocyte surface, but a clone of parasites switches between *var* types (Smith et al. 1995). Switching leads to a diverse population of PfEMP1 variants within a host and even wider diversity among hosts.

The mechanism of *var* switching is not known. It appears that many *var* loci are transcribed during the first few hours after erythrocyte infection, but only a single *var* gene is active when PfEMP1 is translated and moved to the erythrocyte surface (Q. Chen et al. 1998; Scherf et al. 1998). Switching between *var* loci does not depend on the mechanism of gene conversion found in *Borrelia hermsii* and *Trypanosoma brucei*. It may be that some mechanism shuts down expression of all but one locus without modifying the DNA sequence. Scherf et al. (1998) suggest that switches in gene expression do not depend on DNA sequence changes in promoter regions or changes in transcription factors. They argue that regional changes in chromatin structure may control variable expression.

Preiser et al. (1999) found antigenic variation at another stage in the *Plasmodium* life cycle (see also Barnwell 1999). The parasitic forms that invade erythrocytes are called merozoites. In a rodent malaria, *P. yoelii*, the merozoite surface molecule p235 plays a role in attachment or invasion of erythrocytes. There are at least eleven and perhaps as many as fifty discrete genes that encode variants of p235 (Borre et al. 1995). Within an erythrocyte, the parasite develops a multinucleate stage and then divides into new merozoites that burst the host cell. Preiser et al. (1999) found that each of the separate nuclei transcribe a different p235 gene. They suggest that upon division into separate merozoites, each merozoite presents a different p235 protein on its surface. Thus, each clone produces antigenically diverse progeny. The various p235 molecules may facilitate invasion of different classes of erythrocytes.

Other *Plasmodium* species express surface proteins that are distantly related to p235, but in those cases the surface molecules do not arise from an antigenically diverse, multicopy gene family (Barnwell 1999). Some of the *Plasmodium* species have diverged tens of millions of years ago, so it is not surprising that they have different strategies for attachment, immune evasion, and antigenic variation.

In another example, *P. vivax* has an extensive family of variant *vir* genes, estimated to be present at 600–1,000 copies per haploid genome (del Portillo et al. 2001). The parasite expresses only a small subset of these genes in an infected erythrocyte. Del Portillo et al. (2001) expressed the *vir* gene product from two variant loci and tested the proteins for immunogenicity. Sera from twenty-five previously infected hosts provided a panel of antibodies to test for prior exposure to the *vir* gene products. One of the expressed proteins reacted with the serum from only one host, the other protein reacted with sera from two hosts. Thus, *vir* gene products are immunogenic, but each variant appears to be expressed rarely—the hallmarks of antigenic variation from a large archival library.

Sequences related to the *vir* family do not occur in *P. falciparum* or *P. knowlesi*, suggesting that these different lineages have evolved different families of variable antigens. The diversity of gene families in *Plasmodium* that play a role in antigenic variation provides an excellent opportunity for comparative, evolutionary studies.

5.3 New Variants by Intragenomic Recombination

Some parasites store many genetic variants for a particular surface molecule. Usually, each parasite expresses only one archival variant.

New variants of archival copies may be created by recombination. For example, Rich et al. (2001) found evidence for recombination between the archived loci of the variable short protein (Vsp) of *Borrelia hermsii*. They studied the DNA sequences of 11 *vsp* loci within a single clone. These *vsp* loci are silent, archival copies that can, by gene conversion, be copied into the single expression site. The genes differ by 30–40% in amino acid sequence, providing sufficient diversity to reduce or eliminate antigenic cross-reactivity within the host.

Rich et al. (2001) used statistical analyses of *vsp* sequences to infer that past recombination events have occurred between archival loci. Those analyses focus on attributes such as runs of similar nucleotides between loci that occur more often than would be likely if alleles diverged only by accumulating mutations within each locus. Shared runs can be introduced into diverged loci by recombination.

The archival antigenic repertoire of *Trypanosoma brucei* evolves rapidly (Pays and Nolan 1998). This species has a large archival library and multiple expression sites, but only one expression site is active at any time. New genes can be created within an active expression site when several donor sequences convert the site in a mosaic pattern (Pays 1989; Barbet and Kamper 1993). When an active expression site becomes inactivated, the gene within that site probably becomes protected from further gene conversion events (Pays et al. 1981; Pays 1985). Thus, newly created genes by mosaic conversion become stored in the repertoire. Perhaps new genes in silent expression sites can move into more permanent archival locations by recombination, but this has not yet been observed. Recombination between silent, archived copies may also occur, which, although each event may be relatively rare, could strongly affect the evolutionary rate of the archived repertoire.

These examples illustrate the scattered reports of recombination and the evolution of archived repertoires. These preliminary studies show the promise for understanding the interaction between mechanisms that create diversity and the strong forces of natural selection imposed by immune recognition. The combination of generative mechanisms and selection shapes the archival antigenic repertoire.

5.4 Mixing between Genomes

New antigenic variants can be produced by mixing genes between distinct lineages. This happens in three ways.

Segregation brings together chromosomes from different lineages. Reassortment of influenza A's neuraminidase and hemagglutinin surface antigens provides the most famous example (Lamb and Krug 2001). The genes for these antigens occur on two separate RNA segments of the genome—the genome has a total of eight segments. When two or more viruses infect a single cell, the parental segments all replicate separately and then are packaged together into new viral particles. This process can package the segments from different parents into a new virus.

New neuraminidase-hemagglutinin combinations present novel antigenic properties to the host. Rare segregation events have introduced hemagglutinin from bird influenza into the genome of human influenza (Webster et al. 1997). The novel hemagglutinins cross-reacted very little with those circulating in humans, allowing the new combinations to sweep through human populations and cause pandemics.

Intergenomic recombination occurs when chromosomes from different lineages exchange pieces of their nucleotide sequence. In protozoan parasites such as *Plasmodium* and *Trypanosoma*, recombination happens as part of a typical Mendelian cycle of outcrossing sex (Jenni et al. 1986; Conway et al. 1999). Recombination can occur in viruses when two or more particles infect a single cell. DNA viruses may recombine relatively frequently because they can use the host's recombination enzymes (Strauss et al. 1996). RNA viruses may recombine less often because the host lacks specific enzymes to mediate reciprocal exchange of RNA segments. However, many descriptions of RNA virus recombination have been reported (Robertson et al. 1995; Laukkanen et al. 2000; and see chapter 10). In all cases, even rare recombination can provide an important source for new antigenic variants.

Horizontal transfer of DNA between bacteria introduces new nucleotide sequences into a lineage (Ochman et al. 2000). Transformation occurs when a cell takes up naked DNA from the environment. Some species transform at a particularly high rate, suggesting that they have specific adaptations for uptake and incorporation of foreign DNA (Fussenegger et al. 1997). For example, *Neisseria* species transform frequently enough to have many apparently mosaic genes from interspecies transfers (Spratt et al. 1992; Zhou and Spratt 1992; Fussenegger et al. 1997), and *N. gonorrhoeae* has low linkage disequilibrium across its genome (Maynard Smith et al. 1993). Horizontal transfer also occurs when bacteriophage viruses carry DNA from one host cell to another or when two cells conjugate to transfer DNA from a donor to a recipient (Ochman et al. 2000).

5.5 Problems for Future Research

1. Selection of mutation rates. Intense immune pressure favors the generation of antigenic variants. However, variants, like any mutations, may have associated costs. To what extent have molecular attributes of antigenic genes been shaped by the costs and benefits of generating variants? Do microbes under intense immune pressure have higher genome-wide mutation rates compared with similar organisms that do not face immune attack? To what extent have nucleotide sequences of antigens been shaped by the tendency of particular motifs to generate replication errors—a form of local hypermutation?

2. Selection of mechanisms that control switching between archival variants. I described various mechanisms by which gene expression shifts between archived variants. The rate at which switches occur probably affects the parasite's ability to extend infection. If switches happen too quickly, then novel variants will not be expressed after the immune response develops against the many variants expressed early in infection. If switches happen too slowly, then the parasite may be cleared before the variants are expressed. Thus, natural selection can strongly influence the molecular details of the switch process in order to adjust the rate of change between variants. This can be tested by selecting in vitro for faster or slower switch rates. Does an evolutionary response occur in the switch rates? If so, how is the response accomplished at the molecular level?

One could also test the evolution of the switch rate in vivo, comparing situations that imposed different immune pressures on rates of change and on particular orders in which variants are expressed. Such studies allow one to relate the molecular mechanisms of switching to the adaptive significance of switching. Two general questions arise. To what extent do switch rates evolve to enhance parasite fitness? To what extent do mechanistic properties of switching constrain rates of change between variants?

3. Rates of diversification between archival copies. Some parasites have large families of variants archived within the genome. I described studies of *Borrelia hermsii* and *Trypanosoma brucei* in which intragenomic recombination between archival copies generated new variants. This calls attention to the rate at which new variants can be created and the rate of diversification between members of archival gene families.

Rich et al. (2000) argue that all of the antigenic variants of *Plasmodium falciparum* have arisen from a recent common ancestor. A more detailed study by Volkman et al. (2001) estimates that the most recent common ancestor lived less than ten thousand years ago. If this estimate is correct, then the diverse *var* family of antigenic variants must have evolved very rapidly. However, this conclusion remains contentious—Hughes and Verra (2001) argue that the *P. falciparum* lineage is much older.

It would be interesting to compare rates of diversification in these families of variants between the different *Plasmodium* species, *Trypanosoma brucei*, *Borrelia hermsii*, and other microbes with similar families of variants. It would also be interesting to compare *P. falciparum* with another malarial parasite of humans, *P. vivax*. As noted in the text, *P. vivax* has a family of antigenic variants that does not occur in *P. falciparum*. How does the history of variation compare in these two species?

PART III

INDIVIDUAL INTERACTIONS

6 Immunodominance within Hosts

Each parasite presents a large number of epitopes to the host's immune system. The immune response focuses on only a few of the many potential epitopes, a process called *immunodominance.* Immunodominant focus determines which epitopes are favored to vary antigenically to escape immune pressure. In this chapter, I describe how immunodominance develops by competition among B and T cell lineages with different specificities.

The first section reviews antibody immunodominance. The diverse, naive B cells secrete IgM antibodies that bind to nearly any epitope. On initial infection, B cells that bind epitopes with relatively high equilibrium affinity divide rapidly and dominate the early phase of the immune response by outcompeting other B cells. However, antibodies that bind too strongly clear the matching antigens quickly and prevent feedback stimulation to their B cells. The later phases of B cell competition and maturation of IgG favor antibodies with increased on-rates of association to epitopes rather than increased equilibrium binding affinity.

The second section discusses cytotoxic T lymphocyte (CTL) immunodominance. Aspects of specificity such as MHC binding and avoidance of self-recognition determine which epitopes could potentially be recognized. Among this potential set, some epitopes dominate others in stimulating a CTL response. Earlier stimulation of T cell lineages in response to infection rather than more rapid T cell division seems to determine the dominance of lineages. Dominant lineages may repress subdominant lineages by pushing the abundance of pathogens below the threshold needed to trigger weaker, subdominant responses.

The third section describes original antigenic sin, in which the specificity of the immune response depends on the sequence of exposure to antigenic variants. If a host first encounters a variant A and then a later variant A', the second variant will sometimes restimulate the initial response against A rather than a new, specific response against A'. In this case, A' recalls the memory against an earlier cross-reacting epitope rather than generating a primary, specific response against itself. Sometimes the cross-reaction is rather weak, causing the host to respond weakly to the second antigen because of interference by its memory against the first variant. Original antigenic sin has been observed in both antibody and CTL responses.

The final section takes up promising issues for future research.

6.1 Antibody Immunodominance

I emphasize Rao's (1999) studies of B cell competition, one of the few empirical analyses of the dynamics of antibody immunodominance.

BROAD IgM AND NARROW IgG RESPONSE

Kumar et al. (1992) engineered a recombinant polypeptide with 100 amino acids that contained several epitopes from the envelope of hepatitis B virus. They called this polypeptide MEP-1. The initial antibody response, detected one week after injection into a mouse, contained heterogeneous IgM against several epitopes that collectively spanned the entire 100-amino-acid sequence. By contrast, the IgG response four weeks after injection was highly specific for a single epitope. These observations support the idea that the naive antibody repertoire can bind almost any epitope, but that only a subset of the initially binding antibodies stimulate their B cell clones to expand significantly and make the transition to IgG production.

REVIEW OF PROCESSES BY WHICH ANTIBODY RESPONSE DEVELOPS

Major expansion of a B cell clone and transition to IgG production typically depend on stimulation from helper T cells, although some nonprotein antigens can stimulate IgM response without T cell help (Janeway et al. 1999). The interaction between B cells and T cells happens roughly as follows. The B cell receptor (BCR) is an attached form of antibody, which has specificity for particular epitopes. Each B cell expresses many BCRs on its surface, each with the same specificity. When a BCR binds antigen, it may pull the antigen into the cell. If the antigen is a protein, the B cell processes the antigen into smaller peptides, binds some of those peptides to MHC class II molecules, and presents the peptide–class II complexes on the cell surface.

If a helper (CD4$^+$) T cell has a T cell receptor (TCR) that binds the peptide–class II complex, then the T cell sends a stimulatory signal to the B cell. Thus, B cell stimulation requires binding to an epitope of an antigen, processing the antigen, and finding a helper T cell that can bind an epitope of the same antigen. The epitopes recognized by the BCR and TCR may differ, but must be linked on the same antigen molecule to provide matches to both the BCR and TCR (Shirai et al. 1999). T cell stimulation causes B cells to divide more rapidly, to undergo somatic hypermutation, and to switch from IgM to IgG production. Immuno-dominance arises when some B cells receive relatively greater stimula-tion from helper T cells. Signal strength depends on the dynamics of antigen binding for BCRs and TCRs.

The vertebrate host has specialized organs to facilitate interaction be-tween B and T cells. The initial interaction occurs when antigen-binding B cells are trapped in a zone of lymphoid tissue that has a high density of T cells. Some of the stimulated B cells differentiate into antibody fac-tories, whereas others migrate along with matching T cells to primary follicles of the lymphoid tissue. There, if the B cells receive sufficient stimulation from T cells, they undergo rapid division to form germinal centers. At these centers, the B cells hypermutate and proceed through affinity maturation.

AFFINITY WINDOW FOR EPITOPE-PARATOPE BINDING

The naive B cell repertoire binds with varying affinity to different epi-topes of an antigen. The relative stimulation of different B cell clones by an antigen determines progression to the next steps in B cell response. Stimulation depends on the affinity of the BCR paratopes (binding sites) for their particular epitopes.

Rao (1999) found an affinity window for stimulation of B cells. Very strong epitope-paratope binding prevents stimulation; weakly binding B cells are outcompeted for stimulatory signals. I discuss in turn these upper and lower thresholds.

Vijayakrishnan et al. (1994) discovered an upper affinity threshold by the study of two epitopes of the MEP-1 peptide described above. One of these epitopes stimulated the immunodominant IgG response; the other was at the opposite end of the peptide. I refer to the immunodominant epitope as D and the subdominant epitope as S. Vijayakrishnan et al. (1994) followed antibody levels against these two epitopes in immunized mice. Surprisingly, the early antibody response was stronger against S than D. However, secreted antibodies against S bound so efficiently to S that they outcompeted the matching BCR and prevented stimulation of the B cell lineage. By contrast, anti-D antibodies bound with lower affinity and did not outcompete the matching BCR, allowing that B cell lineage to receive strong stimulation from the antigen.

Agarwal et al. (1996) found a lower affinity threshold determined by competition between BCRs for stimulation by helper T cells. They began by constructing a peptide that had on one side a known B cell antigen of hepatitis B virus and on the other side a known T cell epitope from the malaria parasite *Plasmodium falciparum*. They injected this chimeric peptide into mice and followed the antibody response. The early IgM response had specificities that spanned the entire hepatitis B segment. By contrast, the later IgG response focused on a single epitope in the hepatitis B segment composed of the four amino acids DPAF.

Single amino acid changes in DPAF destroyed immunodominance by this epitope, causing nearby epitopes to dominate the IgG response. The anti-DPAF antibodies had affinities between 8- and 60-fold higher than antibodies against neighboring epitopes. Agarwal et al. (1996) showed that the high-affinity response against DPAF suppressed B cells initially activated against neighboring epitopes. Immunodominance depended on competition for antigen-specific helper T cells, which are limiting during the initial stages of an immune response. The stronger-binding BCRs take up antigen and present to T cells more efficiently than do the weaker-binding competitors. Insufficient T cell stimulation leads to suppression of B cell clones.

In later experiments, Agarwal and Rao (1997) manipulated the size of the helper T cell pool. Reduced numbers of T cells allowed IgM response but prevented the switch from the IgM stage to the IgG stage. This supports the hypothesis that competition for T cell help is the rate-limiting step in the transition from the broad IgM response to the narrow IgG response.

Equilibrium Binding Affinity May Determine Early Response

Antibody affinity for epitopes influences initial IgM stimulation and subsequent competition for immunodominance during the switch to IgG. What determines antibody affinity to individual epitopes during these early phases of B cell competition? Rao (1999) summarizes studies that rule out mouse MHC genotype and various physical properties of the epitope such as accessibility within the overall peptide structure. This led to the hypothesis that the Gibbs free-energy of binding between epitope and paratope determines antibody affinity, and that the amino acid sequence of the epitope influences the potential free-energy of the bond.

Nakra et al. (2000) used various model peptides to show that the affinity of an epitope-specific response depends on the amino acid composition of the epitope. They suggested that the relative ordering of affinities for particular epitopes could be predicted by the amino acid sequence of the epitope. In particular, the amino acid side chains of an epitope sequence determine the potential free-energy of binding to an antibody paratope.

Chemical determination of free-energy seems particularly important in the early phases of antibody response, when the antibodies have not yet been optimized for binding by affinity maturation. Unoptimized antibodies do not have strong spatial complementarity of binding; thus there is less steric and greater chemical constraint on binding at this stage. After optimization, it may be that greater steric complementarity of antibody-epitope binding places more emphasis on spatial fit and reduces the predictability of binding energy based solely on chemical composition of amino acid side chains.

KINETIC BINDING ON-RATES MAY DETERMINE AFFINITY MATURATION

So far, I have summarized the first stage of antibody selection: IgM-producing B cells from the naive repertoire compete for T cell help, with the winner(s) dividing more rapidly and starting on the path to IgG production. Equilibrium binding affinity drives this first stage of antibody competition.

I now turn to the next stage, called *affinity maturation* (Janeway et al. 1999). During this stage, B cells congregate in germinal centers of the lymphoid tissue and mutate their antibody paratopes at a high rate. A selection process favors those mutated paratopes that bind relatively strongly to antigen, driving affinity maturation of antibodies for the particular epitopes.

Rao's (1999) group studied affinity maturation by continued analysis of the DPAF epitope in the chimeric hepatitis B and *Plasmodium* antigen mentioned above. Agarwal et al. (1998) found that the equilibrium binding affinity of antibodies did not increase over time, supporting observations in two earlier studies on other systems (Newman et al. 1992; Roost et al. 1995).

Rao's group modified their model antigen by substituting cysteine amino acid residues in the two sites flanking the DPAF epitope (Nayak et al. 1998). This changes the conformation of the DPAF peptide and influences the antibody-epitope binding reaction. Nayak et al. (1998) raised antibodies through affinity maturation against DPAF in the native antigen and in the cysteine-modified antigen. They then compared binding of each of the two antibody types against the native and modified antigen.

Antibodies raised against the native antigen bound with approximately equal equilibrium affinity to native and modified antigen. Antibodies raised against the modified antigen also bound at equilibrium approximately equally against the two antigens. By contrast, the kinetic on-rates of binding were 50-fold higher for native antibody to native antigen than for native antibody to modified antigen. Kinetic on-rates were 14- to 25-fold higher for modified antibody to modified antigen than for modified antibody to native antigen.

Kinetic on-rates measure rates at which bonds form, whereas equilibrium affinity measures the ratio of on-rates to off-rates. Selection during affinity maturation apparently favors faster rates of interaction with increases in both on-rates and off-rates: the on-rates rise, but the equilibrium affinity does not change.

In this model system, it appears that B cells compete by rate of antigen acquisition during affinity maturation. B cells with paratopes that bind more quickly to antigen receive stronger stimulatory signals to divide and to dominate the population in the germinal centers. Thus, the optimized antibodies bind more quickly to antigen than unoptimized precursors, but optimized antibodies do not necessarily increase their equilibrium binding affinity.

In summary, Rao proposed an integrated, dynamic view of how the specificity of an antibody response develops. The particular details may turn out to vary in different cases. However, in all cases, progress will require study of the interactions between molecular structure, the kinetics of binding, regulatory control of cellular competition, and immunodominance.

6.2 CTL Immunodominance

CTL immunodominance is not well understood, because it has been difficult to measure the abundance of CTLs specific for particular epitopes. The technical limitations for quantitative assay of specific T cells may soon be overcome with recently developed methods (Yewdell and Bennink 1999; Doherty and Christensen 2000).

I mentioned in chapter 4 several factors of antigen processing that affect CTL immunodominance. These factors include CTL repertoire shaped by selection against MHC and self-peptide complexes, timing and quantity of intracellular antigen production by pathogens, uptake of extracellular antigen by antigen-presenting cells, proteolytic cleavage of antigens, intracellular transport of peptides, binding to MHC, and specificity of T cell receptors. In this section, I focus on the relative abundance of T cell populations with different recognition specificities.

BREADTH AND SPECIFICITY OF CTL RESPONSE

The CTL response can be described by breadth, the number of different CTL clones expanded, and by specificity, the number of pathogen epitopes recognized by the expanded CTL clones (Gianfrani et al. 2000). The current literature provides varying conclusions about CTL breadth and specificity. This partly reflects the technical difficulties mentioned above, but may also occur because the CTL response is variable.

The timing and methods of measurement may influence five aspects of the observed CTL response (Gianfrani et al. 2000). First, some studies measure primary CTL response, whereas other studies measure memory CTLs stimulated by secondary challenge. W. Chen et al. (2000) found that mouse primary response against influenza is more highly focused on a few epitopes than is the secondary response. By contrast, Busch et al. (1998) observed similar kinetics of primary and secondary responses against four epitopes of *Listeria*.

Second, persistent viral infections may evolve within a host, causing the host to develop a sequence of focused CTL responses.

Third, some methods measure relatively rare CTL-epitope combinations better than other methods. Relatively insensitive measurement leads to observations of narrow response. Relatively sensitive methods may pick up relatively weak CTL responses. The existence of a response does not mean that the response was a significant fraction of the total CTL expansion.

Fourth, it is often necessary to choose a priori a relatively small panel of epitopes as probes for the presence of matching CTLs. As the methods improve to predict CTL epitopes, the number of epitopes observed to stimulate CTL response will rise.

Fifth, some studies measure CTL response aggregated over several hosts. Each host may have a relatively narrow response, but hosts may differ in their choice of epitopes.

With these issues in mind, we can make some sense of the contrasting reports on the diversity CTL response. On the one hand, studies of influenza (Bednarek et al. 1991; Morrison et al. 1992) and Epstein-Barr virus (Callan et al. 1998) report a large fraction of CTLs focused on a single epitope. These studies emphasize the dominance of certain CTL clones at a particular time during infection within a single host (Murali-Krishna et al. 1998; Sourdive et al. 1998; Callan et al. 1998). On the other hand, observed human CTL responses were broad and multispecific against hepatitis B and C viruses and against HIV (Chisari 1995; McMichael and Phillips 1997; Rehermann et al. 1996). These pathogens tend to be genetically heterogeneous within a single host and may evolve by escape mutants in dominant epitopes. Thus, CTL focus may change over the course of infection within a single host.

Gianfrani et al. (2000) found a broad and multispecific human CTL memory response against influenza A. However, their measurements were aggregated over several hosts. Each host tended to respond strongly to a dominant epitope associated with one of its class I MHC alleles and to have memory CTLs for a small number of other epitopes for that dominant class I allele and for another class I allele. It seems that a few CTL clones prevail numerically within each host, but other clones may be stimulated and hosts may vary in which clones react to a particular epitope.

TIME OF CTL RECRUITMENT

Three factors influence the relative abundance of expanded T cell clones: frequency in the naive repertoire, rate of cell division, and time of initial expansion. Bousso et al. (1999) studied expansion of CTL clone abundances in mice against the human MHC allele HLA-Cw3. The response was dominated by a few clones. Those dominant clones were not particularly frequent in the naive repertoire. The relative abundances did not change between dominant and subdominant CTL clones that increased in abundance from the early to late stages of the T cell response, suggesting that expanding clones did not vary in their rate of cellular division.

The dominant CTL clones began their numerical expansion earlier than subordinate clones. CTL clones double every six to eight hours; thus a one-day advance in clonal activation causes an 8- to 16-fold difference in cellular abundance. The timing of initial clonal expansion appears to control immunodominance in this case. Bousso et al. (1999) did not determine whether the earlier proliferation of certain clones arose from binding properties to epitopes that triggered faster activation or from other causes.

INITIAL STIMULATION BY ENDOGENOUS VERSUS EXOGENOUS ANTIGEN

Naive CD8⁺ T cells must be activated to proliferate and to become armed with killer function as CTLs. Naive CD8⁺ cells are also confined to the blood and lymph systems and generally do not pass outside to most tissues, whereas the armed CTLs can exit to infected tissues.

The confinement of naive CD8⁺ cells raises a paradox (Reimann and Schirmbeck 1999). To be activated, the CD8⁺ cells must bind peptide-MHC class I complexes on the surface of cells with foreign antigen. But if the infection is not in the blood or lymph compartments, the naive T cells cannot reach the site of infection. Somehow, the naive CD8⁺ cells must encounter peptide-MHC class I complexes within the blood or lymph compartments even though the site of infection may be outside those compartments.

One possible solution depends on the distinction between endogenous and exogenous antigen (Schumacher 1999; Sigal et al. 1999). The CD8⁺ T cell is traditionally thought to bind primarily to pathogen antigens created endogenously within infected host cells. Those antigens are digested within the cell and transported to the endoplasmic reticulum, where they bind MHC class I molecules. The peptide-MHC complex is then transported to the cell surface, where it becomes available to roving T cells. Endogenously generated antigen is confined to the surface of the cell in which it was produced; thus endogenous antigen cannot be transported from infected tissues that exclude naive CD8$^+$ cells into the lymph nodes, where CD8$^+$ cells are common.

When an infected cell dies, pathogen antigens become liberated and exist exogenously. Sigal et al. (1999) showed that naive CD8$^+$ stimulation against a viral infection of peripheral tissue required transport of exogenous antigen by macrophages or dendritic cells into the lymph nodes. Dendritic cells are known to take up exogenous antigen in peripheral tissues and then to move to lymph nodes (Banchereau et al. 2000; Watts and Amigorena 2000). In addition, dendritic cells can process exogenous antigen and present it bound to MHC class I alleles (Reimann and Schirmbeck 1999). Thus, dendritic cells may serve as scouts in the peripheral tissue, bringing exogenous antigen to lymph nodes when stimulated by signs of infection or tissue damage.

How does this scouting network influence antigenic variation? For pathogens that infect peripheral tissue, CTL stimulation may focus on those antigens likely to be released exogenously and taken up by dendritic cells (or perhaps macrophages). Thus, abundant and stable pathogen proteins may be particularly likely to stimulate CTL response. For example, the capsid proteins of viruses may be more abundant than replicase enzymes and therefore more likely to be taken up as exogenous antigen.

COMPETITION AND INTERFERENCE BETWEEN CTL CLONES

Immunodominant CTL clones suppress the abundance of subdominant clones, a phenomenon called *immunodomination* (see the excellent review by Yewdell and Bennink 1999). Subdominant CTL clones responded more strongly with alteration or deletion of either the epitope stimulating the dominant CTL clone or the class I MHC molecule that presents the dominant epitope, or with direct inhibition of the dominant CTL clone (Zinkernagel et al. 1978; Doherty et al. 1978).

Yewdell and Bennink (1999) compare two explanations for immunodomination. First, the dominant epitope may interfere with the subdominant epitope for binding and presentation by MHC class I molecules. Such competition within antigen-presenting cells seems unlikely because CTL recognition of subdominant epitopes is not affected by coexpression of dominant epitopes (Mylin et al. 1995; Weidt et al. 1998). The abundance of epitopes (pathogen peptides) is usually so low that competition for binding to MHC class I molecules seems very unlikely (Yewdell and Bennink 1999).

Second, dominant CTL clones may directly or indirectly suppress subdominant clones. This may occur because dominant CTLs clear infected cells and associated subdominant epitopes too quickly for the weak CTL stimulation by subdominant epitopes to generate a strong CTL response (Nowak et al. 1995; Nowak and May 2000). Alternatively, the CTLs may compete directly at antigen-presenting cells for stimulation. Finally, the dominant CTLs may be able to suppress subdominant clones by competition for resources or by expressing suppressive cytokines.

On the whole, the evidence supports the second explanation, in which dominant clones suppress subdominant clones. Weidt et al.'s (1998) detailed study of lymphocytic choriomeningitis virus (LCMV) showed that immunodomination in that system arose from CTLs against dominant epitopes suppressing the viral population to a low level such that the suppressed viral population in the host stimulates only a weak CTL response against subdominant epitopes. This supports Nowak et al.'s (1995) model, in which immunodomination arises by the population dynamic consequences of birth and death rates for specific CTL clones and for viral populations that express matching epitopes.

In particular, Weidt et al. (1998) analyzed CTL response against two viral strains. The strain WE stimulated a dominant response against the epitope $NP_{118-126}$, whereas the strain ESC lacked this dominant epitope and stimulated response against various minor epitopes including $GP_{283-291}$. Class I MHC presents the minor epitopes in WE-infected cells, but does not stimulate significant CTL response. Importantly, CTLs specific for the subdominant epitope $GP_{283-291}$ lyse WE and ESC target cells to the same extent, suggesting that the subdominant epitope is presented effectively equally on the surfaces of WE and ESC cells. Thus, the strength of the CTL response is not caused by numerical differences in epitope presentation on cell surfaces.

The $NP_{118-126}$-specific CTLs do not directly suppress CTLs against minor epitopes, because coinfection by WE and ESC produces a significant CTL response against both $NP_{118-126}$ and $GP_{283-291}$, suggesting that ESC generates a CTL response against $GP_{283-291}$ without interference by the WE-induced CTLs against $NP_{118-126}$.

Although the dominant CTLs did not directly interfere with the subdominant CTL population, further evidence suggests indirect competition. Expansion of the dominant CTL clone against $NP_{118-126}$ and clearance of WE infection occurred more rapidly than did expansion of the subdominant CTL clone against $GP_{283-291}$ and clearance of ESC infection. Either WE or ESC infection activated $CD8^+$ T cells against the minor epitope, but in WE infection those minor-epitope T cells did not expand into a significant CTL response with lytic activity. It appears that, in WE infection, the fast development of CTLs against $NP_{118-126}$ suppressed the viral load quickly enough that the weaker-stimulated $CD8^+$ T cells against $GP_{283-291}$ did not have time to develop into a primary CTL response.

These kinetic processes lead to indirect competition. Kinetic control suggests that immunodomination should be a quantitative phenomenon ordering epitopes into a hierarchy. An immunodomination hierarchy has been demonstrated by Wettstein (1986). In addition, factors that alter the rate of CTL expansion against particular epitopes should be able to change the dominance hierarchy. Such changes in the hierarchy occur when the immune system has previously experienced an epitope. For example, if epitope A dominates epitope B in a naive host, then prior exposure only to B can reverse the dominance ranking and cause B to dominate A (Bennink and Doherty 1981; Jamieson and Ahmed 1989; Cole et al. 1997). This switch apparently occurs because secondary challenge causes a more rapid CTL response, allowing CTLs against B to reduce antigen load quickly enough to suppress a CTL response against A.

CTL REPERTOIRE

Why are CTL responses stronger against some epitopes than others? It could simply be that the immunodominant epitopes are expressed more commonly on cell surfaces than subdominant epitopes. However, Yewdell and Bennink (1999) summarize various lines of evidence arguing against a simple correlation between the abundance of presented epitopes and immunodominance, for example, the study by Weidt et al. (1998) described above. Thus, immunodomination of CTL clones appears to be influenced by biases in the $CD8^+$ repertoire.

Three important questions arise concerning $CD8^+$ biases in the naive repertoire (Yewdell and Bennink 1999). First, does immunodomination arise because more CD8$^+$ cells respond to an immunodominant epitope or because CD8$^+$ clones for immunodominant epitopes divide more quickly upon initial stimulation? The available data cannot distinguish between these alternatives.

Second, how does variation between individuals in naive CD8$^+$ repertoires influence the hierarchical ordering of epitopes? Individual variation can occur in self-peptides, TCR genes, and MHC genes. Negative selection shapes the TCR repertoire to avoid matching to self-peptides. TCR genes form the building blocks for combinatorial generation of TCR variability in each individual. MHC genes influence the presentation of peptides.

Third, independently of self-peptides and TCR genes, do immunodominant epitopes stimulate TCRs more strongly? Favorable structural attributes of immunodominant epitopes could interact with relatively constant features of the TCR.

A few studies have compared immunodominance in humans with that in transgenic mice expressing the same human MHC alleles. Both humans and transgenic mice recognized the same immunodominant epitopes when injected with viruses (Engelhard et al. 1991; Man et al. 1995; Shirai et al. 1995). Humans and mice that recognized the same peptide-MHC class I complex used TCRs composed of different Vα and Vβ germline components (Man et al. 1994). Thus, different self-peptides (mouse versus human) or variable TCR genes do not necessarily influence immunodominance, although this is a rather weak conclusion. Instead, immunodominance may depend on interactions between structural properties of the epitopes and relatively constant features of TCRs (Yewdell and Bennink 1999).

Negative selection against self-peptides can influence CD8$^+$ response to particular epitopes. This was shown in a study of human infection by Epstein-Barr virus (Burrows et al. 1994, 1995). Individuals with the MHC class I allele B8 typically have immunodominant responses against EBNA3A$_{325-333}$. The CTLs in this immunodominant response have a high proportion of the same germline TCR genes; that is, the response is composed of a very narrow set of CD8$^+$ clones.

CTL response against EBNA3A$_{325-333}$ cross-reacts to the MHC class I allele HLA B*4402 when the host lacks this HLA allele. Individuals with both B8 and B*4402 produce a relatively weak CTL response against EBNA3A$_{325-333}$. This weaker CTL response does not cross-react with

B*4402 and has a TCR gene composition that differs from the TCRs in the strong CTL response of the B8-positive and B*4402-negative individuals. Self-reactivity apparently reduced the CTLs that cross-react with B*4402. Reduction of those dominant CTLs allows other CD8$^+$ clones to expand, suggesting that the dominant CTLs in the B*4402-negative individuals suppress those CD8$^+$ clones that expand in B*4402-positive individuals.

ALTERED PEPTIDE LIGANDS

A CTL response depends on binding of the TCR to a peptide-MHC complex. An altered parasite peptide sometimes interferes with or enhances a CTL response against the original peptide, a phenomenon known as altered peptide ligand (APL) (reviewed by Sette et al. 1994; Jameson and Bevan 1995; Franco et al. 1995; Moskophidis and Zinkernagel 1995; Davis et al. 1998; Price et al. 1998; Germain and Štefanová 1999; Madrenas 1999; Abrams and Schlom 2000).

Disruption of the lytic activity in an active CTL response provides one example of APL antagonism. In this case, the CTL response against the original epitope can be influenced by the presence of an altered epitope (peptide) with a small number of amino acid substitutions. The altered peptide prevents CTL lytic activity against cells expressing the original epitope. Reduced lytic activity has been observed in HIV (Klenerman et al. 1994) and hepatitis B virus (Bertoletti et al. 1994). Antagonism by APLs lowers the clearance rate of viruses carrying the original peptide, potentially allowing longer survival and greater success of the protected genotypes within infected individuals.

Gilbert et al. (1998) studied the effects of APLs on the distribution of strains in a population of *Plasmodium falciparum* infecting humans in The Gambia. They examined four variant peptides of the circumsporozoite protein. The peptides cp26 and cp29 have CTL epitopes that bind the MHC class I molecule HLA-B35, the most frequent MHC class I molecule in their study area. The other two peptides (cp27 and cp28) do not bind HLA-B35.

The octamers cp26 and cp29 differ only in a single amino acid substitution. Peptide cp26 antagonizes cp29-specific CTLs and cp29 antagonizes cp26-specific CTLs. Interference occurs even when the antagonist occurs in relatively low concentration and is presented on different cells from the partner epitope. In addition, in vitro studies of T cells from hosts unexposed to malaria show that cp26 and cp29 mutually interfere with induction of primary CTL responses (Gilbert et al. 1998). In vivo studies in mice also show the same mutual interference of primary CTL induction (Plebanski et al. 1999).

Mutual interference suggests that hosts jointly infected with cp26 and cp29 will be less effective in clearing parasites than singly infected hosts or hosts with other combinations of strains. Gilbert et al. (1998) found hosts jointly infected with cp26 and cp29 more frequently than expected from population frequencies, suggesting that mutual interference of CTL response favors joint survival and transmission of these strains.

It is clear that APLs sometimes reduce CTL response. In the case of *Plasmodium falciparum*, it appears that variant peptides interfere with immunity sufficiently to influence the distribution of antigenic variation in the parasite population. It is not clear at present whether APLs have a significant influence on the antigenic diversity of other parasites.

6.3 Sequence of Exposure to Antigens: Original Antigenic Sin

The host amplifies specific B and T cell lineages in response to challenge by foreign antigen. Often the host has several B and T cell specificities that match the various antigens of a parasite, but the host amplifies only a subset of matching specificities. I discussed in earlier sections various factors that influence immunodominance—the particular subset of antigens that stimulate an immune reaction from among the broader set of antigens that could potentially stimulate a response.

The sequence in which the host encounters antigenic variants influences the specificity of the immune response. The first observations of sequential effects were made on influenza infections (Francis 1953; Fazekas de St. Groth and Webster 1966a, 1966b). These authors called sequential effects *original antigenic sin* because the first antigenic exposure influenced response to later antigens.

Sequential effects in B and T cell responses can occur in various ways. Figure 6.1a shows the most commonly described pattern. Consider two variant epitopes, A and A', at the same antigenic site. The specific immune response a against the original epitope A cross-reacts with the

		original order		reversed order	
		antigens	*immune response*	*antigens*	*immune response*
(a)	primary exposure:	A	a	A'	a'
	secondary exposure:	A'	a	A	a'
(b)	primary exposure:	A	a	A'	—
	secondary exposure:	A'	a	A	a
(c)	primary exposure:	A B	ab	A'B	a'b
	secondary exposure:	A'B	_b	A B	_ b

Figure 6.1   Three different patterns of original antigenic sin, as described in the text.

antigenic variant A'. If the host encounters A first, then secondary infection with A' stimulates a secondary immune response, a, with relatively higher specificity for A and weaker specificity for A' (original order). If the host encounters A' first, then secondary infection with A stimulates a secondary response, a', with higher specificity for A' and weaker specificity for A (reversed order). This form of cross-reactive interference occurs in CTLs (Good et al. 1993; Klenerman and Zinkernagel 1998) and antibodies (Fazekas de St. Groth and Webster 1966a; Barry et al. 1999).

Figure 6.1b shows a second pattern of cross-reactive effects between variants at the same epitope. This case is similar to the first, in which sequential stimulation by A and then A' causes a cross-reactive response a against secondary challenge by A' (original order). However, primary stimulation by A' does not elicit a response (reversed order). Thus, initial priming of cross-reactive memory cells by first exposure to A is required to generate a response to secondary challenge by A'. Fish et al. (1989) have demonstrated this pattern for antibody response.

The third pattern of sequential effects occurs when parasite challenge raises a specific immune response against several epitopes (fig. 6.1c). In this example, the first challenge with a pair of different epitopes, AB, raises a specific response ab against both epitopes. Secondary challenge by $A'B$, in which epitope A is altered, yields a robust immune response b against the original variant B but only a weak or absent response against the modified epitope A' (original order). Thus, a strong response against a constant epitope represses the response against the changed epitope. This pattern has been observed in sequential influenza infections (Janeway et al. 1999, p. 411).

It is not known how memory B or T cells reduce stimulation of naive clones during a secondary challenge. The rapid response from memory cells may keep parasite density below the threshold required to stimulate naive B or T cells. This would be a form of indirect repression mediated by the population dynamics of the parasite and the specific immune cells.

Alternatively, the memory cells may exert a more direct form of repression (Janeway et al. 1999, p. 410). For example, antigen bound to BCRs on naive B cells stimulates the B cells. But if the bound antigen also has a free antibody attached to it, the antibody interacts with the surface receptor FcγRIIB-1 on the naive B cell to repress activity of that naive B cell. By contrast, antibody bound to antigen-BCR complexes does not repress memory B cells.

6.4 Problems for Future Research

1. Molecular structure, binding kinetics, and competition between cellular lineages. Binding kinetics determine winners and losers in the competition between B cell lineages with different antibody specificities (Rao 1999). Equilibrium affinity dominates early in the competition, whereas on-rates dominate later during affinity maturation.

How can one study the biochemical and structural attributes that determine the binding kinetics of antibodies and epitopes? With regard to equilibrium affinity, one can compare structurally the different antibodies from the naive repertoire in relation to their success in binding a particular epitope and stimulating its B cell lineage. With regard to the shaping of on-rates, the hypermutation and selection during affinity maturation produce a lineal sequence of substitutions that enhances on-rates and perhaps also increases off-rates.

The contrast between the early selection of equilibrium affinity (on:off ratio) and the later selection of on-rate may provide insight into the structural features of binding that separately control on-rates and off-rates. This is a superb opportunity to relate structure to function via the kinetic processes that regulate the immune response.

2. Mathematical models and experimental perturbations. Immuno-dominance results from the kinetics of cellular lineages. Quantitative models help to develop hypotheses that can be tested by experimental perturbation. For example, Rao (1999) suggested that competition for helper T cells determines the expansion of B cell lineages. He tested this idea by manipulating the pool of helper T cells, and found that reducing the helper T cell pool did lower stimulation to B cell lineages.

Rao's quantitative model could be expanded into a mathematical analysis, with interactions between binding rates, pool sizes for different B and T cell lineages, and the rules of competition that determine which lineages succeed. Such a model presents clear hypotheses about the quantitative interactions that regulate immunity. Those hypotheses call attention to the sorts of experimental perturbations that should be informative.

3. Nowak's predator-prey model of competition. Nowak et al. (1995) developed a mathematical model of immunodominance. Their model focused on competition between immune cell lineages for stimulation by epitopes. Immune cells receive relatively stronger stimulation as their matching epitopes increase in numbers. The strongest immune-epitope match leads to the largest, immunodominant population of immune cells. That immunodominant lineage expands until its killing effect reduces the parasite population within the host down to a point of balance.

At that balance point, the parasite population stimulates division of the immunodominant population of immune cells just enough to match the tendency of the immune cell population to die off. In turn, the immunodominant immune cells reduce the parasites just enough to balance their births and deaths and hold the parasite population at a constant level. Other immune cell lineages receive weaker stimulation by the parasites because of their weaker binding characteristics to epitopes. Those subdominant lineages decline because the dominant lineage pushes parasite abundance down to the point where the weaker stimulation received by the subdominant lineages cannot overcome their tendency to decline.

The bottom line from this mathematical analysis matches the simplest, standard theory of predator-prey population dynamics: the most efficient predator reduces the prey down to a level where less efficient predators cannot survive.

Can such idealized mathematical models capture the complex molecular and kinetic details of the immune response? The answer depends on one's point of view. On the one hand, immunodominance is shaped in part by competition between lineages of immune cells, and thus the population dynamics of competition contribute in some way to the patterns of immunodominance. On the other hand, the model abstracts away many aspects of regulatory control, such as the role of helper T cells, the distinction between equilibrium binding affinity and kinetic on-rates of binding in different phases of the immune response, and structural properties that govern affinity and cross-reactivity.

The mathematical abstraction pays off as long as one understands the goal: to bring into sharp focus a hypothesis about how essential processes shape immunodominance. For example, Nowak et al.'s (1995) model predicts that essential properties of population dynamics and stimulatory thresholds matter. Some of the studies described in the text support this prediction. If one suspects that the distinction between equilibrium affinity and kinetic on-rates matters in an essential way for immunodominance, then an extended mathematical model would provide testable predictions about that aspect of the system.

I emphasize these issues here because the dynamics of immune cells and parasite populations within each infected host provide one of the few subjects that has been developed mathematically (Nowak and May 2000). The simple principles from those models do seem to be important, if only because the rules of population dynamics must play a key role in shaping how populations of immune cells and parasites interact.

One can, of course, make more specific mathematical models to predict the dynamics of particular parasites or the role of particular molecular mechanisms. Those specific models require empirical study of their specialized predictions. And that is exactly what we want: tests of clearly and logically formulated quantitative predictions.

4. Helper T cell epitopes in an antibody response. Helper T cells provide an important stimulus in the development of an antibody response. As B cells bind antigen to their BCR, they often pull the antigen into the cell. The B cells process protein antigens into small peptides, bind those peptides to MHC class II molecules, and present the peptide-MHC complexes on their cell surfaces. Helper T cells with matching specificity in their TCRs bind the peptide-MHC complexes and stimulate the B cells. Thus, an antigen must have two epitopes to stimulate a robust B cell response with affinity maturation. One epitope binds the BCR, and a second must survive digestion and be presented on the B cell surface bound to a class II molecule for the TCR of a helper T cell.

Several factors likely affect the degree to which helper T cell epitopes modulate the immunodominance of B cell epitopes. These factors include the proximity of the two epitopes, the binding kinetics of the T cell epitope to the TCR, the nature of the helper T cell signal that provides stimulation to the B cell, and the population dynamics of the helper T cell lineages with different TCR specificities. For example, Shirai et al. (1999) showed that the proximity of a helper T cell epitope to a B cell epitope can influence development of the antibody response. In particular, a helper T cell epitope near the hypervariable region of the hepatitis C virus envelope gene aids in generation of antibodies to the hypervariable region.

5. CTL versus antibody response. Antibody attack favors antigenic variation in parasites' surface molecules. By contrast, CTLs favor variation in any parasite molecule that can be presented by the host's MHC system. The balance of antibody versus CTL defense affects the population dynamics of the parasites within the host, the time before clearance, and the memory properties of host immunity against reinfection (Seder and Hill 2000). The factors that tip an immune response toward antibody, CTL, or a mixture of the two are not fully understood (Constant and Bottomly 1997; Power 2000). Studies of model systems sometimes show a sharp dichotomy between CTL and antibody response controlled by a simple variable such as antigen dosage (Menon and Bretscher 1998). But the immune response to many viruses includes robust antibody and CTL attack (Knipe and Howley 2001).

As more parasite genomes are sequenced, it may be useful to look at which potential antigenic sites do in fact show significant variation. Those highly variable sites can be studied to determine if they are CTL or antibody epitopes, providing clues about which type of immunity imposes the strongest selective pressure on the parasite.

7

Parasite Escape within Hosts

Specific immunity favors parasites that change their epitopes and escape recognition. In this chapter, I summarize examples of parasite escape and the consequences for antigenic diversity within hosts.

The first section presents HIV and hepatitis C virus (HCV) as two pathogens that evolve within hosts to escape specific immunity. HIV variants escape recognition by CTLs, whereas HCV variants escape recognition by specific antibodies. HIV also diversifies its surface molecules in order to attack different cell types. Changing tissue tropisms over the course of an infection provide an additional force to drive the evolution of parasite diversification within hosts. HIV and HCV are both RNA viruses, which mutate frequently and evolve rapidly. The importance of within-host immune escape by random mutations in DNA-encoded pathogens remains to be studied.

The second section describes how parasites interfere with host immunity. For example, viruses may disrupt MHC presentation of antigens, send misleading signals to natural killer cells, block programmed cell death (apoptosis) of infected cells, or express cytokines that alter immune regulation. In some cases, parasite antigens may lack variation because the parasite repels immune attack by interfering with host immunity rather than altering the specificity of its epitopes.

The third section focuses on parasites that escape host immunity by switching gene expression between variants stored within each genome. A single parasite expresses only one of the variants from the archival genomic library. Each parasite lineage changes expression from one stored gene to another at a low rate. As host immunity builds against a common variant, one or more newly expressed variants can rise. The host must then build another specific immune response against the new variants. Parasites that switch variants in this way may gain by extending the total time of infection. Additionally, switching may help to avoid the immunological memory of a previously infected host.

The fourth section introduces processes that enhance or retard the coexistence of antigenic variants within hosts. If antigenic variants compete for a common resource, such as host cells or a limiting nutrient, then one competitively dominant variant tends to drive the other variants extinct. Resource specialization allows different variants to coexist, for example, when each variant attacks a different cell type. Spatial variation in the density of resources can allow different variants to dominate in different compartments of the host's body.

The final section takes up promising issues for future research.

7.1 Natural Selection of Antigenic Variants

In several pathogens, a changing profile of antigenic variants characterizes the course of infection within a single host. Natural selection favors variants that escape immune recognition, although escape is often temporary. Selection may also favor diversification of the pathogens for the ability to attack different types of host cells. I briefly summarize a few examples.

SIV AND HIV

Soudeyns et al. (1999) identified the regions of the HIV-1 envelope under strong selective pressure by analyzing the pattern of nucleotide changes in the population. They compared the rate of nonsynonymous (d_N) nucleotide replacements that cause an amino acid change versus the rate of synonymous (d_S) nucleotide replacements that do not cause an amino acid change. A high d_N/d_S ratio suggests positive natural selection favoring amino acid change; a low d_N/d_S ratio suggests negative natural selection opposing change in amino acids (Page and Holmes 1998; see chapter 15 below).

Soudeyns et al. (1999) found that regions of the envelope gene under strong positive selection corresponded to epitopes recognized by CTLs. The nonsynonymous substitutions in these epitopes typically abolished recognition by a matching CTL clone. The population of viruses accumulated diversity in the dominant epitopes over the course of infection within hosts. These results suggest that CTL attack based on specific recognition drives the rapid rate of amino acid replacements in these epitopes.

Kimata et al. (1999) studied properties of simian immunodeficiency virus (SIV) isolated from early and late stages of infection within individual hosts. The early viruses infected macrophages, replicated slowly, and the viral particles were susceptible to antibody-mediated clearance.

The late viruses infected T cells, replicated more than 1,000 times faster than early viruses, and were less sensitive to antibody-mediated clearance.

Kimata et al. (1999) did not determine the viral amino acid changes that altered cell tropism of SIV. Connor et al. (1997) found that changes in the host cell coreceptors used by early and late HIV-1 correlated with changes in cell tropism, but it is not yet clear which changes are essential for the virus's tropic specificity. Connor et al. (1997) did show that the population of early viruses used a narrow range of coreceptors, whereas the late viruses were highly polymorphic for a diverse range of host coreceptors. Clearly, the virus is evolving to use various cell types.

The relative insensitivity of late SIV to antibody apparently depended on increased glycosylation of the envelope proteins (Chackerian et al. 1997). The late viruses with increased glycosylation were not recognized by antibodies that neutralized the early viruses. Viruses that escape antibody recognition gain significant advantage during the course of infection (Chackerian et al. 1997; Rudensey et al. 1998). Kimata et al. (1999) showed that, when injected into a naive host, the late SIV did not stimulate as much neutralizing antibody as did the early SIV. Additional glycosylation apparently reduces the ability of antibodies to form against the viral surface. Presumably the glycosylation also hinders the ability of the virus to initiate infection; otherwise both early and late viruses would have enhanced glycosylation.

Both the early, macrophage-tropic SIV and the late, T cell–tropic SIV used the host coreceptor CCR5 (Kimata et al. 1999). That observation contrasts with a study of early and late HIV-1 isolated from individual hosts, in which Connor et al. (1997) found that early, macrophage-tropic viruses depended primarily on the CCR5 coreceptors, whereas the population of late viruses had expanded coreceptor use to include CCR5, CCR3, CCR2b, and CXCR4.

Many recent studies focus on HIV diversification within hosts (e.g., Allen et al. 2000; Goulder et al. 2001; Saha et al. 2001).

HEPATITIS C VIRUS

Farci et al. (2000) obtained hepatitis C virus (HCV) samples at various stages of infection within individual hosts. They sequenced the envelope genes from these samples to determine the pattern of evolution within hosts. They then compared the evolutionary pattern with the clinical outcome of infection, which follows one of three courses: clearance in about 15% of cases; chronic infection and either slowly or rapidly progressive disease in about 85% of cases; and severe, fulminant hepatitis in rare cases.

Farci et al. (2000) sampled three major periods of infection: the incubation period soon after infection; during the buildup of viremia but before significant expression of specific antibodies; and after the host's buildup of specific antibodies.

The sequence diversity within hosts identified two distinct regions of the envelope genes. The hypervariable region evolved quickly and appeared to be under positive selection from the host immune system, whereas other regions of the envelope genes had relatively little genetic variation and did not evolve rapidly under any circumstances. Thus, the following comparisons focus only on the hypervariable region.

Those hosts that eventually cleared the virus had similar or higher rates of viral diversification before antibodies appeared than did those patients that developed chronic infection. By contrast, after antibodies appeared, chronic infection was correlated with significantly higher viral diversity and rates of evolution than occurred when the infection was eventually cleared. It appears that hosts who cleared the infection could contain viral diversity and eventually eliminate all variants, whereas those that progressed to chronic infection could not control viral diversification. The rare and highly virulent fulminant pattern had low viral diversity and rates of evolution. This lack of diversity suggests either that the fulminant form may be associated with a single viral lineage that has a strong virulence determinant or that some hosts failed to mount an effective immune response.

GENERALITY OF WITHIN-HOST EVOLUTION OF ANTIGENS

HIV and HCV share several characters that make them particularly likely to evolve within hosts. They are RNA viruses, which have relatively high mutation rates, relatively simple genomes, simple life cycles, potentially high replication rates, and potentially high population sizes within hosts. HIV and HCV also typically develop persistent infections with long residence times in each host. If the mutation rate per nucleotide per replication is 10^{-5} and the population of viruses is on the order of 10^{10} within a host, then there are 10^5 point mutations at every site in every generation. For every pair of sites, there will usually be at least one virus that carries mutations at both sites. Thus, there is a tremendous influx of mutational variation.

Other RNA viruses such as influenza also have high mutation rates and potentially large populations within hosts, but the hosts typically clear infections within two weeks. Some within-host evolution very likely occurs, but it does not play a significant role in the infection dynamics within hosts.

DNA-based pathogens produce much less mutational variation per replication. But large population sizes, long infection times, and hy-permutation of epitopes could still lead to significant evolution within hosts. At present, the persistent RNA infections have been studied most intensively because of their obvious potential for rapid evolutionary change. As more data accumulate, it will be interesting to compare the extent and the rate of within-host evolutionary change in various pathogens.

7.2 Pathogen Manipulation of Host Immune Dynamics

Pathogens use several strategies to interfere with host immunity. A parasite's exposed surface antigens or candidate CTL epitopes may lack variation because the parasite can repel immune attack. I do not know of any evidence to support this idea, but it should be considered when studying candidate epitopes and their observed level of antigenic varia-tion.

Several reviews summarize viral methods for reducing host immunity (e.g., Spriggs 1996; Alcami and Koszinowski 2000). Some bacteria also interfere with immune regulation (Rottem and Naot 1998). I list just a few viral examples, taken from the outline given by Tortorella et al. (2000).

Some viruses interfere with MHC presentation of antigens. Cases oc-cur in which viruses reduce MHC function at the level of transcription, protein synthesis, degradation, transport to the cell surface, and main-tenance at the cell surface.

The host's natural killer (NK) cells attack other host cells that fail to present MHC class I molecules on their surface. Viruses that inter-fere with normal class I expression use various methods to prevent NK attack, for example, viral expression of an MHC class I homolog that interferes with NK activation.

Host cells often use programmed suicide (apoptosis) to control infection. Various viruses interfere with different steps in the apoptosis control pathway.

The host uses cytokines to regulate many immune functions. Some viruses alter expression of host cytokines or express their own copies of cytokines. Other viruses express receptors for cytokines or for the constant (Fc) portion of antibodies. These viral receptors reduce concentrations of freely circulating host molecules or transmit signals that alter the regulation of host defense.

7.3 Sequence of Variants in Active Switching from Archives

Some parasites store alternative genes for antigenic surface molecules. Each individual parasite usually expresses only one of the alternatives (Deitsch et al. 1997; Fussenegger 1997). Parasite lineages change expression from one stored gene to another at a low rate. In *Trypanosoma brucei*, the switch rate is about 10^{-3} or 10^{-2} per cell division (Turner 1997).

Antigenic switches affect the dynamics of the parasite population within the host. For example, the blood-borne bacterial spirochete *Borrelia hermsii* causes a sequence of relapsing fevers (Barbour 1987, 1993). Each relapse and recovery follows from a spike in bacterial density. The bacteria rise in abundance when new antigenic variants escape immune recognition and fall in abundance when the host generates a specific antibody response to clear the dominant variants.

Many different kinds of parasites change their surface antigens by altering expression between variant genes in an archival library (Deitsch et al. 1997; Fussenegger 1997). This active switching raises interesting problems for the population dynamics and evolution of antigenic variation within individual hosts. I briefly describe some of these problems in the following subsections.

STOCHASTIC SWITCHING VERSUS ORDERED PARASITEMIAS

In *Trypanosoma brucei*, lineages switch stochastically between variants. Turner and Barry (1989) measured the switch probability per cell

Table 7.1 $\log_{10}$ of probability of switching between antigenic variants in *Trypanosoma brucei*

	1.22	1.3	1.61	1.62	1.63	1.64
1.63	−2.7		−2.7			−2.3
1.64	−3.4		−3.4		−3.4	
1.64	−3.0		−3.8		−3.1	
1.64	−3.4	−2.6		−4.0		
1.64	−2.7	−2.2		−5.7		

Values are from Turner and Barry (1989). The numbers in the column headings and row labels are names for particular antigenic variants. Table entries show $\log_{10}$ of the switch probability per cell per generation.

per generation for changes between particular antigenic types. Each entry in table 7.1 shows $\log_{10}$ of the probability that a cell expressing a particular variant, designated by a number in the left column, switches to another variant designated by a number in the column headings.

The different rows in table 7.1 summarize data from five separate experiments. Overall, it appears that each type can potentially switch to several other types, with the probability of any transition typically on the order of 10^{-4} to 10^{-2}. *Trypanosoma brucei* stores and uses many different antigenic variants, perhaps hundreds (Vickerman 1989; Barry 1997). Thus, the limited sample in table 7.1 does not provide a comprehensive analysis of switch probabilities between all types.

Switches between types within a cellular lineage occur stochastically. But the sequence of variants that dominate sequential waves of parasitemia tends to follow a repeatable order (Gray 1965; Barry 1986). For example, figure 7.1 shows the date at which different variants first appeared in *Trypanosoma vivax* infections of rabbits. Some separation occurs between variants that arise early versus late.

Temporal separation in the rise of different antigenic variants allows trypanosomes to continue an infection for a longer period of time (Vickerman 1989). If all variants rose in abundance early in the infection, they would all stimulate specific immune responses and be cleared, ending the infection. If the rise in different variants can be spread over time, then the infection can be prolonged.

The puzzle is how stochastic changes in the surface antigens of individual parasites can lead to an ordered temporal pattern at the level of the population of parasites within the host (Agur et al. 1989; Frank 1999;

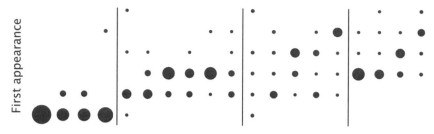

Antigenic variants

Figure 7.1 The sequence of appearance for nineteen antigenic variants of *Trypanosoma vivax* in rabbits. Each column shows a different antigenic variant. The rows are the day since inoculation at which a variant was first detected during an infection. The days of measurement are, from bottom to top, 12, 19, 26, 33, 40, and 47/55, where data from days 47 and 55 are combined in the top row. Barry (1986) collected data from six rabbits. The diameter of each circle shows, for each variant, the frequency of rabbits in which a variant first appeared on a particular day following inoculation. I discarded variants for which there were observations from fewer than five of the six rabbits. I have arbitrarily ordered the variants from those on the left that appear early to those on the right that appear late. The vertical bars crudely group the variants into categories defined by time of appearance.

Turner 1999). Four hypotheses have been developed, none of which has empirical support at present. I briefly describe each idea.

First, the antigenic variants may differ in growth rate. Those that divide more quickly could dominate the early phases of infection, and those that divide more slowly could increase and be cleared later in the infection (Seed 1978). Computer studies and mathematical models show that variable growth rates alone can not easily explain wide separation in the times of appearance of different variants (Kosinski 1980; Agur et al. 1989). Only with a very large spread in growth rates would the slowest variant be able to avoid an immune response long enough to develop an extended duration of total infection. Aslam and Turner (1992) measured the growth rates of different variants and found little difference between the variants.

Second, parasite cells may temporarily express both the old and new antigens in the transition period after a molecular switch in antigenic type (Agur et al. 1989). The double expressors could experience varying immune pressure depending on the time for complete antigenic replacement or aspects of cross-reactivity. This would favor some transitions to occur more easily than others, leading to temporal separation in the order of appearance for different antigenic variants. This model is rather complex and has gained little empirical or popular support, as discussed in several papers (Barry and Turner 1991, 1992; Agur 1992; Muñoz-Jordán et al. 1996; Borst et al. 1997).

Third, the switch probabilities between antigenic variants may be structured in a way to provide sequential dominance and extended infection (Frank 1999). If the transition probabilities from each variant to the other variants are chosen randomly, then an extended sequence of expression cannot develop because the transition pathways are too highly connected. The first antigenic types would generate several variants that develop a second parasitemia. Those second-order variants would generate nearly all other variants in a random switch matrix.

The variants may arise in an extended sequence if the parasite structures the transition probabilities into separate sets of variants, with only rare transitions between sets. The first set of variants switches to a limited second set of variants, the second set connects to a limited third set, and so on. Longer infections enhance the probability of transmission to other hosts. Thus, natural selection favors the parasites to structure their switch probabilities in a hierarchical way in order to extend the length of infection.

Turner (1999) proposed a fourth explanation for high switch rates and ordered expression of variants. The parasite faces a trade-off between two requirements. On the one hand, competition between parasite genotypes favors high rates of switching and stochastic expression of multiple variants early in an infection. On the other hand, lower effective rates of switching later in an infection express variants sequentially and extend the total length of infection.

Many *Trypanosoma brucei* infections in the field probably begin with infection by multiple parasite genotypes transmitted by a single tsetse fly vector (MacLeod et al. 1999). This creates competition between the multiple genotypes. According to Turner (1999), competition intensifies the selective pressure on parasites to express many variants— variation allows escape from specific immunity by prior infections and helps to avoid cross-reactivity between variants expressed by different genotypes. These factors favor high rates of stochastic switching.

The effective rate of switching drops as the infection progresses because the host develops immunity to many variants. Effective switches occur when they produce novel variants, and the rate at which novel variants arise declines over the course of infection. Those novel variants, when they do occur, can produce new waves of parasitemia, promoting parasite transmission.

Turner's idea brings out many interesting issues, particularly the role of competition between genotypes within a host. But his verbal model is not fully specified. For example, delayed expression of some variants and extended infection depend on the connectivity of transition pathways between variants, an issue he does not discuss. The problem calls for mathematical analysis coupled with empirical study.

ROLE OF PRIOR EXPOSURE

Hosts that have recovered from an infectious parasite that switches antigenic type may retain immune memory for many antigenic variants. Successful reinfection would require a parasite to express a variant for which the host lacks specific memory. Antigenic variants expressed from an archival library can help a parasite to overcome immune memory of previously infected hosts.

The role of antigenic variation in avoiding immune memory from prior infections depends on several factors. How many variants stimulate memory during a typical infection? What percentage of infected hosts recover and survive? What is the rate of death among surviving hosts (population memory decay) relative to the rate at which naive, newborn hosts enter the population? What percentage of hosts suffer a primary infection? What percentage become reinfected?

Again, these interacting quantitative factors can be combined into a mathematical model. A model would suggest what conditions must be met for archival antigenic variation to be an effective strategy to avoid host immune memory.

7.4 Ecological Coexistence of Variants within a Host

Two or more antigenic variants may coexist within a host during a persistent infection. Various processes tend to promote or destroy coexistence.

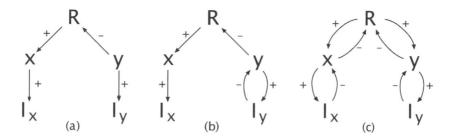

Figure 7.2   Pathways of interaction between a host resource, R, two populations of parasites with different antigenic types, x and y, and two populations
of specific immune cells, I_x specialized for x, and I_y specialized for y. (a) The
various direct effects of an increase in y. Effects over more than one step are
obtained by multiplying the signs along the paths. For example, an increase in
y has a negative effect on R, which in turn has a positive effect on x, which has
a positive effect on I_x. Thus, an increase in y depresses I_x because the product
of the two positive arrows and one negative arrow is negative. (b) An example
of an indirect feedback effect. A change in y has an additional, indirect effect
on I_x via its pathway to I_y. The path to I_y from y is positive, and the return
path to y is negative, yielding a net negative effect. Continuing on from y to
I_x produces another negative component, so the product of the entire indirect
pathway is positive. (c) Additional feedback loops and indirect effects.

PREDATOR-PREY FEEDBACK WITH SPECIFIC IMMUNE CELLS

Consider two variants, x and y, each variant attacked by specific immunity, I_x and I_y. In the simplest case of persistence, each matching pair
fluctuates independently. Thus, as x increases, I_x rises and causes x to
decline. A decline in x lowers stimulation and causes I_x to fall, which
allows x to rise, and so on. A similar cycle happens with the predatory
immune type, I_y, preying on the antigenic type, y.

RESOURCE COMPETITION

It could be that the two cycles progress independently, with coexistence of the antigenic types. Or there can be various forms of coupling
between the cycles. For example, the parasite types x and y may compete for a host resource, R, such as host cells to infect or the uptake of
a limiting nutrient (Smith and Holt 1996).

Direct competition between the parasite variants creates indirect interactions between the specific immune types. Consider what happens

if y increases. Figure 7.2a shows that a rise in y stimulates I_y and reduces the available host resources, R. A drop in R depresses x, which in turn lowers stimulation to I_x. Overall, if we ignore all feedbacks, an increase in y enhances I_y, and depresses x and I_x.

Feedbacks occur, and their consequences must be followed. Continuing with the example, figure 7.2b shows that a rise in I_y grazes y to a lower value, allowing host resources, R, to recover, which enhances x and stimulates I_x. Figure 7.2c shows that several other feedbacks exist even in this highly oversimplified network of interactions—to trace all consequences is beyond normal intuition. Analysis requires mathematical models (Nowak and May 2000).

For this particular example, it turns out that resource competition by itself typically reduces the potential for coexistence of antigenic variants compared with the case in which no competition occurs. If I_y drives y to extinction in the absence of competition, then additional competition for resources will usually not save y. Rather, the competition from x further decreases y's chances for survival.

Several studies suggest that resource competition between parasites may sometimes influence the within-host dynamics of infection. In persistent malaria infections, competition between *Plasmodium* for susceptible erythrocytes apparently plays an important role (Gravenor et al. 1995; Hetzel and Anderson 1996; Gravenor and Lloyd 1998). Wodarz et al. (1999) proposed that the spread of human T cell leukemia viruses (HTLV-1) between host cells is limited by availability of susceptible, uninfected T cells.

Turner et al. (1996) inferred density-dependent effects on the growth rate of the blood-borne parasite *Trypanosoma brucei*. Although Turner et al. (1996) did not demonstrate parasite competition for host resources, it seems likely that some resource limitation arises because of the very high parasite densities that occur at peak parasitemia, on the order of 10^6 to 10^7 parasites per ml of blood. These studies did not directly discuss antigenic variation, but they suggest that resource competition may be important.

RESOURCE SPECIALIZATION

Antigenic variants may specialize on different host resources. For example, parasite surface molecules may influence tropism for host cell type or efficiency in uptake of different host nutrients. To the extent that antigenic variants do differ in their use of host resources, coexistence becomes easier to maintain by reducing the direct competition between the variants.

Variation in tissue tropism appears to be associated with antigenically variable surface molecules in *Neisseria gonorrhoeae* (Gray-Owen et al. 1997; Virji et al. 1999). In *Neisseria*, variable cell tropism may be important in sequentially colonizing different tissues as invasion and spread develop, with little direct competition between the antigenic variants.

HIV provides a potential case of competition and resource specialization between variants. Connor et al. (1997) found changes in coreceptor use by early and late HIV-1 correlated with changes in cell tropism. The population of early viruses used a narrow range of coreceptors, whereas the late viruses were highly polymorphic for a diverse array of host coreceptors. As the population of viruses builds and depresses the abundance of commonly infected cell types, diversification to different cell tropisms reduces competition.

Spatial Segregation

Variable resource concentration can also favor antigenic diversity. Consider a contrast between two antigenic variants. The first has a surface antigen that provides superior entry into host cells, but this variant is cleared at a higher rate. The second variant has a lower rate of entry into host cells, but is cleared at a lower rate. The first type interferes with the second when both are common.

This infection-clearance trade-off can promote coexistence by spatial segregation. For example, host compartments with low resource levels cannot sustain the first type—limited host cells reduce the production rate below the high clearance rate. The second, weaker competitor dominates. By contrast, in compartments with high resource levels, the stronger type dominates by outcompeting the weaker type.

Other Factors

There are, of course, many other factors that influence the abundance of antigenic variants and immune cells. The immunogenicity of the antigenic types may differ, varying the rate of parasite killing and the stimulatory signals to the immune cells. Each parasite carries many different antigenic determinants, raising once again issues of immunodominance, which must be understood in terms of populations of parasite variants and populations of immune cells with matching specificities.

Each factor can have complex dynamical consequences. Mathematical studies show that even rather simple interactions often lead to fluctuating abundances because of the nonlinear processes inherent in population dynamics. Thus, fluctuating abundances of antigenic variants and matching immune specificities may often occur in persistent infections (Nowak and May 2000).

7.5 Problems for Future Research

1. Mutational distance required for escape. How many amino acid substitutions are needed for new variants to escape immunity against the original epitope? Does escape usually arise from a single substitution, or are multiple substitutions often required? If laboratory mice can be used as a model, it would be interesting to infect replicates of a common host genotype by a cloned pathogen genotype. One could then study the relative effect of genotype and stochastic factors on the number of substitutions in escape variants and the genetic pattern of diversification in escape. I discuss relevant preliminary studies in later chapters on experimental evolution.

2. Transmissibility of escape variants. Epitopes often occur in key surface molecules used for attachment or in important enzymes such as replication polymerases. Escape variants gain by avoiding specific immunity but may impose costs by lowering other components of parasite fitness. I mentioned earlier that SIV isolated late in infections had increased glycosylation of surface antigens that reduced susceptibility to antibodies. The glycosylation also reduced the degree to which viruses stimulated an antibody response when injected into new hosts. It would be interesting to know if glycosylation reduces transmissibility or some other component of viral fitness.

Escape within a host does not necessarily reduce transmissibility or other components of fitness. Goulder et al. (2001) studied human mothers with the MHC allele B27 infected by HIV-1. B27 recognizes an immunodominant and highly conserved CTL epitope in the viral Gag protein. Escape mutants at this epitope persist and enhance progression to disease. Mothers can transmit this escape variant to their offspring, who then target a subdominant B27 epitope and fail to contain the infection. These escape variants remain stable and do not revert to the original type when passaged in cell culture. It would be interesting to study similar issues with SIV, in which it would be possible to do experiments in vivo and test whether there is a fitness cost associated with CTL escape.

3. Dynamics of infection in parasites that switch between archival variants. Antigenic switching from archival libraries generates interesting dynamics within the host. Typically, the first variants increase rapidly, causing a high density of parasites within the host. Specific immunity then rises against those initial variants, causing a decline in the parasite population within the host. The initial, dense parasitemia generates variants by occasional switching. The variants rise in abundance during or after the decline of the first parasite burst.

These dynamics point to several questions. What is the basic timing for the initial growth of the parasite population, the rise in specific immune cells, and the decline in the initial parasitemia? What are the densities and the diversity of antigenic variants during the initial parasitemia? What are the timings and the shapes of the growth curves for the populations of antigenic variants?

At what parasite density do the variants begin to stimulate a specific immune response? That stimulatory threshold sets the pace at which the host can raise a new wave of immunity to combat the second parasite wave. How many variants rise in the second wave? What is the timing and pattern of new variants generated by parasites in the second wave? How do the coupled dynamics of specific immune cell populations and matching parasite variants together determine the total length of infection and the fluctuating density of parasites available for transmission? What determines the order in which parasite variants rise in successive parasitemias?

4. Immune dynamics in different body compartments. Different parasite surface molecules may cause infection of different body compartments. The surface molecules that affect tissue tropism may also be strong antigenic determinants. I mentioned that diversifying tissue tropisms during the course of an infection can diversify antigenic variation within the host. In addition, the dynamics of host immunity and the ability of immune effectors to attack parasites likely vary among body compartments. Thus, variants with certain tropisms may sequester themselves in refuges from immune pressure. These protected sites may provide a source of chronic infection or generate relapses after apparent clearance of the initial infection.

PART IV

POPULATION CONSEQUENCES

8 Genetic Variability of Hosts

In this chapter, I discuss the ways in which host immune responses vary genetically. Host variability affects the relative success of different parasite epitopes and the distribution of antigenic variants.

The first section reviews host variation in specific recognition. MHC alleles are highly polymorphic—different hosts usually have different MHC genotypes and therefore recognize different spectrums of parasite epitopes. By contrast, limited genetic variability occurs in the germline genes that encode the antibody and T cell binding regions. Instead, variable antibody and T cell binding sites arise by somatic recombination. Somatic mechanisms to generate variation may buffer the need for hosts to vary genetically.

The second section summarizes genetic polymorphisms in immune regulation. Hosts vary genetically in many of the controls of immune response. This variation leads to differences in the thresholds that trigger immunity and in the intensity of particular immune effectors deployed against parasitic attack. Quantitative differences in immune regulation can affect the intensity of selection on antigenic variants and the immunodominance of host responses against different variants. Immunodominance, in turn, defines the selective pressures that shape the distribution of antigenic variants.

A few major polymorphisms have been found in the promoters of cytokines, molecules that regulate key aspects of the immune system. Different promoter genotypes correlate with better or worse success in combating certain pathogens. Regulatory polymorphisms may be maintained by trade-offs, in which a more intense immune response clears parasites more effectively but also causes more collateral tissue damage to the host.

Major regulatory polymorphisms have different alleles at high frequencies, each allele with a significantly different effect on immune response. High frequencies and large effects make such polymorphisms relatively easy to find.

Rare variants of small effect undoubtedly occur throughout the immune regulatory cascade, maintained by a balance between mutation and selection. Each individual probably carries several minor regulatory variants, causing significant quantitative genetic variability between hosts in the regulation of the immune response.

The final section takes up promising issues for future research.

8.1 Polymorphisms in Specificity

MHC

Polymorphisms sometimes occur in host molecules that directly bind to parasites. For example, the MHC class I and II alleles are the most polymorphic of all human genes. The three main class I loci for presenting peptides, designated A, B, and C, currently have 175, 349, and 90 alleles described, respectively.

The class II molecules have separate designations for individual components of each molecule. The highly polymorphic components tend to be in the β_1 chains that contact bound peptides (Marsh et al. 2000). The β_1 chains for the DR, DQ, and DP class II molecules currently have 246, 44, and 86 alleles described, respectively. The IMGT/HLA online database lists recent allelic counts for both class I and class II loci, as described in Robinson et al. (2000; see http://www.ebi.ac.uk/imgt/hla/).

The MHC molecules bind to parasite peptides and present those peptides to T cells. Differences in MHC genotype cause significant variation between hosts in their ability to bind particular antigenic variants (Yewdell and Bennink 1999). Many studies have shown associations between MHC genotype and disease susceptibility (Hill 1998).

The MHC molecules also shape the TCR repertoire. As T cells mature in the thymus, they bind to MHC molecules presenting self-antigens. Those TCRs that bind too strongly cause the associated T cells to die. Those TCRs that bind too weakly fail to provide sufficiently strong reinforcing signals, again causing the associated T cells to die. Less than 1% of T cells pass these checks (Marsh et al. 2000). Thus, the particular MHC alleles of each individual strongly influence the naive TCR repertoire.

Variant naive repertoires lead to different TCR clones being stimulated in different individuals when challenged by the same epitope (Maryanski et al. 1996, 1999). Because helper T cells influence antibody response and other aspects of immune regulation, the variable TCR repertoire may have additional consequences beyond CTL variability.

Proteolysis of antigens and transport of peptides determine the peptides available for MHC binding. Strong challenge by a particular parasite could lead to selection favoring or disfavoring specific patterns of proteolysis. However, I am not aware of any evidence for polymorphism in proteolytic enzymes. The peptide transporter, TAP, is polymorphic: the two subunits, TAP1 and TAP2, have six and four sequences listed in the IMGT/HLA database (Robinson et al. 2000). So far, no functional differences between alleles have been found (Marsh et al. 2000).

TCR GERMLINE

Different TCR germline loci somatically recombine and mutate to generate the DNA that codes for the variable, antigen-binding part of the TCR (Janeway et al. 1999). These generative mechanisms allow each individual to produce a huge variety of TCR binding specificities.

The intensity of direct selection on germline polymorphisms may be rather weak because specific recognition of antigens depends primarily on somatic mechanisms to create variability. However, the germline alleles do set the initial conditions on which somatic processes build, so it is certainly possible that germline polymorphisms influence individual tendencies to react to particular antigens.

The limited data currently available indicate that some germline polymorphisms exist for the TCR (e.g., Reyburn et al. 1993; Hauser 1995; Moffatt et al. 1997; Moody et al. 1998; Sim et al. 1998; see http://imgt. cines.fr). One interesting study found an interaction between a human germline polymorphism in a subunit of the TCR (VA8.1) and an MHC class II polymorphism (HLA-DRB1) (Moffatt et al. 1997). The authors analyzed two variants of the VA8.1 allele and the six most common HLA-DRB1 alleles. Individuals with enhanced allergic response to a dust mite antigen tended to have one of the two VA8.1 variants combined with the HLA-DRB1*1501 allele.

Moffatt et al. (1997) measured allergic response by the titer of IgE antibodies, which stimulate allergic symptoms (Janeway et al. 1999). Most likely, the TCR and MHC class II polymorphisms influence IgE via helper T cells—TCR binding to antigens presented by MHC class II stimulates helper T cells, which in turn play a role in antibody stimulation. Thus, specific recognition by the TCR and MHC can affect specific recognition by antibodies (Shirai et al. 1999).

Su et al. (1999) compared different TCR germline alleles across several vertebrate species in a phylogenetic analysis. Differences between species do not directly influence antigenic variation in parasites unless the parasites infect different species. But phylogenetic comparisons may illuminate the forces that shape TCR germline variability within species.

BCR Germline

The variable portion of the B cell receptor (BCR) develops by somatic recombination and mutation similar to the processes that generate variable TCRs. Antibodies are secreted forms of the BCR. I found only one report of a major germline polymorphism in the alleles that make up the variable components of the BCR. The same polymorphic alleles at a single BCR germline locus occur in both rabbits and snowshoe hares, suggesting that this polymorphism was inherited from a common ancestor and maintained for a long time in each species (Su and Nei 1999).

Hauser (1995) suggested that somatic hypermutation (affinity maturation) of the BCR provides a buffer between the germline and the matured BCR specific for particular antigens. The TCR has limited somatic mutation after the initial genetic recombinations, perhaps exposing germline TCRs to more intense selective pressures than BCRs. However, lack of observed variability in germline BCR genes may simply reflect limited study.

Match to Variant Cellular Receptors

Major deletions of cellular receptor genes can interfere with parasites that depend on those receptors for binding or entry into cells. For example, the human CCR5 gene encodes a coreceptor required for HIV-1 to enter macrophages. A 32-bp deletion of this gene occurs at a frequency of 0.1 in European populations. This deletion prevents the virus from entering macrophages (Martinson et al. 1997; O'Brien and Dean 1997; Smith et al. 1997).

Hill (1998) reviews cases in which variations in the hosts' vitamin D and other cellular receptors are associated with susceptibility to various diseases. It is not clear whether minor variants of cellular receptors occur sufficiently frequently to favor matching variation of parasites for attachment to those receptors.

8.2 Polymorphisms in Immune Regulation

EXAMPLES OF QUANTITATIVE VARIABILITY

Stimulation of naive $CD4^+$ helper T cells leads to proliferation of either T_H1 or T_H2 helper T cells. T_H1 response typically stimulates CTL proliferation, whereas T_H2 response typically stimulates antibody production.

Several studies have found genetic variation among hosts in the regulation of T_H1 versus T_H2 response. In mice, the actions of multiple genetic loci combine to determine regulation of T_H1 versus T_H2 against *Leishmania* infections (Coffman and Beebe 1998; Power 2000). Mice that develop a T_H1 response control infection because *Leishmania* can be cleared by CTLs. By contrast, those mice that develop a T_H2 response fail to clear infection because *Leishmania* cannot be controlled by a dominant antibody response.

In pigs, polygenic control has been observed for several traits including antibody response, with an important contribution of non-MHC loci; proliferative and cytokine responses of mononuclear blood lymphocytes, such as T cells, B cells, and natural killer (NK) cells; T cell–mediated inflammatory response to innocuous antigens (delayed-type hypersensitivity); and the total number and relative proportions of the various kinds of blood-borne immune cells (reviewed by Edfors-Lilja et al. 1998). High heritabilities have been estimated for several of these traits.

Studies of other organisms have also found polygenic control of quantitative immune responses outside the MHC region (Biozzi et al. 1982). Linkage studies of mice have begun to map locations of genes that influence quantitative variability in components of immunity (Puel et al. 1995; Wu et al. 1996). Many studies of humans report nucleotide polymorphisms in promoters of cytokines and other immune regulatory loci (Daser et al. 1996; Agarwal et al. 2000; Terry et al. 2000). Some human polymorphisms are associated with differential response to particular diseases (Hill 1998; Foster et al. 2000).

INTERLEUKIN 6 (IL6) PROMOTER POLYMORPHISM

IL6 plays a central role in the regulation of immunity (Janeway et al. 1999). It stimulates hepatic acute phase response to infection, induction of fever, differentiation and activation of macrophages and T cells, growth of B cells, and many other functions (Terry et al. 2000). Many cell types release IL6 in response to infection or irritating stimuli.

The rate of gene expression regulates plasma levels of IL6 because this cytokine is cleared rapidly from circulation. Various transcription factors and steroid hormones interact with the promoter region of this gene to produce synergistic combinations of positive and negative stimuli for transcription (Terry et al. 2000).

Terry et al. (2000) sequenced the promoter region of IL6 for 442 haplotypes from 221 humans. They found polymorphisms at three nucleotide sites and a variable-length AT run. These promoter polymorphisms influenced expression level in a nonadditive way—a single nucleotide change may have been associated with higher or lower levels of expression depending on other variable sites in the haplotype. In addition, the IL6 polymorphisms influenced expression in different ways in response to different stimulatory signals and when in different cell types.

The three single nucleotide polymorphisms are separated by 25 and 398 nucleotides. The GGG combination occurs in 54% of haplotypes, AGC in 40%, and GCG in 5%.

It is not clear what processes maintain this polymorphism. I consider a few possibilities in the remainder of this section and in the following sections.

Each haplotype could be associated with a particular variant of the coding region for IL6, thereby linking the pattern of gene expression to different properties of the cytokine. However, Terry et al. (2000) sequenced the coding region from twenty individuals and found no polymorphisms. Thus, positive interactions and linkage between promoters and coding regions seem unlikely in this case.

Alternatively, polymorphisms that affect phenotype are often maintained by a balance between the rate at which deleterious mutation adds variability and the rate at which selection can remove deleterious mutants. Mutation-selection balance probably explains a significant portion of the total quantitative genetic variability observed in populations (Barton and Turelli 1987).

Mutation-selection balance usually matches a high-frequency allele maintained by selection against a distribution of low-frequency mutant variants. Natural selection culls those lower-fitness variants, but mutation maintains a constant flow of new variants. For the IL6 polymorphism, mutation-selection balance cannot explain the similar frequencies of the two dominant haplotypes, because neither haplotype is a rare mutational variant of the other. Mutation-selection balance probably does explain the two rare trinucleotide haplotypes at frequencies of less than 1% observed by Terry et al. (2000).

Daser et al. (1996) and Mitchison (1997) suggested that heterozygosity in cytokine promoters enhances flexibility of the immune response. Enhanced flexibility could occur in heterozygotes by increasing the range of inputs that control the response kinetics of the cytokine.

Heterozygote advantage could explain the observed frequencies of the two common haplotypes if fitnesses are ordered as GGG/AGC > GGG/GGG > AGC/AGC, in which the heterozygote is more fit than either homozygote. However, by this scenario of heterozygote advantage, many individuals would carry lower-fitness homozygote genotypes. Given the three haplotype frequencies listed above, the expected frequency of homozygotes would be the sum of the squared haplotype frequencies, or 45%.

The frequency of heterozygotes would be increased by a larger number of promoter haplotypes. But such diversity would mean that any individual carried two randomly chosen haplotype patterns of regulatory control among the possible haplotypes. It is difficult to image how complementarity between diverse regulatory haplotypes would occur.

MHC CLASS II PROMOTER POLYMORPHISM

Several studies describe promoter polymorphisms of the class II loci (Louis et al. 1993; Reichstetter et al. 1994; Guardiola et al. 1996; Cowell et al. 1998; Mitchison et al. 2000). These regulatory polymorphisms can affect the relative expression of the class II alleles in different cell types. For example, Louis et al. (1994) and Vincent et al. (1997) showed that different class II alleles at the HLA-DRB locus are expressed at different levels. Variable transcription rates were associated with nucleotide polymorphisms in the promoters of these alleles.

The class II molecules present antigens to the helper T cells. Those helper T cells tend to differentiate into type 1 or type 2 (T_H1 versus T_H?) responses. The T_H1 versus T_H2 split influences the balance between several immune effector functions, particularly CTLs favored by T_H1 and antibodies favored by T_H2.

Cowell et al. (1998) and Mitchison et al. (2000) have argued that levels of MHC class II expression, under the control of regulatory polymorphisms, influence the tendency for T_H1 versus T_H2 response. Higher class II expression appears to trigger a cascade leading toward T_H1 helper T cells, whereas lower class II expression favors development of T_H2 helper T cells. Thus, variable regulatory genotypes can influence important aspects of the hosts' immune responses.

Cowell et al. (1998) propose two processes by which heterozygosity in MHC class II regulatory regions might be favored. First, they suggest that in a heterozygote "one pattern of expression could favor differentiation of T_H1 cells while another could favor T_H2's, so that the two in combination together would generate a balanced immune response."

Heterozygote advantage imposes a severe cost, because a binary trait such as high or low expression causes at least 50% of the population to be homozygous and therefore at a disadvantage. Tissue-specific expression or intermediate expression does not require heterozygosity with the associated cost of frequent, disadvantaged homozygotes.

Cowell et al. (1998) propose a second explanation in which promoters are advantageously linked to particular MHC alleles. They argue that "the T_H1-favoring [pattern of expression] might become associated with exons involved in resistance to infections best dealt with by T_H1 cells, and the T_H2-favoring pattern with resistance to infections needing T_H2's."

The available data do not provide a clear test of synergism between particular promoters and class II alleles. The most interesting information comes from sequences of the promoter regions linked to different class II HLA-DRB1 alleles. Louis et al. (1993) found that divergence of promoters followed the phylogenetic history for the linked structural alleles.

Continuous divergence of promoters as a function of phylogenetic distance suggests drifting changes constrained by the balance between mutational input and selection to maintain functional integrity. There may also be a tendency for compensatory nucleotide changes, in which one slightly deleterious substitution is compensated by a second substitution at a different site (Hartl and Taubes 1996; Burch and Chao 1999).

Phylogenetic divergence does not rule out Cowell et al.'s (1998) hypothesis of functional synergism between promoter and allele. Common phylogeny provides the background for all evolutionary divergence, but other processes can occur. For example, functionally synergistic associations may exist between nucleotides in promoter and structural regions that cannot be explained by common phylogeny.

BENEFITS AND COSTS OF CYTOKINE EXPRESSION

Increased expression of the immune response can have both benefits and costs. On the positive side, a more intense immune response may clear infections more rapidly. On the negative side, immune effectors can often be harsh medicine, causing collateral damage to host tissues.

Promoter polymorphisms may be maintained by the balance between effective clearance and tissue damage. For example, the human IL1 promoter polymorphism affects expression of the pro-inflammatory cytokine IL1β. Increased expression of this cytokine plays an important role in stimulating the inflammatory immune response against the widespread gastric pathogen *Helicobacter pylori* (Jung et al. 1997). Host genotypes with stronger IL1β responses probably clear the infection more effectively, but also suffer greater gastric tissue damage and a higher risk of gastric cancer (El-Omar et al. 2000).

A different trade-off occurs between high and low expression of IL10 during HIV-1 infection (Shin et al. 2000). Humans homozygous for a more active promoter variant of IL10 had a significantly delayed onset of AIDS relative to hosts either heterozygous or homozygous for a less active promoter. IL10 inhibits macrophage proliferation (Kollmann et al. 1996; Schols and De Clercq 1996), possibly reducing the number of activated macrophages available for viral replication. In this case, down-regulation of an immune effector, the macrophages, appears to reduce viral spread. Against other pathogens that do not replicate in macrophages, high IL10 expression and reduced macrophage proliferation may favor the pathogen.

MAJOR POLYMORPHISMS VERSUS RARE VARIANTS

The examples of variable regulatory control all have major polymorphisms in promoters, with two or more alternative haplotypes at significant frequencies. Initial screening would naturally turn up major polymorphisms rather than rare variants, which would be harder to detect. But each regulatory element inevitably has some rare variants in the population. Mutation provides a constant influx of such variants;

natural selection culls those variants slowly in proportion to their negative effects on fitness.

The balance of mutation and selection almost certainly creates quantitative variability in every aspect of immune regulation. Each individual likely has several rare mutants spread across different regulatory steps, causing variable quantitative genetic profiles for the thresholds to trigger responses and the intensities of responses.

The balance of mutation and selection sets the amount of quantitative variability in each regulatory component. The influx of quantitative variability depends on how mutations translate into quantitative effects on regulation. The culling of variation depends on the intensity of natural selection acting on the particular regulatory step. Steps that affect fitness relatively weakly will accumulate relatively more variation, until a balance of mutation and selection occurs. Steps that affect fitness strongly will accumulate relatively less variation. In each case, the variation in fitness will be roughly the same.

The major polymorphisms likely arise by processes in addition to mutation-selection balance. In those cases, various trade-offs between immune control of parasites and collateral damage probably balance the fitnesses of different variants. The collateral damage may be inflammatory or other negative effects of a hyperimmune response, as in the gastric tissue damage promoted by IL6. Or more rarely, the damage may arise from reducing the proliferation of immune cells that normally control pathogens but also can be the target of parasitic attack. This latter trade-off appears to occur in IL10 control of macrophages in the context of HIV-1 infection.

Regulatory variability may sometimes alter immunodominance because cytokines modulate positive and negative stimulation of T and B cell clones. Badovinac et al. (2000) provide a hint of how regulatory cytokines influence immunodominance of a CTL response in mice. In their study, normal levels of interferon-γ were associated with about a 5-fold ratio of immunodominant to subdominant T cell clones for two *Listeria monocytogenes* epitopes. By contrast, reduced interferon-γ was associated with roughly equivalent clonal expansion of CTLs specific for these two epitopes.

Badovinac et al.'s (2000) study shows that variations in nonspecific components of immune regulation may affect immunodominance. Immunodominance, in turn, affects the intensity of selection on particular pathogen epitopes. Thus, variations in immune regulation may influence patterns of antigenic variation.

8.3 Problems for Future Research

1. Effects of antigenic variation on MHC diversity. Parasites may favor change in the frequencies of host MHC alleles. For example, the human class I MHC molecule B35 binds to common epitopes of *Plasmodium falciparum*'s circumsporozoite protein (Gilbert et al. 1998). The B35 allele occurs in higher frequency in The Gambia, a region with endemic malaria, than in parts of the world with less severe mortality from malaria.

It would be interesting to know if variant epitopes influence the frequency of matching MHC alleles. For example, one epitope variant may be common in one location and another variant common in another location. Do those variants affect the local frequencies of MHC alleles in the host population? This question focuses attention on the kind of selection pressure parasites impose on MHC alleles.

Each MHC allele may have a qualitative relationship with each particular epitope, in that one amino acid substitution in the epitope can have a large effect on binding. But over the lifetime of an individual, each MHC type meets many potential epitopes from diverse parasites. Thus, MHC alleles vary quantitatively in the net benefit they provide by their different matches to the aggregate of potential epitopes. It may be rather rare for a single parasite to impose strong, sustained pressure on a particular MHC allele. Perhaps only major killers of young hosts can cause such strong selection. Mathematical models could clarify the nature of aggregate selection imposed on MHC alleles.

2. Effects of MHC diversity on antigenic variation. Does the distribution of MHC alleles in the host population shape the distribution of antigenic variants?

It would be interesting to compare parasites in two locations, each location with hosts that have different frequencies of MHC alleles. In principle, differing host MHC profiles could influence antigenic variation. But the pattern of selection may be complex. Each epitope could potentially interact with several MHC alleles. The net effect depends on the balance of fitness gains by an escape substitution against one MHC allele and the potential costs of that substitution in terms of functional performance and the possibility of creating enhanced binding to other MHC alleles.

It would also be interesting to compare parasites that attack only a single host species with those that attack multiple vertebrate species. The generalist parasites face variable selective pressures in the different hosts.

3. Regulatory variability of immune response. I described a few major polymorphisms in immune regulatory promoters. I also listed several hypotheses to explain those polymorphisms: linkage with synergistic coding regions, mutation-selection balance, and heterozygote advantage. These explanations lack empirical support, and the case of heterozygote advantage may also have logical flaws.

I reviewed two cases in which the costs and benefits of a more potent regulatory stimulus may favor polymorphism. In one example, host genotypes with stronger IL1β responses probably clear infection by *Helicobacter pylori* more effectively, but also suffer greater gastric tissue damage and a higher risk of gastric cancer.

In another example, humans with a more active promoter of IL10 had a significantly delayed onset of AIDS. IL10 inhibits macrophage proliferation, possibly reducing the number of activated macrophages available for HIV-1 replication. Against other pathogens that do not replicate in macrophages, reduced macrophage proliferation may favor the pathogen against the immune system.

Mathematical analysis could establish the necessary conditions to maintain polymorphism for controls of the immune response by trade-offs between high and low expression. Such models would clarify the kinds of experiments needed to understand these polymorphisms.

4. Effects of regulatory variability on antigenic diversity. Two possibilities come to mind. First, different patterns of immune regulation may affect immunodominance (Badovinac et al. 2000). Second, immune regulation may affect the intensity and duration of memory. Immunological memory shapes antigenic diversity because a parasite often cannot succeed in hosts previously infected by a similar antigenic profile.

5. Regulatory variability as model for quantitative variability. The widespread genetic variability of quantitative traits forms a classical unsolved puzzle of genetics. To solve this puzzle, one must understand the links between nucleotide variants, the regulatory control of trait development and expression, and fitness. The immune system is perhaps the most intensively studied complex regulatory system in biology. This chapter provided a glimpse of how it may be possible to link genetic variation to immune regulatory control and its fitness consequences. The studies done so far focus on major polymorphisms. But it may soon be possible to study rare variants and their association with regulatory variability and susceptibility to different pathogens. This may lead to progress in linking quantitative genetic variability and the evolution of regulatory control systems.

9   Immunological Variability of Hosts

A host often retains immunological memory of B and T cells stimulated by prior infections. Upon later inoculation, a host rapidly builds defense from its memory cells. Each host acquires a unique memory profile based on its infection history.

In this chapter, I discuss the immune memory profiles of the host population. The following chapter describes how the structuring of immunological memory in the host population shapes the structuring of antigenic variation in parasite populations.

The first section reviews the immune processes that govern immunological memory. I emphasize the rate at which a host can generate a secondary immune response and the rate at which immune memory decays. These rate processes determine how immunological memory imposes selective pressure on antigenic variants.

The second section discusses the different consequences of immunological memory for different kinds of parasites. For example, antibody titers tend to decay more rapidly in mucosal than in systemic locations. Thus, selective pressures on antigenic variation may differ for parasites that invade or proliferate in these different compartments. Cytopathic viruses, which kill their host cells, may be more susceptible to antibodies, whereas noncytopathic viruses may be more susceptible to CTLs that kill infected host cells. The different memory responses of antibodies and CTLs may impose different selective pressures on antigenic variation of cytopathic and noncytopathic viruses.

The third section describes the immunodominance of memory. The memory profile may differ from the pattern of immunodominance during primary infection. The immunodominance of memory affects the ease with which new parasite variants can spread. If each host has narrow memory immunodominance with protection against one or a few epitopes, then a small number of mutations can escape memory. By contrast, if hosts have broad memory profiles, then the parasites have to change simultaneously at many epitopes in order to avoid the hosts' memory responses.

The fourth section focuses on the cross-reactivity between the antigens of a primary and secondary infection. Sometimes a host first develops a memory response to a particular antigen, and then is exposed secondarily to a variant of that antigen. If the secondary variant cross-reacts with memory cells, then the host may produce a memory response to the first antigen rather than a primary response to the second antigen. This original antigenic sin can prevent the host from mounting a vigorous immune response to secondary challenge. It can also prevent a host from expanding its memory profile as it becomes infected by different antigenic variants.

The fifth section summarizes the distribution of immune profiles among hosts. This distribution determines the ability of particular antigenic variants to spread. Older hosts tend to have broader profiles because they have experienced more infections. Maternal antibodies provide short-term protection to infants, and certain antibody and T cell responses may provide temporary protection to recently infected hosts. Finally, the hosts may vary spatially in their prior exposure to different epitopes, creating a spatial mosaic in the selective pressures that favor different antigenic variants.

The final section takes up promising lines of study for future research.

9.1 Immunological Memory

Immunological memory causes different immune responses between primary and secondary exposure to an antigen. Differences include the speed, intensity, and breadth of reaction. I focus on the consequences of immunological memory for antigenic variation of parasites. Thus, I am mostly concerned with how memory affects replication and transmission of the parasite.

Memory Cells

The state of internal memory influences whether secondary response rapidly clears or only partially reduces secondary infection (reviewed by Zinkernagel et al. 1996). The X-Y-Z model (Byers and Sercarz 1968) captures the essential features: X represents a specific, naive B or T lymphocyte clone; Y represents a partially differentiated, long-lived memory state for the specific lymphocyte; and Z represents the short-lived, fully armed effector cells that do the work of clearing infection.

Studies have supported different components of this model for some experimental systems. But many conflicting results have been obtained, and controversy continues. A recent symposium (McMichael and Doherty 2000) and many reviews summarize empirical details and opposing views (Ahmed and Gray 1996; Zinkernagel et al. 1996; Dutton et al. 1998; Ada 1999; Farber 2000; Gray 2000; Seder and Hill 2000).

AN EXAMPLE

In an antibody response, Y represents the long-lived memory B cell clones and Z represents the short-lived plasma B cells that secrete antibody. Ochsenbein et al. (2000) studied B cell memory against vesicular stomatitis virus (VSV) infections in mice. They found that memory cells did in fact live a relatively long time compared with antibody-secreting plasma cells. The antibody-secreting cells had a half-life of 3–10 days.

Memory cells persisted in the absence of recurrent antigenic stimulation. By contrast, the maintenance of plasma cells and circulating antibodies required continued stimulation by antigens. Circulating antibodies often protect against secondary infection by VSV, whereas memory cells alone do not.

This example highlights several questions. Are effector cells generally short-lived or long-lived? Does the maintenance of effectors require recurrent antigenic stimulation? How long do memory cells live in the absence of repeated stimulation? How long does it take for memory cells to differentiate into effector cells? Is there always a sharp distinction between memory and effector cells, or do some cell types have some memory attributes (long-lived, easily stimulated) and effector attributes (directly involved in killing)?

These issues play a crucial role in shaping the immunological structure of host populations and consequently in the evolution of antigenic variation. The various conflicting details do not provide a clear picture at present. But it is possible to discuss how particular memory processes may affect the evolution of parasite diversity. The next subsection provides one example.

RECURRENT ANTIGENIC STIMULATION OF ANTIBODY PRODUCTION

How does a host maintain antibody titers after an infection has apparently been cleared? Zinkernagel et al. (1996) and Ochsenbein et al. (2000) favor the need for internal storage of antigen as a source of recurrent stimulation, with perhaps repeated infection as a booster in some cases. Others studies have implicated a subset of long-lived plasma cells as a potential source of continuous antibody production without the need for recurrent stimulation by antigen (Manz et al. 1998; Slifka et al. 1998). For our purposes, we can take the following relatively safe position.

The ratio of plasma to memory cells likely rises with recurrent antigenic stimulation. A higher concentration of plasma cells and antibodies provides greater protection and more rapid clearance. The benefit for maintaining plasma cells depends on how rapidly the infection develops within the host. Slow infections may allow memory cells to differentiate into an antibody response sufficiently rapidly to contain the infection. Fast infections may spread so quickly that memory cells cannot differentiate antibody-secreting plasma cells fast enough to contain the infection, but memory cells may aid in eventual clearance.

The immunological structure of host populations as it affects parasite transmission depends on plasma:memory ratios, which in turn may be affected by recurrent stimulation by internally stored antigen or extrinsic reinfection. Plasma:memory ratios more strongly influence parasites that grow relatively quickly within hosts.

HELPER T CELL MEMORY

Memory B cells have higher densities of MHC class II molecules on their surfaces than naive B cells (Janeway et al. 1999). Presumably this allows antigens taken up by the B cell receptor to stimulate more strongly helper T cells, which in turn signal the memory B cells to differentiate into antibody-secreting plasma cells.

The $CD4^+$ helper T cells themselves appear to differentiate into a memory form after sufficient initial stimulation (Janeway et al. 1999). Memory $CD4^+$ helper T cells provide stronger stimulation to B cells than do naive $CD4^+$ cells (Scherle and Gerhard 1986; Croft and Swain 1992; Swain 1994; Marshall et al. 1999).

The speed of an antibody response may be enhanced by $CD4^+$ memory cells. This raises some interesting questions concerning the selective pressures that influence antigenic variation in parasites. Suppose, for example, that during initial exposure a host produces a dominant immune response to a parasite's B cell epitope, b, and to a $CD4^+$ T cell epitope, t. Thus, we can write the initial parasite genotype as b/t.

In a host with memory against the b/t parasite, how well would anti-genically variant parasites succeed with genotypes b'/t, b/t', or b'/t', where the primes denote variants? For example, how much advantage does the host gain by CD4$^+$ memory against a parasite with an altered B cell epitope, or from the parasite's point of view, what is the fitness of the parasite genotype b'/t relative to b'/t' in a host previously exposed to b/t? If the difference in fitness is sufficiently large, then the selective intensity on the epitope t may be strong. This would be interesting to know because most attention currently focuses on the obviously strong selective pressure for changes in the epitope b.

Zinkernagel et al. (1996) summarize limited evidence suggesting that helper T cell memory does not play an important role in shaping anti-genic variants of parasites. Helper T cells cross-react between influenza strains (Hurwitz et al. 1984; Mills et al. 1986; Scherle and Gerhard 1986) and between vesicular stomatitis virus (VSV) strains (Gupta et al. 1986; Burkhart et al. 1994). This cross-reactivity does not protect hosts against secondary infection, but it can accelerate antibody response and reduce the time until clearance (Scherle and Gerhard 1986; Marshall et al. 1999).

In influenza infections, the dominant epitopes of helper T cells focus on hemagglutinin, a major surface molecule of influenza. The T cell epitopes are very near the B cell epitopes that dominate protective im-munity (Wilson and Cox 1990; Thomas et al. 1998). It may be that amino acid changes in hemagglutinin between antigenically variant strains are sometimes selected by memory helper T cells. However, for amino acid replacements in hemagglutinin, it is difficult to separate the potential role of memory helper T cells from the obviously strong effects of anti-body memory.

The level of memory helper T cells can be measured by the time re-quired for naive B cells to switch from initial IgM secretion to later IgG se-cretion. When assessed by this functional response, helper T cell mem-ory appears to be short-lived for influenza (Liang et al. 1994) and VSV (Roost et al. 1990). In mice infected with VSV, memory T cell help that ac-celerated the IgM to IgG switch lasted only fourteen to twenty-one days. Other assays find that memory helper T cells remain for several months after initial infection (Gupta et al. 1986); it appears that eventually the number of memory cells drops below a threshold or the memory cells lose a complementary signal. It will be interesting to learn whether limited functional helper T cell memory applies generally to all vertebrates or varies for different hosts or host-parasite combinations.

CD4$^+$ cells have other functions in addition to stimulating B cells. For example, CD4$^+$ cells influence CTL response and the response of other effectors such as macrophages. The limited evidence available does not demonstrate a strong role for CD4$^+$ memory with regard to these effector-stimulating functions (Stevenson and Doherty 1998); however, the potentially diverse memory effects for these cells must be considered (Whitmire et al. 2000).

CTL Memory

Important attributes of memory include the speed and intensity of response to antigen and the time decay of these quantitative responses (Seder and Hill 2000). CTL memory has been measured in various ways, for different hosts and different kinds of parasites (Zinkernagel et al. 1996; Dutton et al. 1998; Stevenson and Doherty 1998). Preliminary data suggest that patterns of immunodominance in the primary response do not necessarily carry through to the memory pool (Belz et al. 2000; Rickinson et al. 2000; Seaman et al. 2000). In some cases, it seems that T cell clones increased to high abundance in the primary response suffer greater reductions as the cellular populations are regulated in the memory phase (Rickinson et al. 2000).

A few general conclusions arise from this work: secondary CTL responses are typically faster and more intense than primary response, and the strength of the secondary response can decay over time. More important, the relations between CTL response and clearance depend strongly on the kinds of parasites.

9.2 Kinds of Parasites

"Every infection is a race" (Mims et al. 1993). The parasites race against immune effectors, which may eventually kill parasites faster than they are born. Each kind of parasite has its particular site of infection, pattern of spread between tissues, and rate of increase. Immunological memory therefore influences the host-parasite race in a different way for each kind of parasite.

In this section, I highlight some of the interactions between immunological memory and parasite attributes. I discuss memory-parasite interactions with regard to the type of immune cell involved, the kinetics
of parasite spread, and the kinetics of immune effector response.

There are four main classes of immune cells that can be enhanced by
primary infection to provide greater protection against later infections:
plasma B cells, memory B cells, effector T cells, and memory T cells
(Ahmed and Gray 1996).

The plasma cells secrete antibody. These effector B cells usually produce mature immunoglobulins such as IgG in systemic sites and IgA
on mucosal surfaces. Circulating IgG often remains at significant titers
throughout life. IgG can sometimes prevent infection by binding to inoculum before the parasites replicate in the host. IgG causes most cases
of long-lived protective immunity against pathogens such as measles,
yellow fever, polio, mumps, smallpox, and many other viruses and bacteria (Plotkin and Orenstein 1999; Knipe and Howley 2001).

IgA is often raised to high titers on mucosal surfaces in response to
infection. IgA antibodies provide effective protection against pathogens
that initially invade mucosal sites, such as influenza through the nasal
mucosa, rotaviruses and many bacterial pathogens via the intestinal mucosa, and gonorrhea via the urethral epithelium (Mims 1987; Ada 1999).
However, IgA titers decline relatively rapidly after infection, lasting on
the order of months rather than years, as is often the case for IgG.

Memory B cells proliferate and differentiate into plasma cells upon
secondary infection. If the pathogen is not immediately cleared by existing antibodies and the pathogen's initial replication is relatively slow,
then the memory B cells may have time to differentiate into plasma cells
and clear the pathogen before widespread infection develops. Differentiation of memory B cells into plasma cells depends on stimulation by
$CD4^+$ helper T cells (Ochsenbein et al. 2000).

Once widespread infection becomes established, memory B cells can
help to produce a more specific, rapid, and intense antibody response.
However, the relative roles of antibodies and T cells in clearing established infection vary depending on the attributes of the pathogen (Mims
1987; Janeway et al. 1999). For example, Zinkernagel et al. (1996) emphasized the distinction between cytopathic (cell-killing) and noncytopathic
viruses. They also distinguished between viruses exposed to antibody

in the blood or mucosa and those hidden from antibody in peripheral tissue.

Antibodies play a key role in clearing cytopathic viruses on mucosa or circulating in the blood. CTLs may be relatively ineffective against cytopathic viruses when the rate at which viruses infect, replicate, and kill a cell is greater than the rate at which CTLs kill viruses in infected cells. The dynamics of this race could be analyzed by mathematical models that compare the viruses' birth and death rates in light of the killing action mediated by antibodies and effector T cells.

For viruses that circulate in systemic infections, memory IgG antibodies may often protect against infection. By contrast, for mucosal infections such as those by rotaviruses and many bacterial pathogens, memory IgA antibodies often decline below protection level, but memory B cells can play an important role in defense by differentiating IgA-secreting plasma cells (Ahmed and Gray 1996).

Effector CTLs dominate clearance of noncytopathic intracellular pathogens and infected peripheral tissue that limits access to antibody (Zinkernagel et al. 1996). Effector T cells typically have a short half-life when not stimulated by antigen. Thus clearance before significant infection develops can occur by various scenarios. First, recent stimulation by antigen can boost effector T cell density to protective levels. Stimulation can occur by persistent antigen maintained in the host or by recurrent infection. Second, slowly spreading infections may allow differentiation of effector T cells from memory T cells in time to control initial spread of the pathogen. Third, memory antibody may clear the pathogen before the initial infection becomes established.

Lack of symptoms during secondary infection may result from rapid clearance of the parasite or from control of the infection that still allows some parasite replication and transmission. It is important to distinguish between clearance and controlled infection when studying the population dynamics and evolution of the parasite.

In summary, parasite attributes determine the type of host memory that impedes secondary infection. I mentioned the site of initial invasion (e.g., mucosal versus systemic), the site of widespread infection (e.g., epithelial, systemic, peripheral), and the lifetime of infected cells for intracellular parasites (e.g., cytopathic versus noncytopathic). Other parasite factors can tip the balance between clearance and widespread infection of a secondarily inoculated host. For example, the number of parasites in the inoculum frequently influences whether an infection is cleared quickly or spreads widely.

These various parasite attributes and the rate parameters that govern parasite birth and death within hosts must be measured against the kinetics of immunological memory and the response to secondary infection. The quantitative outcome influences the selective pressure imposed on various parasite epitopes by host memory. Such selective pressure, in turn, shapes the distribution of antigenic variation in parasite populations.

9.3 Immunodominance of Memory

A host's immunological memory profile depends on three factors. First, which parasite variants have infected that host in the past? Second, to which epitopes did the host respond?—the immunodominance of primary response. Third, to which of the primary epitopes has the host retained memory?—the immunodominance of the memory profile.

The immunological profile of each host and the variation of profiles between hosts influence the selective pressures imposed on parasite antigens. For the profile of each host, consider as a simple measure of immunodominance the number of epitopes to which a host retains protective antibody. If a host retains protection against n epitopes, then a variant parasite strain must differ in at least n sites to avoid all memory. If the mutation rate per site is μ, then the probability is μ^n that a progeny of the original strain is an escape variant with all of the n necessary differences.

Several laboratory experiments of influenza have studied the origin of escape variants when neutralizing antibody pressure is imposed against viral epitopes (Yewdell et al. 1979, 1986; Lambkin et al. 1994). For antibodies against only a single epitope, escape variants arise often because only a single mutation is needed. The mutation rate of influenza is on the order of $\mu = 10^{-5}$ per nucleotide per generation. Thus, a moderate-size population of viruses likely has at least a few escape mutants. By contrast, antibody selection against two or more epitopes rarely yields escape mutants, because the probability of multiple mutations, μ^n, becomes small relative to the effective size of the population.

These laboratory experiments show that a broader antibody response against multiple epitopes impedes the origin of new variants. By contrast, a more focused immunodominant response allows the rapid evolution of escape variants.

Similarly, persistent viral infections within hosts respond differently to narrow versus broad CTL pressure (Wodarz and Nowak 2000). A highly immunodominant CTL response allows rapid evolution of escape mutants and continuing change within hosts. By contrast, a broad CTL response against multiple epitopes impedes the origin of escape variants and leads to relatively slow evolution of viruses within a host.

To determine the selective pressures imposed on parasite populations, the immunodominance of each host's memory profile must be placed in the context of variation in memory profiles between hosts. Suppose, for example, that a parasite has two distinct antigenic sites. A parasite with genotype A/B at the two sites sweeps through the population, infecting all hosts. One-half of the host population maintains memory against both antigens, one-quarter has immunodominant memory against A only, and one-quarter has immunodominant memory against B only.

Now consider how this distribution of memory profiles influences the success of antigenic variants. A mutation at a single site, for example B, yields an altered parasite, A/B'. This mutant can attack the quarter of the host population with memory only against B. As the parasite spreads, a second mutation to A'/B' allows attack of the remaining hosts.

This example shows that strongly immunodominant host profiles limited to one or a few sites allow parasite mutants with few changes to succeed. Once the variant parasite begins to spread between susceptible hosts, additional mutations allow attack against hosts with different immunodominant profiles or against hosts that developed broader immunity against multiple antigenic sites.

Influenza evolution may proceed by this sort of sequential accumulation of variation, with new epidemic strains differing from the previous epidemic strain at several sites (Natali et al. 1981; Underwood 1984; Wang et al. 1086; Wilson and Cox 1990, Lambkin and Dimmock 1996; Cleveland et al. 1997; Nakajima et al. 2000). Surveys of human populations and laboratory studies of mice and rabbits support this hypothesis by showing that individuals often have narrowly focused antibody responses and that individuals vary in the antigenic sites to which they develop antibodies.

In the laboratory, studies show that individual mice infected with human influenza often produce antibody responses focused on a limited number of antigenic sites—probably just one or two sites (Staudt and Gerhard 1983; Underwood 1984; Thomas et al. 1998). Individual mice differed in the antigenic sites to which they raised antibodies. Individual variation in antibody response probably occurs because stochastic recombinational and mutational processes generate antibody specificity (Staudt and Gerhard 1983).

Surveys of human populations find that individuals previously exposed to influenza vary in antibody memory profiles (Natali et al. 1981; Wang et al. 1986; Nakajima et al. 2000). Wang et al. (1986) studied immune memory profiles of individuals when measured for three nonoverlapping sites of the hemagglutinin surface glycoprotein. For samples collected from the early years of the Hong Kong influenza subtype epidemics (1969 and 1971), 33% of individuals had antibodies to all three sites, 50% had antibodies for two sites, and 17% had antibodies for only one site. Approximately equal numbers of individuals lacked antibody to any particular site, suggesting that each site was equally likely to stimulate an antibody response. Most individuals sampled in 1978 had antibodies for all three sites. It appears that after several years of repeated exposure to various strains of the Hong Kong subtype, individuals had acquired a wider repertoire of antibodies.

Human children tend to have particularly narrowly focused antibody profiles against influenza (Natali et al. 1981, 1998; Nakajima et al. 2000). This may occur either because of children's relatively smaller number of exposures or because of their narrower response per infection.

These observations on mice and humans support the hypothesis that individuals have narrowly focused antibody memory and that individuals vary in the antigenic sites to which they respond. This combination of individual focus and population variability creates a heterogeneous pattern of selection on parasites. After a widespread epidemic by a single parasite type, the parasite must acquire several new mutations before it can again spread widely through the population. Stepwise changes can occur by first changing at one site and attacking a subset of the population with a dominant response against that site. The new mutant strain can then accumulate a second change that provides access both to hosts with a dominant antibody response to the second mutant site and to hosts with antibodies against both the first and second mutant sites. Additional mutations allow attack against broader sets of immunological profiles.

This description certainly oversimplifies the actual process. However, the immunodominance of individual hosts for particular epitopes and the population variability of immune profiles can create important selective pressures on parasites.

9.4 Cross-Reactivity and Interference

A host's secondary response to an antigen depends on immunological memory to that antigen. Typically, memory leads to a faster and more vigorous secondary response. Suppose, however, that a host first develops a memory response to a particular antigen, and then is exposed secondarily to a variant of that antigen. If the secondary variant cross-reacts with memory cells, then the host may produce a memory response to the first antigen rather than a primary response to the second antigen. A memory response to the first antigen rather than a primary response to the variant is called *original antigenic sin.* I reviewed aspects of this phenomenon in chapter 6.

A memory response based on previously encountered, cross-reactive antigens has three consequences for the immunological structure of host populations. First, cross-reaction may aid protection or clearance against secondary challenge. This occurs if the cross-reactive memory effectors have sufficient affinity for the variant antigen (Kaverin et al. 2000; Roden et al. 2000; Sonrier et al. 2000; Stalhammar-Carlemalm et al. 2000).

Second, cross-reaction may interfere with the secondary response. This occurs when cross-reactive memory effectors do a poor job of clearing secondary challenge but respond sufficiently to repress a new, primary response against the variant antigen (Good et al. 1993; Klenerman and Zinkernagel 1998; Nara and Garrity 1998; Ferguson et al. 1999).

Third, the host may fail to develop an increasingly broad memory profile over the course of repeated exposures to different variants. This occurs when a new variant stimulates cross-reactive memory rather than a specific primary response, preventing memory particular for the new variant (Fazekas de St. Groth and Webster 1966a, 1966b; Smith et al. 1999).

9.5 Distribution of Immune Profiles among Hosts

The distribution of immune profiles influences selective pressures on antigenic diversity. Several factors shape the distribution of immunity. I have already mentioned the immunodominance of individual immune profiles and the tendency for the pattern of immunodominance to vary among individuals. I also discussed how cross-reactivity can affect clearance of secondary challenge and the development of memory over a host's lifetime. In this section, I add a few more factors that affect the distribution of immune profiles.

AGE STRUCTURE OF HOSTS

An individual becomes exposed over time to an increasingly diverse array of parasite genotypes. Thus, older individuals typically have a broader memory profile than do younger individuals. Age-related patterns have been measured by serological surveys, which describe the presence or absence of circulating antibodies to a particular strain of parasite or to a particular antigen. Many surveys have been published for a wide variety of parasites and hosts (Anderson and May 1991, pp. 49–54).

Here are just a few example pathogens for which broader immunological profiles have been reported in older hosts compared with younger hosts: influenza (Dowdle 1999), *Plasmodium* (Gupta and Day 1994; Barragan et al. 1998), human T cell leukemia virus type 1 (HTLV-1) (Larsen et al. 2000), and hepatitis A, B, and C viruses (Chapman et al. 2000).

The best data on age effects come from studies of the influenza A virus. Most neutralizing antibodies against influenza bind to hemagglutinin, the virus's dominant surface molecule (Wilson and Cox 1990). Three major subtypes of hemagglutinin have circulated in human populations since about 1890, labeled H1, H2, and H3. Antibodies to one subtype cross-react relatively little with the other subtypes. Significant variation occurs within each subtype. Although antibodies to a particular variant do not always protect against infection by other variants of the same subtype, the antibodies to variants of a subtype do often cross-react to some extent.

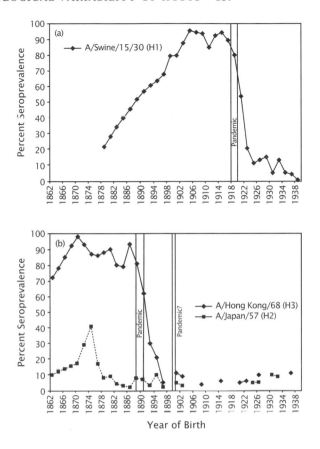

Figure 9.1   Percentage of people having antibodies to the three subtypes of influenza A virus stratified by year of birth. The strains labeled A/strain designation (subtype) were used to test for antibodies to a particular subtype by measuring the degree to which blood samples carried antibodies that reacted significantly against the test strain. Figures were taken from Dowdle (1999), with permission from WHO. Original data for the top panel from Masurel (1976, with permission from Elsevier Science) and for the bottom panel from Masurel (1969, with permission from WHO).

These patterns of cross-reaction allow one to measure immunological profiles of individuals with regard to previous exposure to each of the three subtypes. By measuring individuals of different ages, a picture emerges of the past history of exposure and immunity to the different subtypes.

Figure 9.1a shows the percentage of individuals with antibodies to H1 born in different years. H1 is the subtype that caused the famous 1918

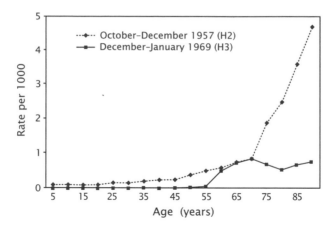

Figure 9.2 Estimated mortality caused by two widely distributed influenza pandemics stratified by age of the host. The 1957 pandemic was caused by an H2 subtype and the 1968-69 pandemic was caused by an H3 subtype. Figure taken from Dowdle (1999), with permission from WHO. Original data from Housworth and Spoon (1971), with permission from Oxford University Press.

pandemic that killed tens of millions of people (Oxford 2000). Note that antibodies against H1 occur in 80–90% of individuals who were less than twenty years old during the pandemic years, suggesting widespread distribution of the disease. The drop in the seropositive level for individuals born before 1900 may be explained by the typically lower percentage of adults than children infected by influenza epidemics (Nguyen-Van-Tam 1998). There may also be some decay in immune memory among older individuals. The large drop in seroprevalence after 1922 suggests that H1 declined in frequency after the pandemic. Perhaps because of widespread immunity to H1, variants of this subtype had difficulty spreading between hosts.

Figure 9.1b shows a similar picture for the H3 subtype associated with a pandemic in 1890. Cohorts born in the years before the pandemic had very high seroprevalence, suggesting widespread infection. Seroprevalence declined sharply in those born just after the pandemic, implying that H3 had nearly disappeared from circulation. Figure 9.1b also shows data on H2 seroprevalence and a possible pandemic in 1900, but those data are more difficult to interpret.

Figure 9.2 illustrates the estimated mortality rate associated with influenza infection in two severe (pandemic) years. The H2 pandemic of

1957 caused relatively high mortality among older people compared with the H3 pandemic of 1968–69. Older people often suffer higher mortality from influenza than do younger people (Nguyen-Van-Tam 1998), so the pattern in 1957 appears to be typical. The contained mortality among older individuals in 1968-69 may have been caused partly by immunological memory to the H3 pandemic of 1890 and consequent protection against this subtype.

The age structure of immunity profiles has probably influenced the waxing and waning of the various influenza A subtypes over the past 110 years. Influenza causes uniquely widespread and rapid epidemics; thus the details of age-related immune profiles and antigenic variation likely differ in other pathogens. Malaria is perhaps the only other disease for which existing data suggest interesting hypotheses.

In areas with endemic *Plasmodium falciparum* infection, hosts often pass through three stages of immunity (Gupta and Day 1994; Barragan et al. 1998; Mohan and Stevenson 1998). Maternal antibodies provide significant protection for newborns up to six months of age. After maternal antibodies fade, high infection rates with severe disease frequently occur until the age of two to three years. Acquired immunity develops gradually over the following years, with significant reduction in the severity of symptoms. However, even healthy adults often have subclinical infections. Maintenance of protection requires repeated exposure. Individuals who depart and live in malaria-free areas for many months become significantly more susceptible upon return (Neva 1977; Cohen and Lambert 1982).

The slow buildup of immunity partly depends on the high antigenic variation of *Plasmodium falciparum* (Marsh and Howard 1986; Forsyth et al. 1989; Iqbal et al. 1993; Gupta and Day 1994). An individual apparently requires exposure to several of the locally common variants before acquiring a sufficiently broad immunological profile to protect against disease (Barragan et al. 1998).

Transmission of Maternal Antibodies

The rate at which susceptible hosts enter the population plays an important role in the dynamics of parasite strains. Newborns, memory decay, and migration provide the main sources of new susceptible hosts.

The susceptibility of newborns is complicated by maternal transmission of antibodies (Zinkernagel et al. 1996). Offspring of mice and humans obtain IgA antibodies in milk and IgG antibodies through the placenta (Janeway et al. 1999, pp. 326–327). IgA protects the gut epithelium and mucosal surfaces. The newborn inherits circulating IgG titers in the blood that match the mother's antibody levels. The infant receives the particular antibody specificities generated by the mother's history of exposure to particular antigens. Thus, the infant has a temporary memory profile that matches its mother's.

Maternal antibodies have a half-life of 3–6 months (Nokes et al. 1986; Anderson and May 1991, pp. 49-54). Infection of a baby early in life may be cleared by maternal antibody, thereby failing to stimulate an immune response and generate long-lasting memory (Albrecht et al. 1977).

Other vertebrates also transmit maternal antibodies to newborns (Zinkernagel et al. 1996). For example, bovines produce highly concentrated antibodies in the first milk (colostrum), which must be absorbed via the calf's gut during the first twenty-four hours after birth (Porter 1972). In this first day, the calf does not digest the immunoglobulins and is able to take up most antibody classes by absorption through the gut epithelium. Birds transmit maternal antibodies through the egg (Paul 1993).

SHORT-TERM PROTECTION FROM RECENT INFECTION

IgA antibodies on epithelia can prevent initial infection by pathogens (Mims 1987, p. 251). For example, IgA may prevent attachment of *Vibrio cholerae* to the intestinal epithelium, gonococcus to the urethral epithelium, or chlamydia to the conjunctiva. IgA titers on epithelia often decay quickly after infection. Thus, protection against infection by IgA typically lasts for a few months or less.

Most vaccines protect by elevating the level of circulating antibodies and perhaps also memory B cells. The need for occasional vaccine boosters to maintain protection against some pathogens suggests that antibody titers or the pool of memory B cells decline in those cases. When long-term protection requires no boost, it may be that a lower threshold of antibodies or memory B cells protects against infection or that some regulatory mechanism of immunity holds titers higher.

In human influenza, T cells stimulated during infection provide some protection against later infection (McMichael et al. 1983b). But that protection wanes over a three-to-five-year period (McMichael et al. 1983a). A study of chickens also showed T cell–mediated control of secondary infection (Seo and Webster 2001). In that case, the secondary infection happened within 70 days of the primary challenge. The time decay of protection was not studied.

Measurements of memory decay have been difficult partly because laboratory mice provide a poor model for long-term processes of immunity (Stevenson and Doherty 1998). Laboratory mice typically live up to two years. It is difficult to separate decay of immunity from aging when immune memory in a mouse declines over many months.

Spatial Structure of Hosts

I discussed above how immune memory profiles may be stratified by age. Memory profiles may also be stratified by spatial location of hosts. At present, few spatial data exist. Thus, I confine my comments to a few conceptual issues.

To begin, consider the temporal pattern of measles epidemics prior to widespread vaccination (Anderson and May 1991, chapter 6). Data from England and Wales in 1948–1968 show a regular cycle of epidemic peaks every two years. The cycle may be explained by the threshold density of susceptible individuals required for an infection to spread. Just after an epidemic, most individuals retain memory that protects them from reinfection. The parasite declines because each infected individual transmits the infection to an average of less than one new susceptible host.

The next epidemic must wait until the population recruits enough newborns who are too young to have been infected in the last epidemic. An epidemic then follows, leaving most of the population protected until the next cycle of recruitment and spread of infection. Probably all parasite populations wax and wane to some extent as protective memory spreads with infection and the pool of susceptibles rebuilds by recruitment or by decay of immune memory.

These temporal fluctuations may also be coupled to spatial processes (Rohani et al. 1999; Earn et al. 2000). Imagine the spatial landscape of a population as a checkerboard of distinct patches. Epidemics may rise and fall synchronously in all patches, or epidemics may occur asynchronously over space. Suppose, for example, that half of the patches, labeled P_1, have epidemics in odd years, whereas the other half of the patches, labeled P_2, have epidemics in even years. One can visualize this dynamic landscape by imagining a peak in each patch rising during an epidemic and falling back to the ground between epidemics. Over an asynchronous landscape, some peaks are rising and others are falling at any time.

Measles virus effectively has only one antigenic type—a host's first infection and recovery provides lifelong protection. The spatiotemporal landscape of measles spread follows the waxing and waning of the numbers of infected individuals, driven by immunological memory, recruitment of newborns, and migration between patches.

Now imagine a parasite with distinct antigenic variants, for which memory to one variant does not provide any cross-protection against the other variants. The variants behave in effect as completely distinct parasites. In a patch, the waxing and waning of one variant may be synchronized with or uncoupled from the dynamics of the other variants. If the variants change asynchronously within patches, then the spatiotemporal landscape is covered by multiple surfaces of rising and falling peaks, the surfaces moving independently of each other.

I have discussed infection landscapes in a rather abstract way. But there is nothing out of the ordinary about hosts spread over space and infected over time by different antigenic variants of a parasite. The difficulty is to identify what general consequences arise from the interaction between antigenic variation and spatial processes. The landscape I have described so far has strains of antigenic variants that do not interact or interfere with each other. Thus, each strain changes independently of other strains, and no interaction occurs between space and antigenic variation.

Now consider antigenic variants for which some pairs of variants cause cross-reactive memory. It is not so easy to imagine the spatiotemporal landscape because the spread of each variant has differing quantitative effects on the dynamics of other variants. One simple analogy with age structure hints at the sort of processes that may occur.

In influenza, it may be that children have immunodominant memory focused on only one or a few antigenic sites. In the simplified example I discussed above, at first a virus strain with two sites, A/B, spreads.

Patch types

	1	2	3	4
Memory:	A/B	A'/B	A'/B'	A/B'
Parasite:	A'/B' → A/B' → A/B → A'/B

Figure 9.3   Spatial connectivity of parasite transmission between patches of hosts with different immunological memory profiles.

Some children develop immunodominant memory against A; other children develop immunodominant memory against B. Adults may have memory for both A and B. Mutant viruses can spread through the entire population in two steps. First, a mutant A'/B can attack children with memory against A. Then a second mutant, A'/B' can attack everyone. The key is that different classes of hosts provide a pathway of connectivity by which single mutations of the virus can eventually spread through the entire population.

Connectivity may also occur over space. Figure 9.3 shows four patch types that have previously been infected by A/B, A'/B, A/B', and A'/B', respectively. This spatial distribution of immunological memory creates a stepwise pathway of connectivity for a parasite. For example, if a parasite A'/B' first invades patch 1, then it can by a single mutation change into A/B' and attack patch 2. Single mutational steps take that parasite to patch 3 and then on to patch 4.

This simplified description of spatial movement highlights two points. First, patches 1 and 3 fluctuate between A/B and A'/B', whereas patches 2 and 4 fluctuate between A'/B and A/B'. These patch identities occur because immunological memory to both antigens imposes a barrier to any variant except the type with changes at both sites. Gupta et al. (1996, 1998) have emphasized the emergence of strain structure caused by this type of immunologically imposed selection. Second, my description extends Gupta et al.'s model to spatially structured host populations. With spatial structure, alternating regions of the host population can be dominated by the different pairwise sets of parasite strains. I will return to these issues in the next chapter, which focuses on the population structure of antigenically variable parasites.

Mathematical models could be developed to explore the interactions between antigenic variation and spatiotemporal dynamics. However, almost no data exist to compare with the models, and so there has been relatively little work along these lines. Some spatial data exist for influenza, but the scale of sampling and the measurement of cross-reactivity probably need to be enhanced before much can be concluded. This will not be easy to do in the short term. But eventually methods will improve for typing strains, and more data will become available.

9.6 Problems for Future Research

The processes that govern immunological memory within hosts and the distribution of immune profiles among hosts remain poorly understood. Throughout this chapter, I have emphasized important topics for further work. Rather than repeat all of those issues, I list here some hypotheses about kinetics that deserve study both empirically and mathematically. Many patterns of antigenic variation turn on these rate processes that drive evolutionary dynamics.

1. Demography. *(a) A higher rate of recruitment into the host population reduces the selective pressure on antigenic variation.* Consider two species, a long-lived species with an average life span of L years, and a short-lived species with an average life span of S years. If $L = 70$, then newborns replace approximately 1/70th of the population per year. By contrast, if $S = 7$, then newborns replace approximately 1/7th of the population each year. Immunological memory decays faster at the population level in short-lived than in long-lived species, perhaps reducing the relative fitness advantage of antigenic variants in short-lived compared with long-lived hosts.

If an antigenic variant has a fitness cost relative to the wild type, then a greater offsetting fitness benefit occurs in the species with longer life span and fewer naive hosts. Thus, a high-cost variant could gain an advantage in long-lived but not in short-lived hosts. Antigenic variation may therefore occur more often in long-lived hosts than in short-lived hosts.

(b) Highly infectious parasites spread more widely in host populations and induce a higher percentage of hosts to have immunological memory against particular antigens. Highly infectious parasites therefore face more severe selective pressure for antigenic change. Here "highly infectious" means a higher basic reproductive number, R_0, that is, a higher number of secondary infections caused by an infected host in a naive population. The density of immunological memory in the host popula-

tion against parasites with different R_0s should be studied mathematically to refine this idea.

(c) Rapidly transmitting parasites face less immunological pressure for change within hosts. If most parasite transmission occurs before the onset of strong, specific immunity, then relatively little pressure for antigenic change occurs within each host. But rapidly transmitting parasites may induce a greater density of immunological memory in the host population as noted in the previous item.

(d) Spatially homogeneous populations develop a higher and more uniform density of immunological memory than spatially heterogeneous populations. All hosts have the same high exposure rate to parasites in a well-mixed, spatially homogeneous population. By contrast, spatially heterogeneous populations may maintain temporarily isolated refuges in which hosts have low exposure. Those refuges could provide a source of hosts with limited immune memory, reducing the intensity of selection favoring antigenic variation.

The dynamics are complex because isolated host populations may have less prior exposure and immune memory but also may be less accessible to invasion by parasites and less able to transmit parasites back into the bulk of the host population. The net effect depends on the spatial connectivity of patches, rates of parasite transmission, and rates at which immune memory builds up and decays.

(e) Heterogeneity in immune memory profiles between age classes or spatial locations favors the stepwise spread of new antigenic variants. In this chapter, I discussed how new variants often need to change in several epitopes in order to spread through a host population with a high density of prior exposure. Heterogeneity enhances the chance of multiple antigenic changes by providing a sequence of susceptible host classes separated by the need for only a single antigenic change.

2. Memory decay. *(a) Faster time decay of immunological memory may reduce the selective pressure on antigenic variation.* Fast decay could potentially reduce the density of immunological memory across the host population. However, the faster the immunological memory decays, the more rapidly the parasites may reinfect hosts. The net effect on memory depends on the balance between these forces.

(b) The effect of immunological memory decay depends on the kind of parasite. The site of initial invasion determines which immune effectors

can potentially block first infection. Epithelial invasion interacts mostly with IgA, a memory class that tends to decline relatively rapidly. By contrast, systemic invasion interacts mostly with IgG, a memory class with a relatively long half-life.

Clearance of extracellular parasites depends mostly on antibodies. If infection spreads primarily to epithelial tissue, IgA plays a key role, whereas IgG dominates against many systemic infections. Antibody memory can increase the rate of clearance.

Once intracellular infection becomes established, the key immune effectors depend on kinetics. Antibodies dominate against intracellular parasites that rapidly kill host cells. In these fast cytopathic parasites, reproduction within cells occurs sufficiently quickly that CTLs cannot reduce the spread of the parasite. Antibody memory, if it does not prevent infection, can increase the clearance rate of fast cytopathic parasites.

Slow cytopathic parasites or noncytopathic parasites that persistently infect host cells must be cleared by killing infected cells. Most killing of infected cells seems to be done by effector CTLs. Thus, the rate of memory decay in CTLs may govern protection against noncytopathic infections that are not blocked during initial invasion by antibodies.

3. Heterogeneity of immune profiles among hosts. The dynamics of immune profiles can be complex because the spread of parasite variants affects the immune structure of the hosts, and the immune structure of the hosts determines the selective pressures on different classes of antigenic variants. Some preliminary theoretical work along these lines has appeared (Gupta et al. 1996; Andreasen et al. 1997; Gupta et al. 1998; Lin et al. 1999). Similar processes of reciprocal coevolution arise when hosts and parasites have multiple genetic determinants that influence the outcome of an attack (Frank 1993, 1994).

4. Examples. Measles apparently can vary its dominant surface antigen, hemagglutinin, and limited variation does occur (Griffin 2001). So it is an interesting puzzle why antigenic variants do not to spread. Perhaps the very high R_0 of measles causes the common strain to spread so widely in the host population that no differences occur between hosts in immune memory profiles. Thus, there is no single-step mutational change that allows a variant to spread to some hosts. The only "nearby" susceptible class arises from the influx of naive newborns.

Influenza A may not evolve as quickly and vary antigenically as much in birds as it does in humans (Webster et al. 1992). This suggestion is based on very limited evidence and must be confirmed by further study. If the pattern holds, then many plausible explanations exist. For example, the process of host invasion and spread during an infection probably differs in birds and humans, which may influence the role of immunity in clearance and in subsequent protection. Another possibility is that relatively short-lived species such as many birds have a larger class of naive hosts than comparably long-lived humans, reducing the relative pressure for antigenic variation in birds.

10 Genetic Structure of Parasite Populations

Variant alleles may be grouped together to form discrete parasite strains. For example, some parasites may be of type A/B or A'/B' at two distinct epitopes, with intermediates A/B' and A'/B rare or absent. In this chapter, I consider the processes that group together variants.

The first section reviews different kinds of genetic structure. The example above describes linkage disequilibrium between antigenic loci, a pattern that may arise from host immune selection disfavoring the intermediate forms. Alternatively, allelic variants across the entire genome may be linked into discrete sets because different parasite lineages do not mix. Spatial isolation or lack of sex and recombination can prevent mixing.

The second section asks whether the observed associations between alleles can be used to infer the processes that created the associations. This would be valuable because it is easier to measure patterns of genetic association than to measure processes such as immune selection or the frequency of genetic mixing. However, many different processes can lead to similar patterns of genetic association, making it difficult to infer process from pattern. Detailed data and a careful accounting of alternative hypotheses can allow one to narrow the possible explanations for observed patterns.

The third section describes various processes of genetic mixing between lineages and the consequences for genome-wide linkage disequilibrium. Some parasites have discrete, unmixed lineages, whereas other parasites recombine frequently and have little linkage between different loci. The degree of mixing determines the pace of antigenic recombination. New antigenic combinations have the potential to overcome existing patterns of host immunity.

The fourth section presents one example of antigenic linkage disequilibrium, the case of *Neisseria meningitidis*. Variants at two antigenic loci group together nonrandomly. Mixed genotypes occur at low frequency, suggesting some recombination. The immune structure of the host population could disfavor recombinant types, explaining the observed linkage between antigenic loci. Alternatively, recent epidemics or linkage with favored alleles at nonantigenic loci could also produce the observed patterns of antigenic linkage.

The fifth section proposes that hosts form isolated islands for parasites (Hastings and Wedgwood-Oppenheim 1997). Island structure confines selection within hosts to the limited genetic variation that enters with initial infection or arises de novo by mutation. Island structure also enhances stochastic fluctuations because each host receives only a very small sample of parasite diversity. As the number of genotypes colonizing a host rises, selection becomes more powerful and stochastic perturbations decline in importance. Rouzine and Coffin (1999) apply the balance between selection and stochastic perturbation to the observed patterns of genetic variability in HIV.

The final section takes up promising lines of study for future research.

10.1 Kinds of Genetic Structure

Genetic structure describes the statistical pattern of associations between alleles (Wright 1969; Crow and Kimura 1970; Li 1976; Hartl and Clark 1997; Hedrick 2000). It is useful to distinguish different kinds of genetic associations.

LINKAGE DISEQUILIBRIUM BETWEEN ANTIGENIC LOCI

Statistical association between alleles at different loci is called linkage disequilibrium. Linkage disequilibrium arises when alleles occur together in individuals (or haploid gametes) more or less frequently than expected by chance.

Immune pressure by hosts could potentially create linkage disequilibrium between antigenic loci of the parasite (Gupta et al. 1996). Suppose that the parasite genotype A/B infects many hosts during an epidemic, leaving most hosts recovered and immune to any parasite genotype with either A or B. Then genotypes A/B' and A'/B will be selected against, but A'/B' can spread. Thus, host immunity favors strong linkage disequilibrium in the parasites, dominated by the two strains A/B and A'/B'.

GENOME-WIDE LINKAGE DISEQUILIBRIUM

Linkage disequilibrium over the entire genome arises when there is some barrier to genetic mixing between lineages, such as spatial isolation or lack of sex and recombination. When lineages do not mix, then the particular amino acid substitutions in each lineage become locked together by their common pattern of inheritance. Genome-wide linkage disequilibrium has been observed in some parasites but not in others (Maynard Smith et al. 1993; Tibayrenc 1999).

Immune pressure can create associations between different antigenic loci of the parasite. But if the parasite mixes its genome by recombination, nonantigenic loci will often remain in linkage equilibrium and will not be separated into discrete strains. Consider, for example, a third, nonantigenic locus with the allele C causing severe disease symptoms and the equally frequent allele C' causing mild symptoms.

Strong host immune pressure could potentially separate the antigenic loci into discrete strains, A/B and A'/B'. But if recombination occurs, the nonantigenic locus will be randomly associated with each strain, for example, $A/B/C$ and $A/B/C'$ will occur equally frequently. The alleles C and C' will also be distributed equally within the A'/B' antigenic strain. Immunity by itself does not organize the entire parasite genome into discrete, nonoverlapping strains (Hastings and Wedgwood-Oppenheim 1997).

The distinction between antigenic and genome-wide linkage is important for medical applications. If genome-wide linkage occurs, then each strain defines a separate biological unit with its own immune interactions, virulence characteristics, and response to drugs (Tibayrenc et al. 1990; Tibayrenc 1999). Strains can be typed, followed epidemiologically, and treated based on information from a small number of identifying markers of the genome.

ASSOCIATION BETWEEN COINFECTING PARASITES

Several parasite genotypes may infect a single host. A recent survey of the literature found nonrandom associations between parasite genotypes within hosts (Lord et al. 1999). For sexual parasites, nonrandom associations within hosts often affect mating patterns. Mating typically occurs between the parasites within a host or between parasites in a vector that were recently derived from one or a few hosts. Nonrandom mating alters heterozygosity at individual loci and the opportunities for recombination between loci.

Host immunity may influence the distribution of strains within hosts. Gilbert et al. (1998) found a positive association within hosts between two antigenic variants of *Plasmodium falciparum*. Their data suggest that the two variants mutually interfere with T cell attack against the parasite, so both variants do better in the host when they are together. In general, the immunological profile of each host constrains the range of parasite variants that may coinfect that host.

EFFECTIVE POPULATION SIZE

The number of adult genotypes sampled to produce the progeny generation influences the effective size of the population (Wright 1969; Crow and Kimura 1970; Li 1976; Hartl and Clark 1997; Hedrick 2000). Population size affects many statistical properties of genetic structure. For example, suppose a particular parasite genotype sweeps through a host population, causing a widespread epidemic. This epidemic genotype rises to a high frequency as other genotypes fail to spread or decline in abundance.

Descendants of the population after an epidemic will likely come from the epidemic genotype (Maynard Smith et al. 1993). The effective size of the population is small because of the limited number of ancestral genotypes. The spread of an epidemic genotype carries along in strong association the alleles of that genotype at different loci. Consequently, strong genome-wide linkage disequilibrium may appear when descendants of the epidemic genotypes are sampled among genotypes descended from other lineages (Maynard Smith et al. 1993; Hastings and Wedgwood-Oppenheim 1997).

Population size also influences the pattern of genomic evolution by natural selection (Kimura 1983). When the effective population size is small, chance events of sampling can favor one allele over another. This stochastic sampling reduces the power of natural selection to shape evolutionary patterns of antigenic variation.

10.2 Pattern and Process

Recently developed molecular tools, such as polymerase chain reaction (PCR), provide the potential for widespread sampling of parasite populations (Enright and Spratt 1999). Statistical descriptions of the sampled data readily allow calculation of heterozygosity levels at single loci, the linkage disequilibrium between loci within genomes, and the spatial distribution of genotypes.

Can we use the measurable patterns of population structure to infer the underlying process that created the pattern? Yes, but only if we can rule out alternative processes that could lead to the same pattern.

Suppose, for example, that we demonstrate genome-wide linkage disequilibrium. The pattern by itself is interesting, because we have established that the parasites fall into discrete strains. Each strain can be identified by its combination of alleles, allowing the movement of strains to be followed. Each strain can also be studied for its unique antigenic and physiological properties, such as response to drugs.

The pattern of genome-wide linkage does not tell us what process created that pattern. The pattern may be created by frequent epidemics, each epidemic stemming from a limited number of genotypes. The parasite may be asexual, binding together alleles at different loci because no process mixes alleles between genotypes. Or, sex and the physical mixing of genotypes by recombination may occur in every generation, but with all mating confined to the pool of genotypes within each host. If only one parasite genotype typically infects a host, then all mating occurs between members of the same lineage with no opportunity for recombination to break down associations between loci.

One can carefully list all processes that could lead to the observed pattern and then do statistical tests of the data to distinguish between the potential causes. Maynard Smith et al. (1993) and Tibayrenc (1999) present detailed statistical analyses to accomplish such tests.

Most statistical analyses have not focused on antigenic variation. Instead, those analyses have used data on genetic variability from loci sampled across the genome. In some cases, the analyses use common enzyme (housekeeping) loci (Enright and Spratt 1999). Housekeeping loci are likely to evolve relatively slowly compared with other parts of the genome. The relatively slow rates of change provide a good indicator of common ancestry between genomes that have been separated for long periods of time. Other analyses use rapidly evolving loci, which provide more information about recent divergence from common ancestors (Tibayrenc 1999).

I review some population studies of genetic structure. I emphasize only the background needed for understanding antigenic variation, leaving out much of the analytical detail. I start with linkage of alleles across the entire genome. I then turn to linkage at antigenic loci.

10.3 Genome-wide Linkage Disequilibrium

BARRIERS TO GENETIC MIXING

Genome-wide linkage arises when different lineages rarely mix their genes (Tibayrenc 1999). Four different barriers prevent genetic mixing (Maynard Smith et al. 1993, Hastings and Wedgwood-Oppenheim 1997). First, asexual reproduction separates lineages irrespective of geographical or ecological locality. Differentiated strains will occur jointly in the same area. In addition, particular multilocus combinations of genes may disperse widely and be found in different regions without being broken up by recombination with local varieties.

Second, physical separation by geography or habitat prevents genetic mixing. Geographic subdivision is common in many populations. Ecological subdivision may arise if some genotypes occur mainly in one host species, whereas other genotypes are confined to a different host. Sexual species divided by physical barriers will have mixed genomes within local regions and differentiated genomes across barriers. Particular multilocus genotypes are unlikely to be found far from their native region because they will be broken up by recombination with neighboring genotypes.

Third, demography can separate lineages if each host or vector carries only a single parasite genotype. Single-genotype infections prevent physical contact between different parasite genotypes, isolating lineages from each other even when they occur in the same region. Epidemics may cause a single genotype to spread rapidly, limiting most infections to the epidemic strain. This limited variability reduces opportunity for genetic exchange and causes the region to be dominated by the linked set of alleles within the epidemic strain (Maynard Smith et al. 1993). In the absence of epidemics, single-genotype infections can maintain a greater diversity of distinct genotypes within a region. Obligate intracellular pathogens may be able to exchange genetic information only when two distinct genotypes coinfect a cell.

Fourth, mixing may occur occasionally between separated lineages, but mixed genotypes fail. Hybrid incompatibility separates eukaryotes into distinct, reproductively isolated species. In segmented viruses, certain pairs of segments may be incompatible, causing the absence of some genotypic combinations (Frank 2001). Recombining viruses and bacteria present more complex possibilities. Certain genomic regions may be able to pass from one lineage to another, whereas other genomic regions may be incompatible. Thus, some genomic regions may exhibit linkage disequilibrium between lineages, whereas other regions may be well mixed.

Sexual, diploid species will be primarily homozygous when different lineages do not mix because most matings will be between the same genotype. Asexual species may maintain significant heterozygosity even in regions dominated by a single clone.

At the nucleotide level, epidemics tend to reduce genetic variability because extant parasites have descended from a recent ancestral genotype that started the epidemic. By contrast, endemic diseases will often maintain more nucleotide variability within genotypes because those genotypes trace their ancestry back over a longer time to a common progenitor.

Sexual, physical, and demographic barriers to genomic mixing shape patterns of genetic variability. Conversely, those patterns provide information about key aspects of parasite biology.

An Example

The protozoan *Trypanosoma cruzi* causes Chagas' disease. Linkage disequilibrium between loci has been observed in several sampling studies (e.g., Tibayrenc et al. 1986; Tibayrenc and Ayala 1988; Oliveira et al. 1998, 1999). Recently, Michel Tibayrenc's laboratory expanded a long-term analysis of genetic variability by using multilocus enzyme electrophoresis (MLEE), random amplified polymorphic DNA (RAPD), and polymerase chain reaction (PCR) (Barnabé et al. 2000; Brisse et al. 2000a, 2000b).

Tibayrenc's laboratory has classified *T. cruzi* into six groups defined as discrete typing units (DTUs) (Tibayrenc 1999). Each individual in a DTU shares a significant proportion of alleles at several polymorphic loci with other members of the DTU and shares relatively few alleles with members of other DTUs. The discrete, nonoverlapping structure of DTUs is simply another way to describe genome-wide linkage disequilibrium—the association of particular sets of alleles within genomes.

The different methods, MLEE, RAPD, and PCR, give similar results for the classification of *T. cruzi* isolates into DTUs. Because each method measures genetic variability in different parts of the genome, the concordance between methods further supports the overall classification into separate DTUs.

The DTUs provide a taxonomy to identify new samples. To the extent that DTUs truly capture genome-wide linkage, each DTU will likely have unique properties. Several studies have compared traits such as growth rate, virulence in mice, and sensitivity to drugs (e.g., Revollo et al. 1998; de Lana et al. 2000). The trait values for different isolates of a DTU often vary widely, with the average values of the isolates differing between DTUs. Thus, there appears to be considerable genetic diversity both within and between DTUs.

What processes maintain genome-wide linkage? The previous section classified barriers to genetic mixing as sexual, physical, demographic, or genetic. Tibayrenc and his colleagues have argued that sexual reproduction occurs rarely in *T. cruzi* and that the lack of sex explains the observed patterns of genetic linkage. They review many lines of evidence, but perhaps the most telling observation concerns repeated occurrences of particular multilocus genotypes.

Barnabé et al. (2000) showed that certain multilocus genotypes recur in samples. Some of the repeated multilocus genotypes were found in widely separated geographic locations. The probability of obtaining the same set of alleles across multiple polymorphic loci would be very small if the loci recombined occasionally.

Epidemics stemming from a single genotype could possibly cause the spread and repeat occurrence of a genotype. But some of the repeated genotypes were found in areas surrounded by other genotypes, far from the geographic foci of their highest frequency. In addition, the high genetic diversity within locations argues against local regions being swept by epidemic strains.

Rare sex seems to be a reasonable explanation given the limited data. Eventually, additional studies will collect more data and develop a clearer picture of genetic structure.

Is a Clonal Population Structure Common?

Tibayrenc et al. (1990, 1991) concluded from the available data that many parasites have genome-wide linkage disequilibrium, suggesting that different lineages rarely mix genes. Tibayrenc et al. use the word "clonal" to describe the observed pattern of genomic linkage, without implying any particular cause such as asexuality or lack of mating between different sexual lineages.

Several recent analyses infer a clonal population structure, including studies of the protozoan *Trypanosoma cruzi* (citations above), the protozoan *Cryptosporidium parvum* (Awad-El-Kariem 1999), and the yeast *Candida albicans* (Xu et al. 1999). However, data from other species present a complex picture, suggesting a wide diversity of genetic structures. I summarize some of the current ideas and observations in the following subsections.

Bacteria and Protozoa

Bacteria reproduce by binary fission, an asexual process. However, bacteria can mix genomes by taking up DNA from neighboring cells (Ochman et al. 2000). Conjugation directly transfers DNA, transduction carries bacterial DNA with infecting viruses, and transformation occurs by uptake of free DNA that has been released into the environment. Foreign DNA fragments can recombine with the host chromosome, inserting a piece of genetic material from a different lineage into the genome.

Maynard Smith et al. (1993) classified bacterial genetic structure as clonal, panmictic, or epidemic. Rare recombination leads to a clonal structure with strong linkage disequilibrium, as observed in *Salmonella enterica* (Spratt and Maiden 1999).

Frequent recombination leads to a panmictic (widely mixed) genetic structure and relatively little association between alleles within genomes. *Helicobacter pylori* has a panmictic structure (Spratt and Maiden 1999). Recombination occurs so frequently that even variable nucleotide sites within genes are often in linkage equilibrium (not statistically associated) (Suerbaum et al. 1998; Salaun et al. 1998).

Neisseria gonorrhoeae also has a panmictic structure (Spratt and Maiden 1999). However, a strain that requires arginine, hypoxanthine, and uracil (AHU) to grow has maintained a tightly linked genotype over a thirty-nine-year period (Gutjahr et al. 1997). That strain can take up and recombine with DNA in the laboratory. Perhaps the clonal AHU strain remains within the broader panmictic population because it rarely occurs in mixed infections with non-AHU genotypes.

Neisseria meningitidis has an epidemic population structure (Spratt and Maiden 1999). Recombination occurs frequently, and broad samples of the population typically show highly mixed genomes with little or no linkage disequilibrium. However, it appears that epidemics sometimes arise from single genotypes and spread rapidly within a restricted geographic area. When samples include a large fraction of the epidemic strain, this strain shows a clonal pattern of inheritance and strong linkage disequilibrium when compared against other isolates. The epidemics appear to be sporadic and localized, and the epidemic clone probably mixes its genome with other lineages over the span of several months or a few years. As the epidemic clone mixes with other genotypes, its unique pattern of genetic linkage decays.

Escherichia coli has a particularly interesting population structure (Guttman 1997). The first broad studies found strong linkage disequilibrium and an apparently clonal structure. However, early studies of population structure tend to sample widely and sparsely, obtaining just one or a few isolates from each habitat or geographic locality. Later studies of *E. coli* provided finer resolution by sampling repeatedly from the same or nearby localities or by using DNA sequences rather than lower-resolution molecular markers. Those later studies found that recombination does occur.

How can *E. coli*'s recombining genetic system maintain widespread linkage disequilibrium? This remains a controversial question with several possible answers. Recombination may be a weak force, introducing changes into genomes at a rate no higher than the mutation rate. Advantageous genes may occasionally sweep through a local population, carrying along linked genes as in epidemics. Frequent sweeps promote linkage and may overwhelm the mixing effect of recombination. Alternatively, different genotypes may be specific for different habitats, so that most recombinational mixing occurs within habitats. This may lead to weaker linkage within habitats but strong linkage when measured between nonmixing lineages that live in different habitats.

I suspect that the relatively complex structure of *E. coli* reflects the more intensive study of this species at different spatial scales. Many bacteria will likely show different genetic structures when analyzed at different scales. The particular spatial scale over which a species differentiates into nonmixing lineages will vary depending on the relative balance of recombination, genetic drift, selective sweeps, epidemics, and migration.

Recent studies on the protozoan *Trypanosoma brucei* illustrate the varying genetic structures revealed by careful sampling (MacLeod et al. 2000). The human-infective subspecies *T. b. rhodesiense* causes African sleeping sickness, whereas the subspecies *T. b. brucei* cannot infect humans. Both subspecies occur in various domestic animals.

T. brucei can recombine sexually in the laboratory, but the extent of genetic mixing in natural populations has been debated (Tibayrenc et al. 1990; Maynard Smith et al. 1993; Hide et al. 1994). MacLeod et al. (2000) demonstrated that the two subspecies are genetically differentiated and show linkage disequilibrium when compared against each other. Within subspecies, *T. b. brucei* had an epidemic structure, in which recombination occurs but can be overwhelmed by clonal expansion of a few genotypes during epidemics. By contrast, *T. b. rhodesiense* appeared clonal within the Ugandan samples obtained. Further sampling may eventually find that the Ugandan isolates are part of a wider population in which some recombination occurs.

The protozoan *Plasmodium falciparum* has an obligate sexual phase that occurs during transmission in the mosquito vector. In geographic regions where infection is common, the vector frequently picks up multiple genotypes, which then mate and recombine before transmission to a new host. By contrast, regions with sparsely infected hosts have a lower probability of mixed genotypes in the vectors, leading to frequent self-fertilization and limited opportunity for recombination between lineages (Babiker and Walliker 1997; Paul and Day 1998; Conway et al. 1999).

Anderson et al. (2000) studied *P. falciparum* genetic structure with twelve rapidly mutating microsatellite loci in 465 isolates from nine geographic regions. Within areas of low infection intensity, they found strong linkage disequilibrium, low genetic diversity, and high variation between geographic locations. They observed the opposite patterns within areas of high infection intensity. This provides another example in which the genetic structure varies across space.

Reassortment in Segmented Viruses

The segmented RNA viruses provide an excellent model for studying genomic linkage disequilibrium. Genomes are broken up into two or more segments. Each segment replicates independently during cellular infection. The segments act like distinct chromosomes but do not pair and segregate as in eukaryotic cells. Instead, new viral particles form by a sampling process that chooses approximately one segment of each type. When multiple viruses infect a single cell, their replicating segments mix. The progeny form by reassorted combinations of genomic segments.

Reassortment has the same effect as recombination. However, reassorting segments are easier to study because the segments mark discretely and clearly the units of recombination.

Occasional reassortment plays a crucial role in creating new strains. Reassortment of influenza A's neuraminidase and hemagglutinin surface antigens provides the most famous example (Lamb and Krug 2001). The genes for these antigens occur on two separate RNA segments of the genome—the genome has a total of eight segments.

It appears that rare reassortments have occasionally introduced hemagglutinin or neuraminidase from bird influenza into the genome of human influenza (Webster et al. 1997). The novel antigens cross-reacted very little with those circulating in humans, allowing the new combination to sweep through human populations and cause pandemics.

Lack of reassortment maintains discrete strains with strong linkage disequilibrium between segments. Rare mixing can be traced back phylogenetically to one or a few events. This is another way of saying that, after reassortment, discrete lineages accumulate new mutations on different segments and keep those new mutations together within the lineage, creating linkage disequilibrium.

Common reassortment reduces linkage disequilibrium between segments by bringing together genetic variants that arose in different individuals. Reassortment causes differences in the phylogenetic history of different segments within a virus.

Reassortment may be common between viruses within a population, but that population may not mix with viruses from another population. Measured within each population, linkage disequilibrium will be low, and there will be a weak correlation between phylogenetic patterns of different segments. But isolated populations do not share the same associations between genetic variants and thus exhibit linkage disequilibrium relative to each other. Equivalently, the segments within each isolated population have a common phylogeny that differs relative to the phylogenetic history of the segments in other populations.

No studies have sampled over different spatial and temporal scales or studied the processes that cause barriers to reassortment. The best studies I found examined the phylogenetic histories of the various segments of influenza. Influenza occurs in three major types: A, B, and C.

Several papers describe reassortment between segments of influenza C (Buonagurio et al. 1985; Peng et al. 1994, 1996; Tada et al. 1997). A phylogenetic tree of the NS (nonstructural protein) segment showed that thirty-four isolates over 1947–1992 split into two distinct lineages. Recent isolates had one NS lineage, whereas older isolates had the other NS lineage. Thus, the newer NS lineage seems to have replaced the older lineage. By contrast, phylogenies of the other six segments identify three or four distinct lineages, in which each lineage contains older isolates as well as recent isolates. Alamgir et al. (2000) suggest that the newer NS type has reassorted with the other segments and replaced the older NS type, perhaps because the newer NS type has a functional advantage that enhances its spread.

The phylogenetic patterns for seven of the eight influenza B segments show clear patterns of reassortment (Lindstrom et al. 1999; Hiromoto et al. 2000). Figure 10.1 illustrates the phylogenetic patterns and putative reassortments for segments based on eighteen isolates obtained over twenty years. Concordant phylogenetic patterns between segments suggest cotransmission of those segments. Such concordance may arise by selection of functionally compatible segments, for example, between the PB1 and PB2 segments that encode components of the polymerase complex (Hiromoto et al. 2000). However, the sample size is small, and the observed concordances may simply be the chance outcome from a small number of reassortment events.

Lindstrom et al. (1998) sequenced all eight segments from ten isolates of influenza A. The isolates were collected over the years 1993–1997. The hemagglutinin (HA) and neuraminidase (NA) segments encode the surface glycoproteins known to determine the main components of antigenicity and interaction with human immunity. These two segments accumulated amino acid changes sequentially over the 5-year period,

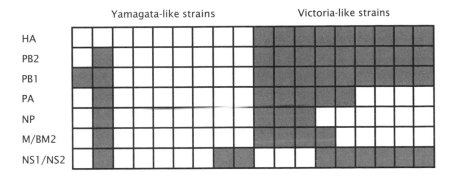

Figure 10.1   The phylogenetic affinities for seven of the eight influenza B segments. Each row shows a particular segment. The columns show the segment type for each of eighteen isolates, with each segment separated into two types and assigned primary affinity for either the Yamagata-like or Victoria-like strains. The dominant antigenic hemagglutinin (HA) defines the strain classification for each isolate. The appearance of Victoria-like segments in some Yamagata-like isolates demonstrates reassortment, as does the appearance of Yamagata-like segments in some Victoria-like isolates. From table 4 of Hiromoto et al. (2000), which includes some data from Lindstrom et al. (1999).

the isolates from each year apparently replacing those from the prior year in a single, nonbranching lineage. Thus, these isolates do not show any reassortment between HA and NA.

The six influenza A segments encoding internal proteins reassorted relative to the HA-NA lineage. Those internal genes did not accumulate changes sequentially over time in a single lineage. For example, the basic polymerase-1 protein, the nucleoprotein, and the matrix protein isolated in 1997 were phylogenetically closer to isolates from 1993–1994 than to isolates from 1995.

This study shows linkage of the antigenic determinants but reassortment of other genetic components. Influenza strains are defined by the common procedure of using antigenic determinants, in this case by HA-NA combinations. The reassortments of the internal segments against HA-NA strain definitions mean that the strain definitions do not describe distinct genotypes.

Lindstrom et al. (1998) point out that HA-NA strains often appear about three years before they expand into epidemics (see also Bush et al 1999). They suggest that new antigenic determinants, arising by mutation primarily in HA, may sometimes require reassortment into a more virulent genetic background before a genotype can initiate an epidemic.

However, that leaves open the question of why mutations would often arise in weak genetic backgrounds and require reassortment into strong backgrounds.

RECOMBINATION IN VIRUSES

Reassortment is a special case of the more general process of recombination. DNA viruses and many RNA viruses have only a single segment, so genetic exchange typically occurs between similar (homologous) segments. Several cases of recombination have been described (summarized by Worobey and Holmes 1999), for example, between vaccine and wild-type polio strains (Guillot et al. 2000).

Recombinants may strongly affect evolutionary patterns even when the frequency of recombination per generation is very low. Occasional recombinants can create the mosaic progenitors of successful lineages (Worobey and Holmes 1999). In addition, recombination means that a particular virus does not have a single phylogenetic history—instead, each part of the genome may trace back to a different ancestral lineage. This may preclude an unambiguous viral taxonomy based on phylogeny.

Recombination can occur only when host cells are coinfected by different viral genotypes. Preliminary reports suggest that some viruses can recombine frequently when genetic variants coinfect a cell (Martin and Weber 1997; Fujita et al. 1998; Bruyere et al. 2000; Hajós et al. 2000; Jetzt et al. 2000; Zhang et al. 2000). Many viruses may be similar to the *Plasmodium* example cited above, in which the frequency of multiple infection by different genotypes determines the degree of genetic mixing between lineages.

The frequency of recombination between genetic variants undoubtedly varies among viruses. Worobey (2000) has shown that isolates of the DNA-based TT virus have mosaic genomes generated by recombination. Recombination is sufficiently frequent that a small subset of the genome provides a poor indicator of the phylogenetic history for the entire genome. Thus, strain typing may have little meaning because highly diverged variants merge by recombination into a single gene pool. A similar study of the RNA-based dengue virus found seven genotypes created by recombination events between seventy-one isolates (Worobey et al. 1999).

Distinct strains do not exist under frequent recombination. By contrast, rare recombination leaves most lineages identifiably intact as discrete strains. With discrete strains, occasional recombinant mosaics can be identified as the mixture of known strains.

HIV isolates across the world have been sequenced (http://hiv-web. lanl.gov/). Most isolates appear to have a phylogenetic affinity for a particular clade, but multiple recombination events and genomic mosaics also occur frequently (Bobkov et al. 1996; Cornelissen et al. 1996; Robertson et al. 1999). The opposing aspects of discrete strains and widespread recombination probably reflect heterogeneous histories in different locations, the temporal and spatial scales of sampling, and the rapidly changing nature of the viral populations as the infection continues to spread.

I briefly speculate about the history of HIV to illustrate the sort of processes and patterns that may occur in viral evolution. The epicenter of HIV diversity and the probable origin of the pandemic occur in central Africa (Vidal et al. 2000). Based on sequences from the V3–V5 *env* region of the genome, all known HIV-1 subtypes occurred in a sample of 247 isolates from the Democratic Republic of Congo. Analysis of the *gag* genomic regions and longer sequences in the *env* region showed a high frequency of recombination within this population.

Overall, the Democratic Republic of Congo population had all known subtypes, a high degree of diversity within each subtype, and significant mosaicism across different genomic regions. This suggests a relatively old and large population that has accumulated diversity and probably been the source for many lineages that have colonized different parts of the world (Vidal et al. 2000).

Different lineages dominate different geographic regions of the world (http://hiv-web.lanl.gov/). For example, subtype B has spread throughout the Americas, Europe, Australia, and parts of eastern Asia. Subtype A is relatively common in the eastern African countries around the Ivory Coast, and subtype C dominates southern Africa. These broad patterns probably represent the initial spread from central Africa into those regions, each region founded by a narrow slice of the worldwide HIV diversity.

Each subtype divides more finely into variants. Such variants may dominate smaller localities. For example, a distinctive B subtype is particularly common in the heterosexual population of Trinidad and Tobago (Cleghorn et al. 2000). Another variant B (Thai B) is common in Thailand.

Each region may accumulate significant diversity within its dominant subtype, with frequent recombination between subtype variants. However, as HIV spreads, a region initially pure for a subtype will eventually be colonized by other subtypes. Recombination between subtypes then mixes the distinct phylogenetic histories of the subtypes. Such recombinations probably have become increasingly common, for example, the admixtures of subtypes occurring along the routes of intravenous drug user transmissions in China (Piyasirisilp et al. 2000). Drug users in Greece and Cyprus also appear to be fertile sources of recombinants between subtypes (Gao et al. 1998).

These studies suggest that recombination may be relatively common. Such recombination between antigenic sites can strongly influence the evolutionary dynamics of antigenic variation because new genotypes can be generated by combinations of existing variants rather than waiting for rare combinations of new mutations.

10.4 Antigenic Linkage Disequilibrium

The previous section described studies of distinct strains caused by epidemics or barriers to genetic mixing between lineages. Those studies defined strains mainly by measurement of genetic variability at nonantigenic loci (Enright and Spratt 1999). Methods of measurement include electrophoresis and nucleotide sequencing.

In this section, I focus on genetic variability between lineages when defined by differences at antigenic loci. Immune pressure by hosts can potentially separate the parasite population into discrete, nonoverlapping antigenic types (Gupta et al. 1996, 1999). Suppose that a haploid parasite with alleles at two different loci, A/B, infects many hosts during an epidemic, leaving most hosts recovered and immune to any parasite genotype with either A or B. Then genotypes A/B' and A'/B will be selected against, but A'/B' can spread. Thus, host immunity favors strong linkage disequilibrium in the parasites, dominated by the two nonoverlapping genotypes A/B and A'/B'.

Few data exist on the degree of antigenic overlap between genotypes (reviewed by Gupta et al. 1996, 1999). The best example comes from Feavers et al. (1996), who analyzed variability in the outer membrane

Table 10.1   Linkage disequilibrium between antigens of *Neisseria meningitidis*

VR1 type	VR2 type	Expected percent	Observed percent
5	10	8.2	25.3
7	4	6.5	20.3
19	15	3.2	15.3
other combinations		82.1	39.1

protein PorA of *Neisseria meningitidis*. This protein has two distinct variable antigenic regions, VR1 and VR2. Strong associations occurred between VR1 and VR2 variants in a sample of 222 isolates from England and Wales obtained in 1989-1991. Table 10.1 shows that three combinations account for 61% of the observed genotypes, much higher than the 18% expected for these combinations if the two antigens occurred independently. The "other combinations" include mixtures of the listed types, for example, VR1 type 5 with VR2 type 4, plus other, rarer types not listed.

The existence of uncommon combinations suggests that recombination can occur. Some process apparently opposes recombination to maintain strong linkage disequilibrium between VR1 and VR2. Gupta et al. (1996) favor host immune selection as the force that structures bacterial genotypes into nonoverlapping sets. This is certainly a plausible explanation. But, as with most population genetic patterns, other processes can lead to the same observations. For example, the three common types might just happen to be the strains circulating most widely among the individuals sampled. Those strains might be common because of chance events that led to mild epidemics caused by a few different types. Or those types may have advantageous alleles at other loci, possibly antigenic but not necessarily so. Over time, recombination could break down the associations between advantageous alleles and the VR combinations, but over a few years such associations can be strong.

Gupta et al.'s (1996) work on antigenic strain structure calls attention to several interesting questions. Are different antigenic combinations structured into nonoverlapping sets? The pattern by itself is important for the design of vaccines and the study of epidemiological distributions.

If discrete antigenic strains occur, are they associated with other components of the genome that code for attributes such as virulence? Hastings and Wedgwood-Oppenheim (1997) provide a good introduction to the processes that potentially link antigenic type to other characters.

What processes can potentially structure populations into discrete, nonoverlapping antigenic combinations? Immune selection is one possibility, but any process that reduces gene flow relative to the scale of sampling tends to create nonrandom associations between loci.

How can one differentiate between the various processes that lead to similar patterns? A clear understanding of the processes that reduce gene flow and their consequences (Hastings and Wedgwood-Oppenheim 1997) can help. Direct observations of immune selection disfavoring "recombinant" antigenic types would be useful, but perhaps difficult to obtain.

10.5 Population Structure: Hosts as Islands

Parasite populations often subdivide into Wright's (1978) classical "island model" structure from the theory of population genetics (Hastings and Wedgwood-Oppenheim 1997). Each host forms an island colonized by parasites from one or more sources. The population of parasites within the host undergoes selection that depends on the amount of genetic variation between parasites within the host. The host transmits migrant parasites to colonize new hosts (islands). Each population within a host expires when the host dies or clears the infection.

General Aspects of Transmission and Selection

The number of genotypes colonizing a host may often be small. For example, only a few parasites may colonize a host, or all of the parasites may have come from a single donor that itself had little genetic variation among its parasites. If initial genetic variability is low, then selection within the host depends primarily on de novo mutations that arise during the population expansion of the parasites. By contrast, high initial genetic variability within hosts causes intense selection between coinfecting genotypes.

The island structure of parasite populations resembles the genetic structure of multicellular organisms when taking account of selection within individuals. Each new organism begins as a single cell or, in some clonal organisms, as a small number of progenitor cells. The individual develops as a population of cells, with the potential for selection between cellular lineages that vary genetically. Genetic variation may arise from the small number of progenitor cells or from de novo mutations. The individual transmits some of its cells to form new bodies (islands). Eventually, the individual dies.

There is some general theory on the population genetics of mutation and selection within individuals (Slatkin 1984; Buss 1987; Orive 1995; Michod 1997; Otto and Hastings 1998). Levin and Bull (1994) discussed how selection within and between hosts can shape patterns of parasite life history (reviewed by Frank 1996). But there has been little work on the consequences of island population structure for antigenic variation. Hastings and Wedgwood-Oppenheim (1997) illustrated how a quantitative theory of island-model genetics can be used to understand the buildup or decay of linkage disequilibrium.

I found one study that develops the theory of island population structure for parasites.

GENETIC VARIATION OF HIV WITHIN INDIVIDUAL HOSTS

Rouzine and Coffin (1999) sought to explain the high genetic diversity of HIV within hosts. They developed the theory of island population structure for parasites to compare the relative strengths of natural selection and stochastic processes that can cause genetic variability.

Rouzine and Coffin (1999) focused on the *pro* gene, which encodes a protease that processes other HIV gene products. Analysis of nucleotide sequences for this particular gene suggested that natural selection acts primarily in a purifying way to remove deleterious mutations. Consequently, their model describes the accumulation of nucleotide diversity shaped by two opposing forces. On the one hand, stochastic effects occur because only a small number of viruses invade each host— the founders of that island. Stochastic drift during colonization allows deleterious mutations to rise in frequency. On the other hand, purifying selection within hosts removes deleterious mutations. How do the opposing forces of mutation and selection in parasites play out in the island structure of hosts?

If each new host is colonized by viruses from a single donor host, then the founding population tends to have limited genetic diversity. Low diversity causes natural selection to be weak because there is not much opportunity for competition between genetic variants. Only new mutations that arise within the host provide an opportunity to replace deleterious mutations by genetic variants that restore full fitness.

With colonization from a single donor host, the viruses in each host share a lineage of descent that is isolated from the viruses in other hosts. Isolated lineages and bottlenecks in viral numbers that occur during transmission allow the accumulation of deleterious genetic variation by drift.

Coinfection from different donor hosts mixes lineages, increases genetic variation within hosts, and greatly enhances the power of natural selection to remove deleterious variants. Rouzine and Coffin (1999) estimate that a coinfection frequency higher than 1% provides sufficiently strong selection within hosts to reduce the level of genetic variation relative to the amount of variation that accumulates by drift in isolated lineages.

If coinfection occurs more commonly than 1%, as Rouzine and Coffin (1999) believe to be likely, then some other process must explain the high levels of genetic variability observed. Rouzine and Coffin (1999) discuss an interesting type of selection that purifies within hosts but diversifies between hosts. According to their model, purifying selection within hosts removes T cell epitopes to avoid host immunity. MHC type varies between hosts, causing different T cell epitopes to be recognized by different hosts. Thus, diversifying selection acts between hosts to establish reduced recognition by MHC. Purifying selection within hosts and diversifying selection between hosts may account for the apparently paradoxical observations: nucleotide substitutions leave the signature of purifying selection, yet the viral population maintains significant genetic diversity.

Very few studies have considered how the island population structure of parasites influences the distribution of genetic diversity. As more sequences accumulate, there will be greater opportunity to match the observed patterns to the combined stochastic and selective processes that shape parasite diversity.

10.6 Problems for Future Research

1. Statistical inference. Patterns of genetic structure must be interpreted with regard to alternative models. For example, table 10.1 shows linkage between two antigenic loci of *Neisseria meningitidis*. I mentioned three hypotheses to explain those data: immune selection against recombinants, epidemics, and linkage with favored alleles at other loci.

Each hypothesis leads to a model dependent on several parameters. For example, the rarity of recombinant genotypes under immune selection depends on the distribution of immune profiles in hosts, the intensity of selection against the recombinant genotypes, and the frequency of recombination.

To determine if an observed pattern favors one model over another, one must understand the range of outcomes likely to follow from each model. This requires mathematical development to calculate the predicted outcomes from the different models. Then one must design sampling schemes to obtain data that can differentiate between the models. Theoretical analysis of sampling schemes can compare the information in different sampling procedures with regard to the alternative processes under study.

Technical advances will continue to improve the rate at which samples can be processed and analyzed. Improved technical facilities will allow designed sampling procedures and hypothesis testing.

2. Scale-dependent population structure. Sampling over different distances will often reveal a hierarchy of scale-dependent processes that depend on the epidemiology and demography of the parasite. It may be common to find spatial isolation at longer scales, mixing in dense aggregations at local scales, and occasional swaths of genome-wide linkage at varying scales caused by population bottlenecks or the rapid spread of epidemic strains. The relative scaling of these processes will differ greatly among parasites.

3. Different phylogenetic histories of genomic components. Very intense selection on antigenic loci can occur in parasites. This focused selection can cause different components of the genome to have different genetic structures and phylogenetic histories. I briefly mention one example to provide hints about what may happen and to encourage further work.

I described earlier in this chapter the example of influenza. In that case, Lindstrom et al. (1998) found that the two antigenic segments, hemagglutinin and neuraminidase, cotransmitted in an epidemic fashion over five years of samples. By contrast, the other six segments appeared to mix their lineages relative to the single line of cotransmitted antigenic segments. Thus, epidemically bound linkage groups may occur against a mixing genetic background. More data of this sort might show different genomic components changing their population structures relative to each other over different temporal and spatial scales. Such data could provide insight into the scale-dependent effects of demographic, genetic, and selective processes.

4. Population bottlenecks and genomic diversity. Rich et al. (2000) argue that all of the very diverse antigenic variants of *Plasmodium falciparum* have arisen since a recent population bottleneck that occurred less than fifty thousand years ago. Variant alleles at antigenic loci appear to trace their phylogenetic history back to common ancestors more recent than the putative bottleneck event. This pattern suggests intense natural selection favoring novel diversity at antigenic sites against a background of low genome-wide diversity caused by a recent bottleneck.

Alternatively, the antigenic variants could trace their history back to ancestors that predated the bottleneck (Hughes 1992; Hughes and Hughes 1995; Hughes and Verra 2001). This pattern arises when natural selection strongly favors rare variant antigens, holding diverse antigens in the population through the bottleneck that reduced variation in the rest of the genome. Ancient polymorphisms of this sort suggest that natural selection preserves existing variants rather than favors de novo generation of new variants (Ayala 1995; O'hUigin et al. 2000).

A recent, more detailed study by Volkman et al. (2001) estimates that the most recent common ancestor of *P. falciparum* lived less than ten thousand years ago. If this estimate applies to the *var* genes as well as the loci studied by Volkman et al. (2001), then the diverse *var* family of antigenic variants must have evolved very rapidly. Further studies of different genomic regions will contribute to understanding the speed of diversification in the *var* archival library.

5. Island structure. Many classical genetic models develop the island structure for populations (Wright 1978). However, those general studies of migration, selection, and stochastic perturbation provide little guidance for the genetic structure of parasites. Studies for parasites must account for the density and variability of host immune memory, the longevity of infections, the genetic diversity of inocula, and the patterns of genetic mixing between parasites.

Much insight can be gained by island models focused specifically on the special biology of parasites (Hastings and Wedgwood-Oppenheim 1997). Rouzine and Coffin's (1999) study shows how a clear model of population genetic process can lead to predictions about the expected patterns in the data. This suggests how one could couple process-oriented theory with the problem of statistical inference.

PART V

STUDYING
EVOLUTION

11 Classifications by Antigenicity and Phylogeny

In this chapter, I compare immunological and phylogenetic classifications of antigenic variation. Contrasts between these classifications provide insight into how natural selection shapes observed patterns of diversity. Following chapters take up other methods to infer processes of selection.

The first section describes immunological measures of antigenicity. These measures summarize the ability of specific antibodies to recognize different antigenic variants. The reactivities for various antibodies tested against different antigenic isolates form a matrix of antigenic or immunological distances between parasite variants. These distances can be used to classify antigenic variants into related clusters.

The second section notes that antigenic variants can also be classified by phylogeny. This classification scheme measures relatedness between variants by distance back in time to a common ancestor. Such distances arise from the patterns of nucleotide or amino acid differences in genomic sequences.

The third section defines possible relations between antigenic and phylogenetic classifications. Concordance commonly occurs because antigenic distance often increases with time since a common ancestor, reflecting the natural tendency for similarity by common descent. A particular pattern of discord between antigenic and phylogenetic classifications suggests hypotheses about evolutionary process. Suppose, for example, that phylogenetically divergent parasites are antigenically close at certain epitopes. This suggests as a hypothesis that selective pressure by antibodies has favored recurrent evolution of a particular antigenic variant.

The fourth section presents flaviviruses as an example of concordant antigenic and phylogenetic classifications. This example compares strains that differ by relatively long phylogenetic distances with antigenicity measured by averaging reactivity over many different epitopes. Aggregate antigenicity tends to diverge steadily over time as amino acid differences accumulate (Benjamin et al. 1984). Particular details of natural selection with regard to each amino acid substitution disappear in the averaging over many independent events.

The fifth section shows a mixture of discordance and concordance between antigenic and phylogenetic classifications for influenza A. The classifications cover a history of transfers between different host species. Antigenicity and phylogeny both separate isolates from pigs into two groups, the classical swine types and avian-like swine types more recently transferred from birds to pigs. Two bird isolates group phylogenetically with the avian-like swine types, as expected. However, antigenic measures separate the bird isolates as distinct from the relatively similar classical swine and avian-like swine groups. Perhaps host adaptation influences antigenicity of some epitopes used in this study.

The sixth section suggests that immunological pressure by antibodies drives the short-term phylogenetic divergence of influenza A. If so, then antigenic classifications over the same scale of diversity may match the phylogenetic pattern. Concordance probably depends on the percentage of amino acid substitutions explained by antibody pressure.

The seventh section considers explanations for the discordant patterns of phylogeny and antigenicity reported for HIV. Shared antigenicity over long phylogenetic distances may arise by stabilizing or convergent selection. Stabilizing selection prevents change in particular amino acids because of their essential contribution to viral fitness. Convergent selection causes recurrent evolution of the same antigenic type by repeatedly favoring that type in different times and places. Alternatively, divergent antigenicity over short phylogenetic distances can arise from intense immune pressure. Stabilizing, convergent, and diversifying selection can all occur over different temporal scales, combining to shape the relations between antigenicity and phylogeny.

The final section lists problems for future research.

11.1 Immunological Measures of Antigenicity

Immunological methods measure the reactions of antigens with antibodies or T cells. A particular test can be described by a matrix. One dimension consists of standardized immunological components such as different antibodies; the second dimension lists alternative parasite isolates or molecules to be tested for their antigenic properties. Each matrix entry contains the strength of the immunological response—a measure of antigenicity.

Immunology differentiates antigens only to the extent that the test antigens react differently with the panel of immunological agents. Thus, the measures depend on the immunological panel used for discrimination. This reiterates a key point of chapter 4, that specificity and diversity describe interactions between the host and parasite. The antigenic diversity of a parasite has meaning only in the context of the specificity of host recognition.

Different kinds of immunological panels have been used. Monoclonal antibodies (MAbs) provide a high titer of identical antibodies. Each clone responds to variation in a small region of a parasite molecule. Different clones produce antibodies with different specificities. A panel of MAbs provides a highly specific and repeatable set of determinants.

Polyclonal antibody serum contains the diverse antibody specificities raised by a host against a particular challenge. The host may be challenged with a peptide, with a whole molecule, or with an entire parasite. Polyclonal sera from different hosts form a panel that can be used to test novel antigens. The response of each polyclonal serum aggregates reactions against many antigenic epitopes. Thus, polyclonal measures tend to be broader measures of total differences between antigens when compared with monoclonal measures, but it is harder to know exactly what differences the polyclonal technique measures.

T cell immunity has generally not been used to form an immune panel for discrimination of antigenic diversity. T cell recognition depends on the processing of peptides, their binding to MHC molecules, and the affinity of T cell receptors for peptide-MHC complexes. Until recently, it has been difficult to control these steps in a repeatable and measurable way. A new method, tetramer binding (Altman et al. 1996; Doherty and Christensen 2000), may allow some progress in this area. This method first creates peptide-MHC complexes, then measures the percentage of a host's T cells that bind those peptide-MHC complexes. A test of parasite variability could take the following form: challenge a host with a particular parasite type, then compare the host's T cell response against peptide-MHC complexes with peptides derived from different antigenic variants.

Immunological tests can be conducted with intact parasites, whole molecules, or molecular fragments such as peptides. Each choice has its benefits and limitations. Peptides provide small, controllable, and easily studied variants. However, antibodies normally respond to exposed, three-dimensional conformations rather than naked, sometimes linearized peptides. Whole molecules maintain three-dimensional structure and provide a broader aggregate measure of variation over the entire molecule. The shape of the molecule may, however, be altered when combined into a whole parasite, and many parts of the surface of the naked molecule may be inaccessible when in the intact parasite. Whole parasites provide the most realistic aggregate measure of differentiation. Assays may be technically difficult with the whole parasite, and results from such assays do not focus on specific variant epitopes (Nyambi et al. 2000a).

A completed immunological test fills the matrix of reaction strengths for each immunological agent and parasite isolate. The matrix can be used to classify the parasite isolates into related groups according to the degree of similarity in their immunological reactivity. The classification provides a basis to type new isolates according to immunological properties. The matrix may also be used to identify the major determinants of antigenic differences, which can be helpful in the design of vaccines against antigenically variable parasites.

11.2 Phylogeny

The amount of change between two antigens relative to a common ancestor provides another way to classify antigenic variants. One typically reconstructs the phylogenetic relationships of evolutionary descent by analyzing the patterns of change in the nucleotide or amino acid sequences that encode antigenic molecules (Page and Holmes 1998; Rodrigo and Learn 2000).

Allelic variants of a gene can usually be arranged into a phylogenetic pattern of evolutionary descent—a gene tree. That phylogeny by itself simply describes the lineal history of antigenic variants without regard to the processes that shaped the pattern of descent. The phylogenetic history provides a necessary context for interpreting evolutionary process (Hughes 1999).

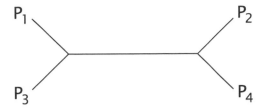

Figure 11.1 Hypothetical relationship of four parasite isolates based on immunological reactions. The clustering shows that the pair P_1 and P_3 reacts in a similar way to immunological agents, the pair P_2 and P_4 reacts in a similar way, and the two pairs differ in their patterns of reactivity.

11.3 Hypothetical Relations between Immunology and Phylogeny

Suppose that we have constructed an immunological classification of four parasite isolates, P_1, P_2, P_3, and P_4. The four parasites group into two clusters, shown in figure 11.1.

Figure 11.2 shows a phylogenetic classification with the same groupings as the immunological pattern in figure 11.1. If a phylogenetic analysis provides the same classification, then immunological distance increases with phylogenetic distance. The parasites may, for example, accumulate genetic differences randomly throughout their genomes. Parasites that diverged from a more distant common ancestor have more genetic differences both inside and outside the tested antigenic regions, with no concentration of differences in the antigenic sites. Alternatively, natural selection on the antigenic sites may be driving apart the clusters. Then both antigenic and nonantigenic sites provide the same phylogenetic pattern, clustering P_1/P_3 versus P_2/P_4, but the differences between the clusters would likely be concentrated disproportionately in the antigenic sites.

A correspondence generally occurs between phylogenetic distance and the differences measured on particular characters, reflecting the natural tendency for similarity by common descent. Sometimes a particular force disrupts this natural concordance.

Figure 11.3 shows a discordant pattern between phylogenetic and immunological distance. In this case, broad similarity over the nucleotide or amino acid sequence phylogenetically groups P_1 with P_2 and P_3 with P_4. The immunological test, which focuses on only a narrow subset

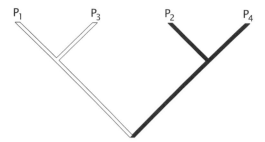

Figure 11.2   Hypothetical phylogenetic relationship of four parasite isolates based on nucleotide or amino acid sequences. The same clustering occurs as in fig. 11.1. The white lineages have the antigenic properties of the P_1/P_3 immunological grouping, and the black lineages have the antigenic properties of the P_2/P_4 immunological grouping shown in fig. 11.1.

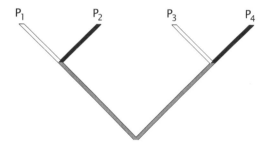

Figure 11.3   Alternative phylogenetic pattern that clusters P_1 with P_2 and P_3 with P_4. The white lineages share the P_1/P_3 immunological grouping and the black lineages share the P_2/P_4 immunological grouping shown in fig. 11.1. The gray lineages show that the immunological type for the ancestors of each phylogenetic group cannot be resolved.

of the total sequence, highlights antigenic divergence within closely related phylogenetic pairs. The pattern shows recurrent evolution of an antigenic type.

Many processes can generate the discordant pattern of figure 11.3. Suppose, for example, that only two variants can occur at a particular epitope because of conformational constraints on the function of the parasite molecule. If an epidemic begins with a parasite in state one, then host immunity will eventually favor the spread of state two. Conversely, an initial epidemic beginning with state two leads eventually to replacement by state one. Pairs of closely related lineages will often be of opposite state.

Functional hypotheses can often be tested by comparison of the predicted and observed phylogenetic patterns. For example, the functional constraint that an epitope can exist only in two alternative, antigenically distinct states predicts a discordant pattern between phylogenetic and immunological classifications. Alternatively, an observed discordance between phylogenetic and immunological classifications may lead to a functional or process-oriented hypothesis. That hypothesis can be tested by using other methods to infer function or process—for example, whether an observed epitope is indeed constrained to two alternative states by structural and functional attributes.

11.4 Immunology Matches Phylogeny over Long Genetic Distances

The flaviviruses illustrate broad correspondence between immunological and phylogenetic distances. This group includes well-known pathogens such as yellow fever, dengue fever, and West Nile virus. Kuno et al. (1998) built a phylogeny from the nucleotide sequences of seventy-two viral strains. These viruses span a diverse group, with nucleotide sequence identities of 69% or higher within the fourteen phylogenetic clades and lower percentages of identities between clades.

The flavivirus clades identified by molecular phylogeny correspond closely to the antigenic classification by Calisher et al. (1989) based on reactions to polyclonal antisera, although the two methods do disagree on the classification of a few strains. Two factors probably contribute to the close match between antigenic classification and molecular phylogeny. First, distinct clades have fairly large nucleotide sequence differences. Thus, both phylogenetic and antigenic groupings measure broad-scale divergence. Second, the antigenic analysis used polyclonal antisera, so that each test agent averaged broadly over many antigenic sites.

11.5 Immunology-Phylogeny Mismatch with Radiations into New Hosts

Influenza A isolates show a mixture of concordant and discordant relations between antigenic distance and phylogeny. Figure 11.4 illustrates the phylogenetic pattern for eleven isolates and an immunological matrix of reactivities to monoclonal antibodies (Brown et al. 1997). The phylogenetic analysis separated three clusters: classical swine types on

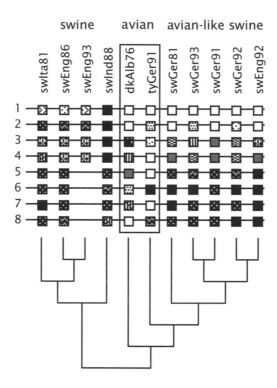

Figure 11.4 Phylogeny of influenza isolates based on nucleotide sequences from the HA1 region of the hemagglutinin (HA) gene. The isolates were obtained from swine (sw), turkey (ty), and duck (dk). The avian isolates were closer to the swine isolates on the right (avian-like swine) than to the swine isolates on the left when measured by nucleotide distances (data not shown). The matrix above the tree shows the intensity of reaction for each isolate to eight monoclonal antibodies. Darker patterns correspond to stronger reactions. All data from Brown et al. (1997).

the left, avian types in the middle, and avian-like isolates obtained from swine on the right.

The immunological reactivities divide the swine and avian-like swine into distinct clusters, matching the phylogenetic classification. The avian isolates are immunologically relatively distant from the other clusters and from each other, creating dissonance between phylogeny and antigenicity. It may be that the avian isolates have differentiated more strongly at the sites recognized by some of the monoclonal antibodies than they have when averaged over the entire sequenced region. It would be interesting to know more about the sites to which the different monoclonal antibodies bind. Perhaps some of those sites are influenced by selective pressures for attachment to host cells or for avoidance of host defense that differ between birds and pigs.

11.6 Short-Term Phylogenetic Diversification Driven by Immunological Selection

Influenza A variants with substitutions in the hemagglutinin molecule rise to high frequency in epidemics, causing a selective sweep through the influenza population. Isolates obtained in a particular year tend to trace their ancestry back to a common progenitor lineage just a few years into the past (Bush et al. 1999). Thus, the temporal sequence of the population is dominated by lineal replacements rather than bifurcating divergence.

Host antibodies mainly attack hemagglutinin. Immune selective pressure on hemagglutinin appears to drive the lineal replacements—put another way, immunological pressure drives change in the population-wide pattern of phylogenetic descent. Thus, the phylogenetic pattern of change may match the immunological pattern of change. Concordance probably depends on the percentage of amino acid substitutions explained by antibody pressure and the degree to which the antibody panel used for classification measures aggregate divergence.

11.7 Discordant Patterns of Phylogeny and Antigenicity Created by Within-Host Immune Pressure

Nucleotide sequences of the HIV-1 envelope divide this virus into eleven lineages within the M (major) group, into an O (outlier) group, and into an N (new) group (Robertson et al. 1999; http://hiv-web.lanl.gov/). The phylogenetic distance between isolates does not predict well the strength of shared immunological response (Vogel et al. 1994; Nyambi et al. 1996, 2000b; Weber et al. 1996; Zolla-Pazner et al. 1999).

Vaccines must stimulate an immune response against most viral genotypes in order to provide sufficient protection. A candidate vaccine might, for example, include isolates from each of the common phylogenetic lineages. This provides good coverage of diverse pathogens when antigenicity corresponds to phylogeny. However, phylogeny does not predict antigenicity for HIV. In order to choose HIV variants for a vaccine, one needs to divide viral diversity into antigenic types that together cover most of the antigenic range.

A few studies have developed antigenic classifications for HIV-1 (Vogel et al. 1994; Nyambi et al. 1996; Zolla-Pazner et al. 1999). Nyambi et al. (2000b) analyzed binding by twenty-eight monoclonal antibodies to twenty-six intact viral particles. The viral genotypes were sampled among eight different clades of the M group.

Nyambi et al. (2000b) grouped viral isolates according to their similarity in binding to the antibodies. Such grouping defines antigenic similarities of epitopes between the viral samples. The twenty-six viral isolates formed three immunological clusters. The immunotypes did not correspond to phylogenetic lineages (genotypes), geographic origin, or tropism for different host-cell receptors (CXCR4 versus CCR5). Thus, diverse genotypes share common epitopes, and similar genotypes can be differentiated by antibody binding, causing a mismatch between phylogeny and antigenicity. Nyambi et al. (2000a) emphasized that many antibodies that bind do not neutralize. Further studies must determine if the observed antibody binding can influence viral fitness in vivo.

Joint studies of phylogeny and antigenicity in HIV call attention to stabilizing, convergent, and diversifying natural selection.

First, shared antigenicity over long phylogenetic distances may be caused by stabilizing selection. Under stabilizing selection, a mutation that changes an epitope has opposing effects. The mutation allows escape from immune recognition but also reduces some functional aspect of the epitope. External viral epitopes sometimes affect binding or entry to host cells. Strong stabilizing selection of epitopes leads to conservation of amino acid composition over all phylogenetic scales of divergence.

In some cases, stabilizing selection may allow certain amino acid replacements that preserve geometric structure and charge. For example, Nyambi et al. (2000a) argue that parts of the genetically variable V3 loop of the HIV envelope have highly conserved structure and antigenicity. Binding affinity to monoclonal antibodies may be a better measure of antigenic conservation than amino acid sequence.

Second, shared antigenicity over long phylogenetic distances may be caused by convergent selection. Suppose a small set of alternative structures for a parasite epitope retain similar function. This functional set constrains the range of acceptable escape mutants. Immune pressure

favors change of epitopes within the acceptable set, eventually return-
ing to the original epitope. Phylogenetic pattern will reveal short-term
changes and occasional long-term similarity. T cell pressure based on
MHC binding may be particularly likely to create such patterns. A parasite that can escape from a particular host's MHC array will be favored.
The next host will likely have a different MHC pattern, perhaps favoring a return to the epitopes lost in the previous host. Testing for this
pattern requires detailed data over different temporal scales.

   Nyambi et al. (2000b) found that the tip of the V3 loop was conserved
antigenically between genotypes, whereas other parts of the V3 loop separated isolates into different antigenic groups. The genetic variants of
the V3 loop may fall into relatively few conformational, antigenic types.
The range of types may be constrained by stabilizing selection, causing short-term phylogenetic fluctuations between types but occasional
convergence to past types within phylogenetic lines of descent.

   Third, distinct antigenicity between phylogenetically close isolates
implies very rapid diversifying selection. Escape mutants within hosts
follow this pattern. For example, Nyambi et al. (1997) studied the temporal pattern of escape mutants and antibody profiles over the course
of a single infection of a chimpanzee by simian immunodeficiency virus
(SIV), a near relative of HIV. They analyzed eleven consecutive serum
(antibody) samples and eight SIV isolates taken at about four-month intervals over a total of forty-one months. They tested the eighty-eight
pairwise reactions between serum antibodies and viral isolates. The
data showed viral escape mutants emerging at intervals of about fifteen
months, each escape followed approximately eight months later by new
antibody responses that matched the escape variants. Several studies of
HIV escape mutants have been published (see references in Beaumont
et al. 2001).

   Combinations of diversifying, stabilizing, and convergent selection
may determine the relationship between HIV phylogeny and antigenicity (Holmes et al. 1992). Diversifying selection within hosts favors escape variants that avoid antibodies or T cells. Diversifying selection
between hosts favors mutants that avoid MHC recognition or immunological memory. Stabilizing selection constrains the range of variants.
Convergent selection causes recurrence of previous antigenic types in
response to diversifying selection and the stabilizing constraints that
limit the range of alternative forms. Together, these factors group HIV

isolates into a limited number of immunological types. The immunological classification does not match the phylogenetic classification.

Holmes et al. (1992) observed both diversifying and convergent selection within a single host infected by HIV. They sequenced the V3 loop of the viral envelope from eighty-nine isolates collected over a seven-year period. The isolates evolved over time through a series of replacements, with different sequences dominating in frequency at different times. Two divergent lineages formed about three years after infection. Most subsequent isolates mapped to one of these two major lineages. The same sequence of 6 amino acids at the tip of the V3 loop evolved convergently in the two lineages.

In summary, phylogeny provides the historical context in which to interpret immunological patterns. Hypotheses about natural selection can be tested by mapping the sequence of immunological changes onto the lineal history of descent.

11.8 Problems for Future Research

1. Adaptation to different hosts. Relations between antigenicity and phylogeny suggest hypotheses about how natural selection shapes antigenic variation. Consider, for example, the data for influenza A in pigs and birds (fig. 11.4). Antigenicity groups isolates according to current host species, whereas phylogeny groups isolates according to the history of transfers between species.

Adaptation to different hosts may shape antigenicity. This could occur by adaptation of viral surfaces to host receptors associated with attachment. Or the nature of immune pressure might differ significantly between birds and pigs. Such hypotheses, suggested by statistical patterns of association between phylogeny and antigenicity, must be tested by molecular studies.

2. Optimal sampling for evolutionary inference. Most antigenic and phylogenetic data were collected for reasons other than analyzing relations between antigenic and phylogenetic classifications. Little thought has been given to the sampling schemes that maximize information about evolutionary process. Ideal studies require analysis of the interactions between evolutionary process, methods of measurement, and statistical inference.

Different sampling schemes may be needed to study different kinds of natural selection. For example, stabilizing selection impedes change. To detect relatively slow antigenic change, one should probably sample over relatively long phylogenetic distances. The average divergence of genomes over long distances sets a standard against which one can detect reduced antigenic change at sites constrained by stabilizing selection.

By contrast, diversifying selection accelerates change by favoring antigenic types that differ from the currently prevalent forms. To detect relatively rapid change, one should probably sample over relatively short phylogenetic distances. This sets a low level of background change against which rapid, diversifying change can be detected.

3. Antigenic selection may shape phylogeny. The degree of match or discord between antigenic and phylogenetic classifications may depend on the demographic consequences of selection. If selection on a few closely linked epitopes determines the success or failure of a parasite lineage, then phylogeny may follow antigenicity. By contrast, selection may strongly influence patterns of antigenic change without absolutely determining success or failure of lineages. In this case, antigenicity does not constrain phylogeny.

Mathematical models would clarify the various relations that may arise between antigenic and phylogenetic classifications. Those relations depend on the time scales of differentiation, the epitopes used for antigenic classification, and the antibodies used to discriminate between variant epitopes.

12 Experimental Evolution: Foot-and-Mouth Disease Virus

Experimental evolution manipulates the environment of a population and observes the resulting pattern of evolutionary change. This allows one to study the selective forces that shape antigenic diversity. For example, one could manipulate immune selection by exposing parasites to different regimes of monoclonal antibodies. The parasites' evolutionary response reveals the adaptive potential and the constraints that shape patterns of antigenic variation.

In this chapter, I describe experimental evolution studies of foot-and-mouth disease virus (FMDV). I also use this virus as a case study to show how different methods combine to provide a deeper understanding of antigenic variation. These approaches include structural analysis of the virion, functional analysis of epitopes with regard to binding cellular receptors, sequence analysis of natural isolates, and experimental analysis of evolving populations.

The first section introduces the antigenicity and structure of FMDV. Structural studies provide the three-dimensional location of amino acids. This allows one to analyze how particular amino acid substitutions affect shape, charge, and interaction with antibodies. Structural information also aids functional analysis of substitutions with regard to binding cellular receptors or affecting other components of viral fitness.

The second section describes antibody escape mutants of FMDV. Most of these escape mutants were generated by application of monoclonal antibodies in controlled experimental studies. Several laboratory escape mutants occur in an exposed loop on the surface of the virion, which is also the site of a key antigenic region identified by sequencing natural isolates. This antigenic loop mediates binding to cellular receptors, an essential step for viral entry into host cells. The pattern of antibody escape mutants identifies varying and unvarying amino acid sites. The unvarying sites play an essential role in binding to host cells.

The third section continues discussion of binding to host cells and tropism for different host receptors. Experimental evolution studies show that in cell culture FMDV can evolve to use alternate cellular receptors.

This switch in receptor tropism relieves the constraint on the previously unvarying amino acid sites in the key antigenic region. Consequently, escape mutants in that conserved region arise readily, demonstrating that the conserved sites play an important role in recognition by antibodies. This highlights the dual selective pressures by antibodies and receptor binding that may shape key antigenic sites.

The fourth section describes an experimental approach to analyze the fitness consequences of amino acid substitutions. Molecular studies can measure changes in binding affinity for antibodies and cellular receptors associated with changes in amino acid shape and charge. But substitutions ultimately spread or fail based on their consequences for the dynamics of growth and transmission. These aspects of fitness can be difficult to measure. I describe one study in which pigs were injected with a wild-type virus and various antibody escape mutants. The relative success of parental and mutant viruses provides clues about how particular amino acid substitutions may influence evolutionary dynamics.

The final section lists problems for future research.

General discussions and examples of experimental evolution can be found in Rose (1991), Bennett and Lenski (1999), Landweber (1999), Crill et al. (2000), and Stearns et al. (2000).

12.1 Overview of Antigenicity and Structure

FMDV is an RNA virus that frequently causes disease in domesticated cattle, swine, sheep, and goats (Sobrino et al. 2001). FMDV belongs to the *Picornaviridae* family of viruses, which includes poliovirus, human hepatitis A virus, and the human rhinoviruses (Racaniello 2001). FMDV populations maintain antigenic diversity in several rapidly evolving epitopes (Mateu et al. 1988; Feigelstock et al. 1996).

Seven major serotypes occur across the world (Sobrino et al. 2001). Phylogenetic distance between serotypes correlates reasonably well with antigenic distance measured by cross-reactivity to polyclonal antisera—in other words, phylogeny roughly matches serology at a broad scale of sequence divergence (Mateu 1995). By contrast, small-scale phylogenetic divergence does not correspond to patterns of antigenicity. One or a few amino acid substitutions within a serotype can greatly alter antibody recognition (Mateu et al. 1994).

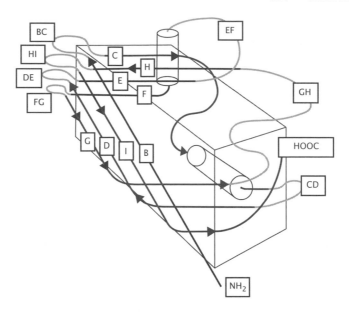

Figure 12.1   Schematic diagram of the foot-and-mouth disease virus surface proteins. Each of the three main surface proteins, VP1, VP2, and VP3, fills a trapezoidal space with eight β chains (arrows) labeled B-I and two α chains (cylinders). The loops connecting the β chains tend to be exposed on the protein surface, sometimes protruding from the protein core. The two-letter codes for the loops name the connected β chains. The carboxyl (HOOC) and amino (NH$_2$) termini may also occur at the surface. Antibodies apparently interact mainly with the loops and termini. The three proteins differ in the location and exposure of various loops, as indicated in fig. 12.2. Redrawn from Haydon and Woolhouse (1998) based on original work in Harrison (1989, with permission from *Nature,* www.nature.com).

Figure 12.1 illustrates the structure of the surface proteins of FMDV. Figure 12.2 shows how the three types of surface proteins combine to form the FMDV capsid. The most widely immunodominant epitopes occur on the GH loop of the VP1 surface protein (see fig. 12.3; Mateu et al. 1994; Mateu 1995; Sobrino et al. 2001). This loop has about 20 amino acids that contribute to several overlapping epitopes. These antibody binding sites appear to be determined mostly by the amino acids in the GH peptide (a continuous epitope). Antibodies that bind to an isolated GH peptide also neutralize intact viruses.

Many antibody escape variants occur in the GH loop, leading to extensive genetic variation in this region. However, a conserved amino acid triplet, Arg-Gly-Asp (RGD), also binds to antibodies. This conserved

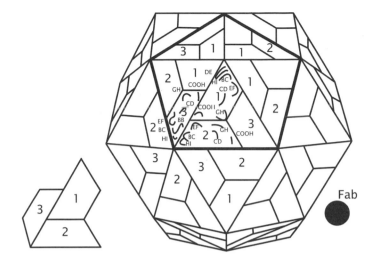

Figure 12.2   Structure of the foot-and-mouth disease virus. There are three surface proteins, VP1, VP2, and VP3, labeled 1–3, respectively. Each protein presents an approximately trapezoidal shape on the surface. The three different proteins group into a structural unit as shown in the lower left. On the capsid, the boldly lined pentagon contains five structural units arrayed in five-fold rotational symmetry about the pentagonal center. Each pentagonal vertex defines the intersection of six structural units aligned in threefold rotational symmetry. The wiggly lines labeled on one unit of the capsid show the location of structural loops that occur on the capsid surface (see fig. 12.3). Those loops are candidates for antibody binding. The black circle at the lower right shows the approximate relative size of an antibody-binding region (Fab), illustrating the potential coverage of capsid protein loops that may be involved in immune recognition. Redrawn from Mateu (1995, with permission from Elsevier Science) based on original work in Harrison (1989, with permission from *Nature*, www.nature.com).

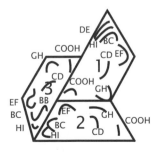

Figure 12.3   An enlarged view of the β loops and carboxyl termini shown in fig. 12.2.

triplet mediates binding to integrin host-cell receptors typically used in FMDV attachment and entry (Berinstein et al. 1995; Neff et al. 1998; Sobrino et al. 2001).

The GH loop of VP1 contains continuous epitopes that together define the hypervariable antigenic site A common to all serotypes. Discontinuous epitopes occur when amino acid residues from widely separated sequence locations come together conformationally to form a binding surface for antibodies. Two antigenic sites of serotypes A, O, and C have discontinuous epitopes that have received widespread attention (Mateu et al. 1994; Feigelstock et al. 1996).

The first discontinuous site occurs near the capsid's threefold axes of symmetry at the vertices of the pentagonal structural units (fig. 12.2). This site includes the BC loop of VP2 and the BB knob of VP3 in serotypes A, C, and O (fig. 12.3). In serotype C, the carboxyl terminus of VP1 also contributes to this site, and in serotype O, the EF loop of VP2 is sometimes involved. This region (antigenic site D) forms the second major immunodominant region of serotype C after antigenic site A in the GH loop of VP1 (Feigelstock et al. 1996).

A second discontinuous epitope occurs in serotype O. The GH loop and the carboxy-terminal (COOH) end of VP1 jointly form the binding region for some antibodies. However, in serotype C, the GH loop and the carboxy-terminal end of VP1 form independent, continuous epitopes. The high specificity of antibodies means that the sequence and conformational differences between serotypes change the detailed antigenic properties of particular regions. Studies focused on natural selection of particular amino acid residues must account for background differences of sequence and conformation among test strains.

12.2 Antibody Escape Mutants

Many antibody escape mutants have been sequenced (references in Martínez et al. 1997). One can develop a map of natural escape variants by comparing changes in sequence with differences in binding affinity to a panel of MAbs.

Two problems of interpreting selective pressures arise from an escape map based on natural variants. First, field isolates do not control the multitude of evolutionary pressures on variation. Mutants may spread either in direct response to antibody pressure, in response to other selective pressures, or by stochastic fluctuations independent of selective forces. Lack of variability may result either from lack of antibody pressure or from constraining selective pressures such as binding to host receptors.

The second problem for interpreting selective pressures from natural isolates concerns lack of control over genetic background. Whether a particular amino acid site affects antibody affinity may depend on conformation-changing variants at other sites.

Site-directed mutagenesis controls amino acid replacements in a fixed genetic background. One can alter sites that do not vary naturally to test for effects on antibody binding. Site-directed mutagenesis has provided useful information for FMDV (Mateu et al. 1998). But this method can only define changes in antibody binding; it does not show how viral populations actually respond to immune pressure.

Several studies have applied monoclonal or polyclonal antibodies to FMDV in laboratory culture (Mateu 1995; Sobrino et al. 2001). This allows direct control of selective pressure by comparing lines with and without exposure to antibodies. In addition, cultures can be started with genetically monomorphic viruses to control genetic background.

Martínez et al. (1997) began laboratory evolution studies from a single viral clone of serotype C. These viruses were grown on baby hamster kidney cells (BHK-21). All host cells were derived from a single precursor cell. Two separate viral lines were established. C-S8c1 developed through three successive plaque isolations. C-S8c1p100 began with C-S8c1 and developed through one hundred serial passages on a monolayer of BHK-21 cells. The host cells were refreshed from independent stock in each passage and therefore did not coevolve with the virus over the passage history.

In natural isolates, extensive sequence variability in the GH loop of VP1 correlates with escape from antibody neutralization. However, the Arg-Gly-Asp (RGD) sequence near the center of this GH loop is invariant in field isolates (Sobrino et al. 2001). Controlled studies of laboratory evolution provide some insight into the evolution of this region.

The monoclonal antibody SD6 binds to an epitope spanning residues 136–147 in the GH loop of VP1. Martínez et al. (1997) applied selective pressure by SD6 after establishment of the separate viral lines C-S8c1 and C-S8c1p100 by growing a cloned (genetically monomorphic) isolate

Table 12.1 Escape mutants of FMDV (from Martínez et al. 1997)

Amino acid substitution	Mutants of C-S8c1	Mutants of C-S8c1p100
Ala-138 → Pro	1	0
Ala-138 → Asp	3	1
Ser-139 → Arg	20	0
Ser-139 → Gly	2	0
Ser-139 → Asn	8	2
Ser-139 → Ile	17	8
Gly-142 → Glu	0	4
Asp-143 → Gly	0	1
Leu-144 → Val	0	5
Leu-144 → Ser	0	8
Ala-145 → Val	0	2
His-146 → Arg	31	0

in the presence of the antibody and sampling escape mutants. Nucleotide sequences of escape mutants were obtained. Each mutant (except one) escaped antibody neutralization by a single amino acid change.

Table 12.1 lists the changed amino acids in the escape mutants, excluding the one double mutant. The different locations of these mutations in the original (C-S8c1) line compared with the serially passaged (C-S8c1p100) line provide the most striking result of this study. The original line conserved the Arg-Gly-Asp (RGD) motif at positions 141–143. By contrast, the serially passaged line had numerous mutations within the RGD motif. Figure 12.4 contrasts the location of mutants for the two lines.

Variants in the RGD motif had not previously been observed in spite of neutralizing antibodies' affinity for this region. The RGD motif was thought to be invariant because of its essential role in binding to the host cell. Yet the serially passaged line accumulated variants in this region. Those variants replicated with the same kinetics as the parental viruses of C-S8c1p100, with no loss in fitness. Baranowski et al. (2000) showed that lineages with an altered RGD motif use an alternative pathway of attachment and entry to host cells.

Martínez et al. (1997) sequenced the capsid genes from the original line, from the serially passaged line, and from an escape mutant of the serially passaged line. The escape mutant from the serially passaged line differed from the parental virus of this line only at a single site in the

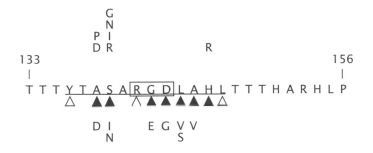

Figure 12.4   Amino acid sequence in the central region of the VP1 GH loop of foot-and-mouth disease virus. The start and stop numbers label amino acid positions. The box shows the RGD motif at positions 141–143. The monoclonal antibody SD6 recognizes the continuous epitope defined by the underlined positions. Black triangles show positions at which most replacement amino acids greatly reduce binding by SD6; in other words, a single replacement at any of these sites creates an escape mutant. The white triangles denote positions that can tolerate certain amino acid replacements without greatly affecting antibody binding.   Unmarked positions in the epitope can vary without much change in binding.   The letters above the sequence summarize the escape mutants of C-S8c1 (original line); letters below the sequence summarize escape mutants of C-S8c1p100 (passaged line).   Letters denote amino acids according to the standard single-letter code.   Table 12.1 shows the full distribution of escape mutants.   Redrawn from Martínez et al. (1997, copyright National Academy of Sciences, U.S.A.).

Table 12.2   Capsid amino acids that differ between C-S8c1 and C-S8c1p100 (from Martínez et al. 1997)

Secondary structure*	Position	Amino acid substitution
VP1 βB strand	41	Lys → Glu
VP1 BC loop	46	Asp → Glu
VP1 C terminus	197	His → Arg
VP3 N terminus	25	Ala → Val
VP3 GH loop	173	Glu → Lys
VP3 C terminus	218	Gln → Lys

*Secondary structure descriptions in Mateu et al. (1994). See figs. 12.2–12.4.

RGD region.   Tolerance to replacements in the RGD region must follow from the differences accumulated by C-S8c1p100 during serial passage. Table 12.2 shows the 6 amino acids that differed between the original and serially passaged lines. Apparently those substitutions changed cell

tropism properties of the virus and allowed variation in the previously
invariant RGD motif.

12.3 Cell Binding and Tropism

Attachment and entry to host cells impose strong natural selection
on some regions of the viral surface. Experimental evolution provides
one approach to analyzing those selective forces, as described in the
previous section. In this section, I briefly summarize further studies
of amino acid variation in the FMDV capsid and the consequences for
attachment and entry to host cells.

Natural isolates of FMDV use cellular integrin receptors for some of
the steps in attachment and entry (Berinstein et al. 1995; Jackson, Sheppard, et al. 2000). Integrins are transmembrane glycoproteins composed
of two different subunits, α and β. Various integrins mediate adhesion
between cells, attachment of cells to the extracellular matrix, and signal
transduction of pathways that affect cell proliferation, morphology, migration, and apoptosis (Springer 1990; Hynes 1992; Montgomery et al.
1994).

The integrin receptors rely on an RGD amino acid sequence of ligands
in order to bind host proteins such as fibronectin, fibrinogen, and type I
collagen (Fox et al. 1989). All field isolates of FMDV have the conserved
RGD motif needed for interaction with the integrin receptors (Berinstein
et al. 1995; Jackson, Sheppard, et al. 2000).

FMDV can evolve changes in receptor usage, as shown by the experimental evolution studies of Martínez et al. (1997) described above. In
their study, certain FMDV lineages mutated in the RGD motif and lost
the ability to use integrin receptors. The altered viruses had a high affinity for heparan sulfate (HS) (Jackson et al. 1996; Sa-Carvalho et al. 1997),
a common carbohydrate component of surface proteoglycans found on
many types of host cells (Salmivirta et al. 1996; Fry et al. 1999; Sasisekharan and Venkataraman 2000).

An affinity for HS has been reported for several viruses, including HIV-
1, human cytomegalovirus, dengue virus, Sindbis virus, vaccinia virus,
and adeno-associated virus type 2 (Schneider-Schaulies 2000). HS may
also play a role in bacterial adhesion (Rostand and Esko 1997; Hackstadt
1999). Some of these cases of increased affinity for HS may be caused by

adaptation of the pathogens to cell culture, as occurred in FMDV, Sindbis virus, and classical swine fever virus (Klimstra et al. 1998; Bernard et al. 2000; Hulst et al. 2000).

These various studies call attention to the complementary processes of attachment and entry (Haywood 1994). In some cases, viruses may first attach to host cells based on the kinetics of binding between viral and host attachment sites. Once viruses bind to host attachment sites, a second-phase kinetic process determines binding between viral and host receptors that initiate viral entry into host cells. For example, FMDV in cell culture may first bind to HS, a widespread component of the host cell surface. The viruses, attracted near the cell surface, may then encounter and bind to the relatively sparser host integrin receptors.

Viral kinetics may be modulated separately for preliminary attachment and secondary binding to the port of entry. Structural and kinetic studies of FMDV variants provide some clues about how modulation of attachment and binding may occur.

FMDV type O adaptation to cell culture favors a histidine to arginine substitution at position 56 of the surface protein VP3 (Fry et al. 1999). This amino acid change increases the positive charge of the viral surface at this site and strongly enhances binding to negatively charged HS. Structural studies show that HS binds near the point of contact between the three surface proteins, VP1, VP2, and VP3 (figs. 12.2 and 12.3), including contact with codon 56 of VP3 on the βB strand (fig. 12.1).

Serotype A_{12} does not acquire HS binding in cell culture, instead modifying amino acids near the RGD sequence that presumably allow tighter binding to integrin (Reider et al. 1994; Neff et al. 1998). Not surprisingly, genetic background affects the binding consequences of amino acid substitutions and the evolutionary changes that occur in different strains.

HS provides a relatively low-affinity receptor at high density on the surface of many cell types. FMDV variants with increased attraction to HS may interact with host cells in two different ways. First, viruses may enter host cells directly from attachment to HS without binding and entering through a second host receptor (Neff et al. 1998; Baranowski et al. 2000). Second, low-affinity and high-density HS may serve as an attractant that brings viruses into proximity of high-affinity and low-density integrins (Jackson et al. 1996; Fry et al. 1999; Baranowski et al. 2000).

Various host adhesion molecules such as vitronectin and fibronectin have affinity for both HS and integrin (Potts and Campbell 1994). HS and integrin are sufficiently close on the host cell surface to interact simultaneously with viral binding sites for HS and integrin (Fry et al. 1999). Studies of other pathogens have inferred a two-step process with low-affinity receptors serving as the first site of adsorption (reviewed in Jackson et al. 1996; Schneider-Schaulies 2000).

HS-binding variants of FMDV derived from cell culture cannot develop virulent infections in vivo (Sa-Carvalho et al. 1997; Neff et al. 1998). Similarly, equine encephalitis virus adapted for cell culture gained enhanced HS binding and subsequently produced relatively weak, rapidly cleared infections in mice when compared with the wild type (Bernard et al. 2000). HS-binding variants of Sindbis virus are also cleared rapidly from hosts (Byrnes and Griffin 2000). HS-binding variants of FMDV with arginine at codon 56 of VP3 reverted to histidine or cysteine in experimental in vivo infections, demonstrating strong selection and rapid evolution of reduced HS affinity (Sa-Carvalho et al. 1997).

Strong binding to HS impedes the spread of infection between host cells. Viral particles may adhere too strongly to cells that cannot be infected, or the rate of clearance may be raised by exposure on tissue surfaces. Fry et al. (1999) speculated that HS-binding variation provides different kinetics of infection and clearance in various tissues and also quantitative modulation of virulence. Thus, pathogens may adapt within the host to different tissues by altering HS affinity. In addition, reduced virulence may sometimes be favored when associated with enhanced persistence of infection, perhaps by sequestering viruses at low abundance in certain tissues. Surface stickiness may therefore influence several aspects of pathogen kinetics within the host and the consequences of infection on host morbidity and mortality.

No evidence presently suggests that HS binding plays an important role in natural isolates of FMDV. Rather, these analyses should be interpreted as a model for studying how particular amino acid substitutions can profoundly alter kinetics and cellular tropisms. In each case, the benefits for increased rates of entry to host cells balance against the costs of reduced spread and faster clearance from certain host compartments. Combined studies of experimental evolution in vitro and in vivo provide a useful tool for studying how selective forces shape parasite characters via particular amino acid substitutions.

Comparisons of HS versus integrin binding form a contrast between two very different types of host receptors interacting with two distinct regions of the FMDV capsid. Recent studies have turned to more subtle variations between FMDV isolates with regard to binding different integrin receptors.

Jackson, Blakemore, et al. (2000) compared the affinity of different viral genotypes for two integrin receptors, $\alpha_v\beta_3$ and $\alpha_5\beta_1$. The standard RGD motif was required for both receptors. The following amino acid at the RGD+1 position influenced relative affinity for the two integrin types. For $\alpha_v\beta_3$, several different amino acids at RGD+1 allowed binding, consistent with this receptor's multifunctional role in binding several ligands. By contrast, $\alpha_5\beta_1$ has narrower specificity, favoring a leucine at RGD+1.

Jackson, Blakemore, et al. (2000) compared two viruses that differed only at RGD+1, the first with an arginine and the second with a leucine. The first virus had relatively higher affinity for $\alpha_v\beta_3$ compared with $\alpha_5\beta_1$. By contrast, the second virus had relatively higher affinity for $\alpha_5\beta_1$ compared with $\alpha_v\beta_3$. For at least some antibodies that recognize RGDL, loss of leucine at RGD+1 abolishes recognition (see fig. 12.4; Martínez et al. 1997).

Thirty type O and eight type A field isolates had leucine at RGD+1. By contrast, five SAT-2 isolates had arginine, two Asia-1 isolates had methionine, and one Asia-1 isolate had leucine (Jackson, Blakemore, et al. 2000). These and other data suggest that most serotypes have leucine at RGD+1 and perhaps a higher affinity for $\alpha_5\beta_1$. SAT-2 may either have greater affinity for $\alpha_v\beta_3$ or its binding may be conditioned by amino acid variants at other sites.

In another study, Jackson, Sheppard, et al. (2000) analyzed FMDV binding to a different integrin, $\alpha_v\beta_6$. This integrin binds relatively few host ligands and depends on an RGDLXXL motif with leucines at RGD+1 and RGD+4. Most FMDV isolates have leucines at those two positions. $\alpha_v\beta_3$ does not have stringent requirements at those sites, suggesting that $\alpha_v\beta_6$ may be an important natural receptor.

Overall, RGDLXXL binds to the widest array of integrins, at least over those studied so far, although relative affinities for different integrins may be modulated by substitutions at RGD+1 and perhaps other sites. It would be interesting to sample isolates from various host tissues that differ in the densities of the various integrin receptors and analyze whether any substitutions appear relative to isolates in other body compartments of the same host.

Viral success in different cell types or in different hosts may depend on variations in nonstructural genes that do not mediate binding and entry to host cells. For example, Núñez et al. (2001) serially passaged FMDV in guinea pigs. FMDV does not normally cause lesions in guinea pigs, but after serial passage, viral variants arose that caused disease. Among the several amino acid substitutions that arose during passage, a single change from glutamine to arginine at position 44 of gene 3A provided virulence. The function of 3A in FMDV is not known. In poliovirus, a distantly related picornavirus, 3A plays a role in virus-specific RNA synthesis.

These studies show the potential power of experimental evolution in studying evolutionary forces, particularly when combined with analysis of naturally occurring variation.

12.4 Fitness Consequences of Substitutions

Antibody escape mutants are typically isolated in one of two ways. First, pathogens may be grown in vitro with antibodies. This creates selective pressure for substitutions that escape antibody recognition. Second, naturally occurring variants from field isolates may be tested against a panel of antibodies. Certain sets of antibodies may bind most isolates, allowing identification of those variants that differ at commonly recognized epitopes.

Escape variants gain a fitness advantage by avoiding antibody recognition targeted to important epitopes. However, those pathogen epitopes may also play a role in binding to host cells, in release from infected cells, or in some other aspect of the pathogen's life cycle. Functional and structural studies of amino acid substitutions provide one method of analysis. That approach has the advantage of directly assessing the mechanisms by which amino acid variants affect multiple components of parasite fitness, such as escape from antibody recognition and altered host attachment characteristics.

Although functional and structural approaches can directly measure binding differences caused by amino acid substitutions in different genetic backgrounds, they cannot provide a good measure of all the fitness consequences associated with changes in genotype.

Carrillo et al. (1998) used an alternative approach to analyze the consequences of amino acid substitutions. They studied the relative fitnesses in vivo of a parental FMDV genotype and three mutant genotypes derived from the parental type. They measured relative fitness by competing pairs of strains within live pigs.

The parental type, C-S8c1, came from a C serotype isolated from a pig. The first monoclonal antibody–resistant mutant, MARM21, arose in a pig infected with C-S8c1. MARM21 differs from C-S8c1 by a single change from serine to arginine at VP1 139 (fig. 12.4), providing escape from the monoclonal antibody SD6.

The second mutant, S-3T$_1$, came from a blood sample of a pig one day after experimental inoculation with C-S8c1. That isolate had a single change from threonine to alanine at VP1 135 (fig. 12.4). Only one of fifty-eight monoclonal antibodies differentiated between the parental type and S-3T$_1$, and the difference in affinity was small. This supports the claim in figure 12.4 that position 135 is not strongly antigenic.

The third mutant, C-S15c1, derived from a field variant of type C1 isolated from a pig. This mutant type had eight amino acid differences in VP1 compared with C-S8c1. C-S15c1 did not react with monoclonal antibody SD6.

One of the three mutants was coinoculated with the parental type into each experimental pig. Two replicate pigs were used for each of the three pairs of mutant and parental types. Fever rose one day after infection and peaked two or three days postinfection. All animals developed vesicular lesions two to four days postinfection. For each animal, between two and seven samples were taken from lesions, and the relative proportions of the competing viruses were assayed by reactivity to monoclonal antibodies.

The small sample sizes do not allow strong conclusions to be drawn. Rather, the following two results hint at what might be learned from more extensive studies of this sort. First, the parental type strongly dominated MARM21 in all seven lesions sampled from the two experimental animals, comprising between 80 and 94% of the viruses in each lesion. The MARM21 mutation appears to confer lower fitness in vivo, at least in the two animals tested. The lower fitness may arise because the mutant was cleared more effectively by antibodies, bound less efficiently to host cells, or had reduced performance in some other fitness component.

Second, S-3T$_1$ abundance relative to the parental type varied strongly between lesions. In the two lesions analyzed from one animal, the parental type comprised 67 ± 3.4 and $3.2 \pm 1.5\%$ (mean $\pm$ standard deviation). In the other animal, the three lesions analyzed had parental-type percentages of 75 ± 4.1, 25 ± 2.8, and 5.9 ± 1.2. Differences in dominance between lesions also occurred between C-S15c1 and the parental type. Variations in dominance may arise from stochastic sampling of viruses that form lesions, from differences in tissue tropism, or from some other cause.

Further studies of this sort may provide a more refined understanding of the multiple fitness consequences that follow from particular amino acid changes, their interactions with the genetic background of the virus, the role of different host genotypes, and the effect of prior exposure of hosts to different antigenic variants.

12.5 Problems for Future Research

1. Escape versus performance. Both antibodies and cellular binding impose strong natural selection on the GH loop of VP1. This leads to a general question: How much does immune pressure impede natural selection of functional performance?

Experimental evolution may provide some insight into this problem. Consider two experimental lineages, one passaged in immunodeficient hosts and the other passaged in immunocompetent hosts. If immune pressure constrains functional performance by improved cellular binding, then the immunodeficient line should respond with amino acid substitutions that improve binding function.

In this context, improved binding function means increased viral fitness rather than increased affinity of the virus for the host receptor. Changes in fitness can be measured by competing the original genotype against the genotype created by selection in immunodeficient hosts. It would be interesting to study how amino acid substitutions affect the kinetics of cellular binding and reproduction and how those kinetics arise from structural changes in shape and charge. One could also compete these same genotypes in the immunocompetent line to study how amino acid substitutions change response to antibodies.

2. Components of fitness. Serial passage experiments impose a complex set of selective pressures on different components of pathogen fitness. For example, collecting pathogens from hosts early after infection favors very rapid reproduction within the host, perhaps at the expense of survival over the entire course of infection. By contrast, collecting pathogens late after infection favors survival within the host rather than rapid growth.

In a naive host without prior exposure to the pathogen, early sampling may pick pathogens before strong antibody pressure develops. This may favor amino acid substitutions that promote improved cellular binding over avoidance of immune pressure. By contrast, late sampling may favor more strongly avoidance of antibody pressure. Early and late sampling in both immunocompetent and immunodeficient hosts would allow comparison of amino acid substitutions under varying selective pressures.

One could also examine evolutionary response in experiments to test the idea that heparan sulfate binding modulates the pathogen's stickiness to different tissues and consequently the dynamics of growth and clearance.

3. Adaptation to new hosts. The passage experiments in guinea pigs showed that small changes in FMDV genotype allow virulent infections to develop in novel hosts. Host adaptation forms the central problem in the study of emerging diseases. Experimental evolution provides a useful tool to identify the amino acid changes required to infect new hosts, to cause virulent infections in those hosts, to transmit between the new hosts, and to transmit back to the original host.

4. Genetic background. Pathogen genotypes that differ by many amino acids can have significantly altered protein shape and charge. It can be difficult to assess how those structural differences affect selection on particular amino acid sites. Experimental evolution studies could analyze a replicated design in which initial pathogen genotypes vary. This approach can identify how genetic background alters selective pressure at particular sites.

Different genotypes may be chosen from natural isolates to study the forces that shape particular variants in the field. Or special genotypes may be constructed to test hypotheses about how structure affects the fitness of amino acid substitutions at particular sites.

5. Experimental evolution of other pathogens. Most experimental evolution studies of pathogens have been conducted on RNA viruses. These viruses often grow easily in culture, grow to large population sizes, mutate frequently, and evolve quickly. RNA viruses also tend to have very small genomes, making it easy to identify and sequence evolving genes.

Experimental evolution will become an important tool for studying other kinds of pathogens. In section 5.5, I proposed an experiment to study programmed antigenic switching in organisms such as *Borrelia hermsii*.

The mechanistic issue concerned whether switch rates between different archival variants within a single genome could be modulated by natural selection, and if so, by what changes in DNA sequence or regulatory control. This highlights experimental evolution's role as a tool to study biochemical mechanism.

The evolutionary problem concerned the extent to which switch rates adapt to enhance bacterial fitness versus the extent to which mechanistic properties of switching constrain rates of switching between variants. This highlights experimental evolution's role in studying the constraints that govern evolutionary adaptation.

13 Experimental Evolution: Influenza

Experimental evolution of influenza has identified amino acid sites that mediate escape from antibody attack. Experimental studies have also located sites that influence binding to host receptors. In this chapter, I put these experimental studies in the context of influenza structure. I also discuss how amino acid substitutions affect the kinetics of antibody binding and neutralization. These rate processes influence the fitness consequences of amino acid variants and the course of evolutionary change.

The first section provides an overview of influenza antigenicity and structure. Detailed structural information exists for hemagglutinin, the key viral surface glycoprotein. Structural analyses also describe hemagglutinin bound to its host receptor and hemagglutinin bound to antibodies. These diverse structural studies set the foundation for evolutionary analyses, allowing one to develop detailed hypotheses about the forces acting on amino acid replacements.

The second section discusses antibody escape variants, many generated in experimental evolutionary studies with controlled antibody pressure. Much of the exposed surface of hemagglutinin responds to antibody pressure with escape mutants.

The third section describes experimental studies of cell binding and receptor tropism. Ancestral lineages of influenza A in birds use an $\alpha(2,3)$-linked form of sialic acid as the host receptor. Derived lineages in humans use an $\alpha(2,6)$ linkage. Experimental evolution studies grew a human $\alpha(2,6)$-tropic form in cell culture with horse serum that binds and interferes with the $\alpha(2,6)$-tropic linkage. A single amino acid change of leucine to glutamine produced an $\alpha(2,3)$-tropic viral receptor. The favored amino acid, glutamine, matches that found in birds at the same site. The reverse experiment began with the avian $\alpha(2,3)$-tropic form and selected for human $\alpha(2,6)$-tropic binding. The avian glutamine changed to leucine, matching the amino acid found in human isolates.

The fourth section analyzes the fitness consequences of amino acid substitutions. Observed substitutions can raise or lower binding affinity for the host receptor. Natural selection of affinity may balance the kinetics of binding and the kinetics of release from the widely distributed sialic acid receptor on host cells. A few studies report the effect of amino acid substitutions on antibody binding affinity. Those studies also relate antibody binding affinity to neutralization of viruses, a measure of the reduction in viral fitness. I describe preliminary studies on the mechanisms and the kinetics by which antibodies interfere with viruses. Those details will be required to understand how amino acid substitutions alter viral fitness.

The fifth section summarizes experimental evolution studies of other pathogens.

The sixth section presents topics for future research.

13.1 Overview of Antigenicity and Structure

Influenza viruses occur as three phylogenetically distinct types (Lamb and Krug 2001; Wright and Webster 2001). Influenza A and B have eight RNA segments, and influenza C has seven segments. Influenza C occurs primarily in humans, has relatively little antigenic variation, and does not cause significant disease. Influenza B occurs naturally only in humans. By contrast, influenza A infects humans, several other mammalian species including pigs and horses, and many avian species. Influenza A has much greater amino acid sequence variability than influenza B, although type B does vary among natural isolates.

The nearly annual human epidemics of influenza A or B cause significant morbidity and mortality (Nguyen-Van-Tam 1998). The yearly outbreaks often spread widely through human populations. Epidemics lead to immunological memory against common strains (Natali et al. 1981; Wang et al. 1986; Dowdle 1999; Nakajima et al. 2000). Immunological memory creates strong selective pressure on the viruses to change antigenic properties, escape immune memory responses within hosts, and initiate new outbreaks (Wilson and Cox 1990; Cox and Bender 1995). Widespread epidemics and the strong selective pressures of host immunity cause influenza A to evolve very rapidly in humans. Individual strains often die out after a few years, replaced by antigenic variants that temporarily escape immunological memory (Bush et al. 1999).

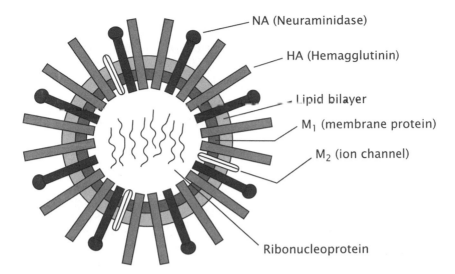

NA (Neuraminidase)

HA (Hemagglutinin)

Lipid bilayer

M_1 (membrane protein)

M_2 (ion channel)

Ribonucleoprotein

Figure 13.1 Influenza A structure. HA and NA spikes dominate the surface and form the main antigenic regions for antibody binding. Complexes of RNA and protein form the ribonucleoproteins. Eight distinct RNA segments make up the influenza A genome. Redrawn from Lamb and Krug (2001), with permission from Lippincott-Raven.

Figure 13.1 shows the organization of the influenza A virus. Hemagglutinin (HA) and neuraminidase (NA) comprise the major surface glycoproteins.

HA and NA reactivities with antibodies define the subtypes of influenza A (Cox and Subbarao 2000). Fifteen different HA antigenic subtypes occur, each subtype cross-reacting relatively little with the other subtypes. Nine distinct NA subtypes are known. The designation HxNy describes an influenza subtype with HA antigenic subtype $x = 1, \ldots, 15$ and NA antigenic subtype $y = 1, \ldots, 9$.

RNA sequences differ more between antigenic subtypes than within subtypes. Sequence similarity falls below 70% between HA subtypes and rises above 80% between isolates of the same subtype (Röhm et al. 1996). Thus, broad measures of antigenic and phylogenetic distances provide similar pictures of divergence. Much antigenic diversity also occurs between different members of an antigenic subtype. At these smaller distances, antigenic measures of differentiation become sensitive to the panel of antibodies and the nature of the test.

The HA and NA genes occur on different RNA segments. The other six segments contain the remaining genes. A host infected with two different viral genotypes can produce hybrid viral progeny with reassorted genotypes (Scholtissek 1998). For example, coinfection with HxNy and HwNz could produce the hybrids HxNz and HwNy in addition to the parental types.

The H3N2 subtype that caused the "Hong Kong" pandemic of 1968 arose by reassortment of the human H2N2 subtype with avian genes. The reassorted genotype had the H3 subtype and the PB1 gene from the bird lineage and the other six segments from the H2N2 human lineage (Kawaoka et al. 1989; Cox and Subbarao 2000). Other reassortments between the major human subtypes have been documented during the past twenty-five years (Cox and Bender 1995). Reassortment between subtypes may not occur frequently, but may be important in creating novel genotypes that have the potential to spread widely through a host population, causing pandemics.

All HA and NA subtypes occur in aquatic birds, suggesting that those avian species were the original host of influenza (Webster and Bean 1998; Cox and Subbarao 2000). Widespread human epidemics have been limited to H1N1, H2N2, and H3N2, although occasional transfers of other subtypes occur from birds or mammals to humans. Pigs harbor H1 and H3, whereas horses have H3 and H7. Other mammals and nonaquatic birds occasionally become infected, but do not appear to maintain stable lineages over time.

Influenza HA and NA molecules mediate viral attachment and entry to host cells and release of progeny viral particles by budding through the membrane of infected cells (Lamb and Krug 2001). Current understanding assigns adsorption and entry functions to HA (Steinhauer and Wharton 1998) and release of progeny to NA (Colman 1998). However, the HA and NA molecules may have multiple active sites and various functions, and the different subtypes of each molecule differ significantly (Lamb and Krug 2001). With those caveats, a brief summary of structure and function follows.

HA binds to sialic acid on the surface of host cells. The HA molecule then cleaves into two parts, the terminal HA1 and the basal HA2 fragments. Cleavage exposes on the surface of HA2 a highly conserved, hydrophobic region that mediates fusion and entry via the host membrane (Wilson and Cox 1990; Skehel and Wiley 2000).

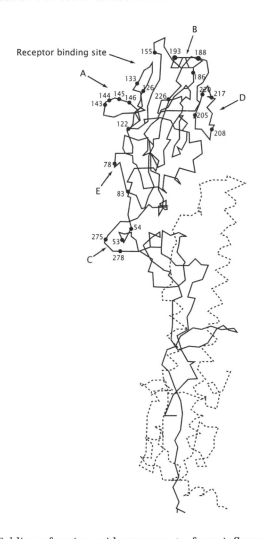

Figure 13.2   Folding of amino acid sequence to form influenza hemagglutinin HA1 (solid line) and HA2 (dotted line) subunits. This drawing is based on structural analysis of H3 hemagglutinin. Inference about other HA subtypes depends on presumed structural similarity with H3. Labeled amino acid numbers for HA1 are a subset of the variable sites listed in Wiley et al. (1981). The sites A–E show common antibody binding regions. Redrawn from Wilson et al. (1981), with permission from *Nature*, www.nature.com.

Figure 13.2 shows a diagram of the HA amino acid chain and its folding into a three-dimensional structure. The sialic acid binding site occurs near the tip of HA1. The letters A–E locate the major regions for

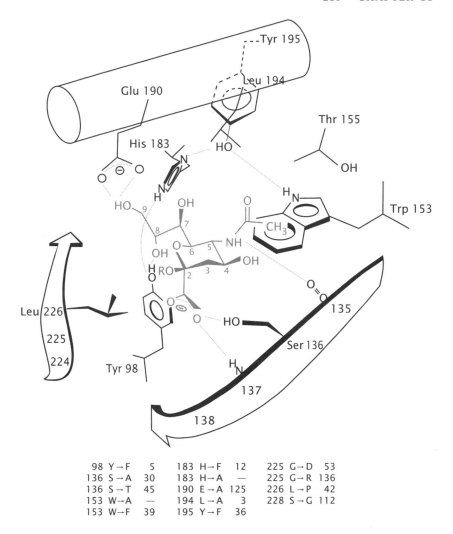

98 Y→F	5	183 H→F	12	225 G→D	53
136 S→A	30	183 H→A	—	225 G→R	136
136 S→T	45	190 E→A	125	226 L→P	42
153 W→A	—	194 L→A	3	228 S→G	112
153 W→F	39	195 Y→F	36		

Figure 13.3 Sialic acid binding site of human influenza A hemagglutinin sub-type H3. Sialic acid bound in the pocket appears in gray. The listing below shows the binding affinities for sialic acid when particular amino acids are changed experimentally by site-directed mutagenesis (Martín et al. 1998). The number on the left defines the amino acid site in HA1, $x \to y$ shows the original and new amino acid, and the number on the right is the binding affinity of the mutant as a percentage of the affinity of the wild type. Dashes show cases in which the receptor site is not properly expressed. Redrawn from Skehel and Wiley (2000), with permission from the *Annual Review of Biochemistry*, www.annualreviews.org.

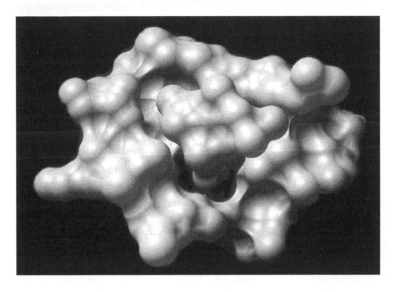

Figure 13.4   Binding of sialic acid (foreground) to the receptor binding site of influenza hemagglutinin (background). The sialic acid has been displaced slightly to show the structure of the fit. From Wilson and Cox (1990).

antigenically variable amino acid substitutions, although some substitutions occur over much of the exposed surface.

Figure 13.3 sketches the arrangement of the binding site and the orientation of sialic acid within the recessed contact region. The amino acids numbered within and around the binding site provide a reference for the location of important residues. The bottom of the figure shows the effect on binding affinity to sialic acid caused by experimental change of particular amino acids.

Figure 13.4 illustrates the fit between sialic acid and the HA1 binding site. This space-filling model has roughly the same orientation as the schematic diagram in figure 13.3, allowing one to locate approximately the structures and particular amino acids shown in figure 13.3 in the spatial view of figure 13.4.

Antibodies bound to HA can neutralize influenza infectivity by physically obstructing the sialic acid binding site. For example, the HC19 MAb binds to HA of strain X-31 (H3 subtype), partially overlapping the sialic acid binding site (Bizebard et al. 1995). The specific antibody-epitope region of direct contact covers 1250 Å^2, including amino acids 134, 136,

153, 155, and 194. Figure 13.3 shows that these residues occur on three of the four edges of the concave receptor binding depression. The depression extends 315 Å^2, of which the antibody binding region covers 167 Å^2. Antibody escape mutants map to the ridge of amino acids that ring the conserved amino acids in the binding pocket.

Bizebard et al. (1995) analyzed only the Fab fragments of antibodies, which contain the antibody paratope that directly binds to epitopes. Antibodies have a Y shape (fig. 2.1). Each upper arm forms an Fab fragment, with the binding region on the tip of the fragment. An antibody molecule can be cleaved to release two identical Fab fragments, each containing a binding region.

Bizebard et al. (1995) established direct overlap of the Fab binding region with the sialic acid binding site. However, other antibody escape mutants map to regions of HA away from the sialic acid binding site. Those sites are too far away to allow overlap of the direct antibody-epitope binding region with the sialic acid binding site.

Fleury et al. (1999) studied binding and neutralization by the HC45 MAb, which binds to a site distant from the sialic acid binding site. The Fab fragment of HC45 bound to its epitope with approximately the same kinetics as HC19 bound to its epitope, but HC19 was an order of magnitude more efficient at neutralization. Presumably this occurs because the Fab of HC19 causes greater obstruction of binding to sialic acid than does the more distantly bound Fab of HC45. By contrast, the full antibody molecules of HC19 and HC45 neutralized virus in proportion to their binding affinity for their respective epitopes. Fleury et al. (1999) suggest that the full antibody molecule is large enough to obstruct sialic acid binding even though the epitope binding site is distant from the sialic acid binding site.

Fleury et al. (1999) also noted a difference between HC19 and HC45 antibodies in their relative affinities for free HA molecules and HA molecules on the surface of viral particles. HC19 binds to the tips of HA molecules away from the viral surface; thus HC19 faces relatively little obstruction when binding to intact HA on viruses. By contrast, HC45 binds away from the tips of HA, toward the viral surface. This requires HC45 to diffuse through the HA spikes, slowing the rate of HA-HC45 association and reducing the net affinity of the binding. Clearly, neutralization depends on the structural environment of intact epitopes.

Other studies have noted differences between antibodies in their relations between binding and neutralization (Dimmock 1993; Schofield et al. 1997b, 1997a; Edwards and Dimmock 2000; Sanna et al. 2000). The site of antibody attachment, the kinetics of antibody binding, and the mechanism by which antibodies interfere with viral success all likely play a role in determining the strength of natural selection on various regions of the HA molecule. (See section 13.4 below, *Fitness Consequences of Substitutions*.)

Various structural mechanisms allow HA escape mutants to reduce binding by antibodies (Fleury et al. 1998). Bulky side chains may cause steric hindrance that interferes with antibody-epitope contact. Glycosylation adds surface carbohydrates that can prevent antibody access to potential epitopes (Caton et al. 1982; Skehel et al. 1984; Cox and Bender 1995). Some substitutions may destroy key hydrogen bonds. Alternatively, amino acid changes sometimes cause physical displacement of various protein loops.

Fleury et al. (1998) compared binding of an antibody to an original HA epitope and to a mutation of that epitope with changed conformation. When the antibody bound to the mutant epitope, the antibody-epitope complex reverted to the same structure as the antibody bound to the original type. However, the energy required to distort the conformation of the mutant epitope during binding reduced the binding affinity of the antibody by 4,000-fold relative to the affinity of the antibody for the original type. These various studies of antibody binding, structure, and kinetics provide necessary background for analyses of evolutionary change at the amino acid level.

I now turn to NA, which has not been studied as intensively as HA (Colman 1998). The function of NA is not completely understood (Lamb and Krug 2001). In general, neuraminidase enzymes cleave certain linkages within sialic acid. Sialic acid components of host cells form the primary site of influenza attachment. Thus, NA appears to cleave the host receptors to which influenza binds. This function seems to aid in releasing progeny viral particles from infected host cells.

It may be that viruses lacking neuraminidase activity enter host cells and replicate, but get stuck on the surface of the cell by attachment to sialic acid (Palese and Compans 1976). Kilbourne et al. (1968) showed that antibodies to NA do not prevent infection and replication, but do slow the rate at which viruses kill host cells—perhaps by reducing viral spread from infected to uninfected cells.

13.2 Antibody Escape Mutants

Several different experimental methods and lines of evidence can be used to infer the nature of antibody pressure on antigenic variation.

First, surface mapping determines which amino acids occur in sites accessible to antibodies. Underwood (1982, 1984) raised a panel of 125 mouse IgG MAbs against HA. Underwood compared the reactivities of the MAb panel against different natural and laboratory sequence variants of HA. Statistical methods identified which changed amino acids caused a reduction in antibody binding. The changed amino acids were located on the three-dimensional HA structure provided by Wilson et al. (1981). Almost the entire distal exposed surface of HA reacted with antibody, suggesting that the exposed regions provide a nearly continuous surface of potential epitopes. Antigenic sites B and D (fig. 13.2) contained a greater proportion of epitopes than other regions and, at least in particular laboratory mice, those sites appear to be more antigenic than other sites.

There are some problems with inferring antibody pressure by mapping surface antigenicity. Different natural and laboratory isolates of influenza may have multiple amino acid differences. This makes it difficult to assign changed antibody binding either to single amino acid substitutions or to the role of the genetic background with variations at other sites. In addition, changed antibody binding at different sites may have different consequences for binding kinetics and viral fitness. Some of the following methods mitigate these limitations.

A second approach applies MAb to either cultured or in vivo influenza (Wiley et al. 1981; Caton et al. 1982; Thomas et al. 1998). This experimental evolution favors escape variants that avoid neutralization. The locations of the escape variants map the potentially variable sites that can mutate to avoid recognition while preserving the ability to remain infectious. This antigenic map can be used to determine whether naturally varying amino acid sites likely changed under antibody pressure or by some other process.

Often, the same amino acid substitution occurs in replicate lineages faced with the same MAb, suggesting that the particular substitution provides the best balance of escape from neutralization and preservation of viral fitness. Sites that do not change under MAb pressure may either lack important contact with the antibody or may be constrained by function. These alternatives can be tested by site-directed mutagenesis, which experimentally changes particular amino acids.

A third experimental technique simultaneously applies antibodies to two or more sites (Yewdell et al. 1979, 1986; Lambkin et al. 1994). This mimics host reactions in which two or more immunodominant sites generate neutralizing antibodies. The frequency of escape mutants to a single antibody is about 10^{-5}, so simultaneous escape against two distinct antibodies occurs at a vanishingly low frequency of 10^{-10}. It appears that host antibodies directed simultaneously to two or more sites can greatly reduce the chance of new escape mutants during the course of a single infection.

A fourth experimental method focuses on escape mutants from low-affinity, subneutralizing antibodies (Thomas et al. 1998). Laeeq et al. (1997) obtained mice that lacked the ability to make the transition from initial, low-affinity IgM antibodies to subsequent, high-affinity IgG. They used those mice to raise low-affinity MAbs against influenza X-31 (subtype H3N2).

In previous studies, high-affinity MAbs applied to influenza typically selected single amino acid changes in one of the major antigenic sites A–E (fig. 13.2). By contrast, low-affinity MAbs selected escape mutants that had two amino acid substitutions, one in the conserved receptor-binding pocket and one in the highly antigenic regions next to the receptor-binding site.

Clearance and protection probably derive from high-affinity IgA and IgG antibodies rather than low-affinity IgM. So results from low-affinity MAbs do not reflect the most common selective pressures on antigenic variation. This study does, however, call attention to the processes by which immunodominance develops within a host. The initial, naive antibody repertoire may span widely over the HA surface, including the receptor binding pocket. The stronger antigenic sites apparently outcompete weaker sites in attracting high-affinity antibodies.

NA escape mutants have been studied less intensively than those for HA (Webster et al. 1984, 1987).

13.3 Cell Binding and Tropism

Influenza binds to sialic acid on host cells (Skehel and Wiley 2000). Sialic acid occurs as the terminal residue attached to galactose on certain carbohydrate side chains. Two common linkages between sialic acid and galactose occur in natural molecules, the $\alpha(2,3)$ and $\alpha(2,6)$ forms.

Different amino acid residues in the HA receptor binding site affect the relative affinity of HA for $\alpha(2,3)$ versus $\alpha(2,6)$ linkage (Matrosovich et al. 1997, 1998). Isolates of influenza A from aquatic birds favor the $\alpha(2,3)$ linkage. This matches the common $\alpha(2,3)$ form on the intestinal tissues of those hosts. All fifteen HA subtypes in aquatic birds share a highly conserved receptor binding site (Webster et al. 1992). The binding site apparently evolved before the evolution of the different subtypes and has been retained during subsequent divergence.

The human influenza A subtypes H1, H2, and H3 derived from avian ancestors (Webster et al. 1992). Each human subtype evolved from the matching subtype in aquatic birds, for example, human H1 from avian H1. In all three subtypes, the binding affinity of human lineages evolved to favor the $\alpha(2,6)$ linkage (Paulson 1985; Rogers and D'Souza 1989; Connor et al. 1994).

The evolutionary pathways differ for the human subtypes with regard to the amino acid substitutions and changes in binding that eventually led to preference for the $\alpha(2,6)$ form. Matrosovich et al. (1997) identified seven amino acid positions of the receptor binding site of aquatic birds that have changed during adaptation to human hosts. Human subtypes H2 and H3 have substitutions at positions 226 and 228 relative to avian ancestors. By contrast, human subtype H1 retains the ancestral avian residues at 226 and 228, but has changes in positions 138, 186, 190, 194, and 225 (see fig. 13.3 for locations of amino acid positions). Thus, different human lineages have followed different pathways of adaptation to receptor binding.

Experimental evolution studies of the H3 subtype support the phylogenetic data. Rogers et al. (1983) grew human H3N2 strains in chicken eggs in the presence of nonimmune horse serum. Horse serum contains $\alpha(2,6)$-linked sialic acid, which binds to human strains of influenza and interferes with the viral life cycle. The horse serum therefore selects strongly for altered binding to $\alpha(2,3)$-linked sialic acid (Matrosovich et al. 1998). After selection, Rogers et al. (1983) found a single amino acid substitution at position 226 of HA1. This substitution changed the leucine of human H3 to a glutamine residue, the same residue found in the ancestral avian H3 subtype. This substitution caused the modified virus to avoid $\alpha(2,6)$ binding and interference by horse serum and allowed binding to $\alpha(2,3)$-bearing receptors as in the ancestral avian type.

Rogers et al. (1989) selected in the reverse direction. They began with a duck H3 isolate that had glutamine at position 226 and favored binding to $\alpha(2,3)$ sialic acid linkages. Binding to erythrocytes selected variants that favor the $\alpha(2,6)$ linkage. Viruses bound to erythrocytes were eluted and used to infect Madin-Darby canine kidney (MDCK) cells, a standard culture vehicle for human influenza isolates. This selection process caused replacement of glutamine at position 226 by leucine, which in turn favored binding of $\alpha(2,6)$- over $\alpha(2,3)$-linked sialic acid.

The same sort of experimental evolution on H1 isolates would be very interesting. If selection of avian H1 for a change from $\alpha(2,3)$ to $\alpha(2,6)$ binding causes the same substitutions as occurred in the human H1 lineage, then the different genetic background of avian H1 compared with H3 would be implicated in shaping the particular amino acid substitutions. By contrast, if experimental evolution favors a change at position 226 as in H3, then the evolution of human H1 receptor binding may have followed a more complex pathway than simple selection for $\alpha(2,6)$-linked sialic acid.

Various steps have been proposed for adaptation of aquatic bird isolates to humans. For example, Rudneva et al. (1996) and Matrosovich et al. (1999) discuss the need to match HA and NA specificities. NA removes sialic acid from HA receptors, apparently facilitating release of viral progeny from the surface of host cells. If a viral lineage switches its HA specificity from the avian $\alpha(2,3)$ to the human $\alpha(2,6)$ form, but NA retains the avian specificity, then the lineage may have difficulty spreading in humans. Complex pathways may be required for joint adaptation of HA and NA (Matrosovich et al. 1999).

These studies raise the general problem of evolutionary pathways by which pathogens change host receptors. If two or more pathogen functions must change simultaneously, then changes in receptor affinity may be rare. The need for joint change may cause significant constraint on amino acid substitutions in receptor binding factors.

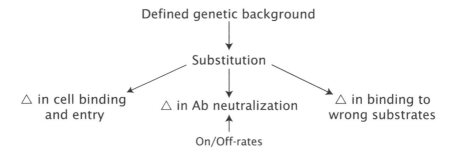

Figure 13.5   Effects of amino acid substitutions on fitness. In an experimental setting, one begins with a particular, defined genotype as the genetic background for further analysis. One then obtains single amino acid substitutions or small numbers of substitutions derived from the original background genotype. Substitutions may be obtained by imposing selective pressures such as antibodies in an experimental evolution regime or by imposing site-directed or random mutagenesis. Substitutions affect various components of fitness as described in the text.

13.4 Fitness Consequences of Substitutions

Surface amino acid substitutions affect fitness in three different ways (fig. 13.5). Each of these processes relates fitness to different kinetic aspects of surface binding.

First, changes in cell binding and entry affect the performance of intracellular pathogens. The relationship between binding kinetics and fitness may be rather complex. For example, figure 13.3 shows that naturally occurring amino acids may promote lower binding affinity than is associated with certain substitutions. In that figure, the substitutions 190 E→A, 225 G→R, and 228 S→G all have stronger binding affinity than the common wild type.

HA has a relatively low affinity for its host-cell receptors (Skehel and Wiley 2000). The fact that some substitutions raise affinity suggests that binding has been adjusted by selection to an intermediate rate. It may be possible to test this idea in various experimental systems by competing viruses with different cell binding kinetics.

Robertson (1993, 1999) reviews experimental evolution work on the adaptation of influenza to culture conditions in chicken eggs and Madin-Darby canine kidney (MDCK) cells. Those in vitro systems allow study of competition between different viral genotypes (Robertson et al. 1995).

Simple in vitro culture conditions may select for higher binding affinity between pathogen and host cells (Robertson et al. 1995). It would be interesting to compare the fitnesses in vivo between wild type and mutants selected for higher binding affinity in vitro.

The second role of substitutions arises from binding that interferes with viral fitness. Too high affinity of HA for the primary host-cell receptor may impair release of progeny viruses. High affinity may also aggregate viruses in localized regions, interfering with infectious spread. Again, it would be interesting to compete variants with different affinities under various in vitro and in vivo conditions.

Receptor binding sites may also be strongly selected to avoid binding molecules similar to the host-cell receptor. For example, the nonimmune component of horse serum attracts influenza particles that bind the $\alpha(2,6)$ linkage of sialic acid (Matrosovich et al. 1998). Selection favors equine influenza strains that both bind $\alpha(2,3)$ linkages and avoid $\alpha(2,6)$ linkages. By contrast, mucins of human lungs contain $\alpha(2,3)$-linked sialic acid, favoring human lineages that avoid the $\alpha(2,3)$ linkage (Couceiro et al. 1993). Thus, host fluids or host tissues different from the primary infection target can cull viruses from circulation. The kinetics of such fitness losses must be balanced against kinetic gains in receptor binding and avoidance of antibodies.

The third fitness effect of surface substitutions arises from changes in antibody binding. A few studies have related different aspects of antibody-virus binding kinetics to the neutralization (killing) of viruses (Schofield et al. 1997a, 1997b; Drescher and Aron 1999; Edwards and Dimmock 2000; Kostolanský et al. 2000; Sanna et al. 2000). This topic stands as a preliminary model for analyzing the relations between binding kinetics and fitness (Dimmock 1993; McLain and Dimmock 1994; Dimmock 1995).

No work has clearly established the roles of various amino acid substitutions in antibody neutralization kinetics. I highlight a few general issues and some particular studies on influenza. I suspect that experimental evolution will be an important tool in understanding the links between fitness, amino acid substitutions, the kinetics of binding to host cells, and the kinetics of antibody neutralization.

ANTIBODY-EPITOPE BINDING

I begin with a few key measures. Consider the simple chemical reaction $[A] + [V] \rightleftharpoons [AV]$, where brackets denote concentration (mol/l) for antibodies, A, viruses, V, and bound antibody-virus complexes, AV. Binding occurs at the on-rate, or rate of association, k_a (l/mol·s), and the breakup of bound complexes occurs at the off-rate, or rate of dissociation, k_d (1/s). The equilibrium binding affinity is

$$K_a = \frac{k_a}{k_d} = \frac{[AV]}{[A][V]}$$

with units l/mol. At equilibrium, the binding affinities can also be given by the dissociation constant, $K_d = 1/K_a$.

Most studies of antibody-parasite binding report equilibrium affinity. This may capture an important aspect of neutralization, but other processes may also be important. For example, equilibrium binding affinity provides no sense of the time course of association because it describes the ratio between on-rate and off-rate. In vivo, the race occurs between the rate of antibody binding and neutralization versus the rate of pathogen attachment and entry into host cells (Dimmock 1993; McLain and Dimmock 1994). Experimental evolution studies could be devised to measure under what conditions selection favors particular changes in rate processes or only an overall change in equilibrium affinity.

NEUTRALIZATION MECHANISMS AND KINETICS

I now turn to a few particular studies. Schofield et al. (1997a) compared equilibrium affinity, K_a, and neutralization strength for five MAbs against influenza HA. They measured neutralization by the rate at which a mixture of antibody and virus loses infectivity when presented with a layer of cultured host cells. For the five MAbs, the rank order of binding affinity approximately matched the rank order of neutralization rate. Thus, binding affinity explains some of the variation in neutralization rate. However, the ratio of affinity to neutralization rate varied by a factor of 125. Affinity alone does not explain all of the variation.

Edwards and Dimmock (2000) studied several aspects by which IgG MAbs H36 and H37 neutralize influenza. H36 binds to site B and H37 to site A on the HA molecule (see fig. 13.2). Antibodies in cell culture may neutralize by blocking viral attachment, by preventing fusion of the virus with the host cell membrane, by inhibiting internalization of the virus, or by interfering with viral replication.

Edwards and Dimmock (2000) found that, when antibodies inhibited infectivity by 50% of viruses, attachment was blocked for only 5 to 20% of viruses. Thus, other neutralizing mechanisms must play an important role. Further studies demonstrated that antibody inhibition of viral fusion increased in proportion to neutralization. Interference with fusion appears to be the primary neutralizing mechanism. However, antibody concentration influenced the relative contributions of blocking attachment versus blocking fusion: increased concentrations enhanced the degree of interference with viral attachment for both H36 and H37 antibodies. At high concentrations, interference with attachment became the dominant mechanism. As in Schofield et al. (1997a), binding affinity alone did not determine neutralization efficiency. H36 neutralized 10-fold more efficiently than did H37, but H37 binding affinity was 1.4-fold higher for H37 than for H36.

Schofield et al. (1997a) observed pseudo-first-order kinetics of influenza neutralization by antibody, defined as a log-linear decrease in infectivity over time. Pseudo-first order kinetics typically occur for antibody neutralization of viruses (Dimmock 1993), although exceptions occur (McLain and Dimmock 1994). Many different underlying mechanisms of reaction can give rise to pseudo-first-order kinetics (Latham and Burgess 1977).

The most commonly proposed mechanism for pseudo-first-order neutralization follows the single-hit model, in which one assumes that a single bound antibody can neutralize a virus (Dimmock 1993). In this model, the probability at time t that a particular virion has not been hit by at least a single antibody is $e^{-\lambda t}$, with an average time until the first hit of $1/\lambda$. The logarithm of the number of antibody-free virions decays linearly in time with a slope proportional to $-\lambda$. This exponential decay typifies models of random waiting times, random decay, and the Poisson distribution for the number of events in a particular time period. In the antibody-virus model, one assumes an excess of antibody so that antibody pressure does not decline over time as antibodies bind to viral surfaces.

In an exponential decay model of binding, there is on average one antibody bound to each virion when $\lambda t = 1$, following a Poisson distribution with an average count of one. Thus, when the average number of bound antibodies per virus is $\lambda t = 1$, the single-hit model for first-order neutralization kinetics predicts a frequency of $e^{-\lambda t} = e^{-1}$ antibody-free virions and $1 - e^{-1}$ bound and neutralized virions. Conversely, $1 - e^{-1} = 63\%$ neutralization predicts an average of one bound antibody per virion.

The observed number of bound antibodies per virion at 63% neutralization varies widely (Dimmock 1993): approximately 1 for polyclonal antibodies neutralizing adenovirus hexon protein (Wohlfart 1988) and poliovirus (Wetz et al. 1986), 4 to $\geq$ 15 for poliovirus with MAb IgG (Icenogle et al. 1983; Mosser et al. 1989), and about 70 MAb IgG per influenza virion (Taylor et al. 1987).

First-Order Kinetics with Multihit Binding

To understand the apparent contradiction between the observed first-order kinetics and multi-hit binding, one must understand the mechanisms by which antibodies neutralize virus. Two possibilities have been discussed (Icenogle et al. 1983; Dimmock 1993; McLain and Dimmock 1994).

First, a particular epitope may occur many times on the surface of a virion. The different sites have the same antigenicity but may differ in the effect of bound antibody on neutralization. Antibody bound to critical sites neutralizes; antibody bound to noncritical sites does not neutralize. Taylor et al. (1987) found an average of 70 HA-binding IgG molecules per virion at 63% neutralization, suggesting a ratio of noncritical to critical sites of 70:1. A virion has about 1,000 HA spikes, implying about 14 critical sites per virion. Thus only one hit in 70 neutralizes. This model is possible, but at present there is no reason to suppose that only a small fraction of apparently identical HA spikes differs in some critical way.

Second, each bound antibody may partially neutralize a virion (Icenogle et al. 1983). Although this process does not yield a perfectly log-linear plot of neutralization versus time, the predicted kinetics are sufficiently close to log-linear (pseudo-first-order) that departures would not be easily noticed in experimental data. This model is attractive because a single antibody bound to one of 1,000 HA spikes on an influenza virion might fractionally reduce infectivity rather than completely neutralize the virus.

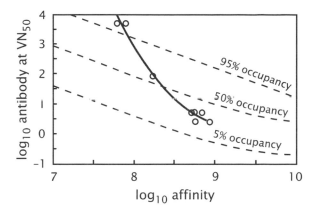

Figure 13.6   The amount (units in ng) of MAb IIB4 required to impose 50% neutralization (VN_{50}) of influenza grown in cell culture. Each observation (open circle) shows the neutralization of a different influenza strain with variant amino acids at the antibody binding site.   The amino acid variants cause different equilibrium binding affinities (K_a) with the antibody (units in l/mol). The percent occupancy describes the fraction of HA spikes occupied by antibody under equilibrium conditions at 50% neutralization. Redrawn from Kostolanský et al. (2000), with permission from the Society for General Microbiology.

Kostolanský et al. (2000) took a different approach to understanding the interaction between the number of bound antibodies and the neutralization of influenza. Earlier studies compared different MAbs directed to different epitopes, so that it was difficult to separate the effects of the different antibodies and epitopes on the relations between affinity, neutralization kinetics, and mechanisms of neutralization. By contrast, Kostolanský et al. (2000) compared binding of a single MAb, IIB4, to different influenza strains. Those strains have variant amino acids in a single epitope located at HA antigenic site B (see fig. 13.2).

By focusing on a single MAb against variants of the same epitope, Kostolanský et al. (2000) could analyze how variations in affinity influence the number of bound antibodies and the degree of neutralization. They measured equilibrium binding affinity (K_a) of MAb IIB4 for HA variants and the ability of IIB4 to neutralize each variant.   They reported neutralization as VN_{50}, the amount of antibody in vitro required to reduce influenza replication rate by 50%.

Higher-affinity epitopes needed less antibody to reach VN_{50} (fig. 13.6). In addition, higher-affinity epitopes had fewer antibodies per virion at VN_{50}. For example, the highest affinity of $K_a \approx 10^9$ l/mol had about

13% of HA spikes occupied by antibody, whereas the lowest affinity of $K_a \approx 10^8$ l/mol had about 98% of HA spikes occupied. These results suggest that neutralization depends on quantitative effects of affinity and the cumulative effects of multihit binding.

The particular mechanism that leads to quantitative effects on neutralization remains unclear. It may be that lower-affinity antibodies primarily interfere with attachment to host cells by covering most viral attachment sites. By contrast, higher-affinity antibodies may interfere primarily with fusion and entry to host cells, and such steric interference at the cell surface requires a lower density of bound antibody.

Kostolanský et al. (2000) measured percent occupancy of free virions. When virions attach to cell surfaces, the lower-affinity epitopes may lose a larger fraction of bound antibody than higher-affinity epitopes. The net effect is that, to achieve VN_{50}, both high- and low-affinity epitopes may have similar fractions of bound antibody during virion-cell binding.

Sanna et al. (2000) found that simultaneous binding by two antibodies to different epitopes acted synergistically to enhance neutralization. Synergism occurs when simultaneous binding by two antibodies causes higher neutralization than expected by adding the effects of each antibody when bound alone. Thus, the fitness effect of an amino acid substitution may depend both on the reduced affinity for the conforming antibody and on the context of other antibody-epitope combinations for that pathogen genotype.

13.5 Experimental Evolution of Other Pathogens

FMDV and influenza distinguish themselves as model experimental systems. Structural studies locate particular amino acid sites in their three-dimensional context. Experimental evolution substitutes amino acids in response to immune pressure, altered cellular receptors, interference with the viral receptor binding site, or changed kinetics that arise in cell culture. Binding affinity and kinetics of neutralization relate amino acid substitutions to components of fitness.

Several other pathogens have been studied by experimental evolution. The range of information for each pathogen tends to be limited when compared with the multiple types of evidence for FMDV and influenza. In this section, I briefly list a few additional studies of experimental evolution.

Ciurea et al. (2000) manipulated in vivo the components of the mouse immune response against cytopathic lymphocytic choriomeningitis virus. Experimental reduction of CD8$^+$ T cell response greatly enhanced the production of escape mutants from neutralizing antibody, suggesting that antibodies play a greater part in controlling the virus in the absence of CD8$^+$ T cells. Experimental deletion of the B cell response led to an absence of amino acid substitutions in the presumed antibody epitopes, demonstrating that substitutions in surface proteins arise in response to antibodies rather than cell tropism.

Hepatitis B virus (HBV) can cause severe liver damage in humans. Liver transplants following damage by HBV infection require suppression of HBV to prevent harm to the transplanted organ (Gow and Mutimer 2000). One suppressive method treats patients with antibody directed at the HBV surface antigens. This treatment creates an in vivo selection experiment in the patient, favoring HBV escape mutants. Not surprisingly, escape mutants do arise frequently with amino acid substitutions in the immunodominant surface antigens (Gow and Mutimer 2000).

HBV encodes surface antigens and nucleotide polymerases in different reading frames of the same nucleotide genomic sequence (Shields et al. 1999). Antigenic change in response to antibody pressure can change polymerase function, and substitutions in the polymerase in response to nucleoside analog drugs can change antigenic properties of surface proteins. The mapping of amino acid substitutions to fitness may be rather complex in this case. Ghany et al. (1998) showed that antibody escape mutants reverted to wild type after antibody pressure was removed, suggesting that the escape mutants had reduced polymerase function.

Liebert et al. (1994) studied measles encephalitis in a rat model. MAbs injected in vivo reduced neurovirulence and selected escape mutants that were isolated from brain tissue. MAb escape mutants selected in vitro produced altered and variable patterns of neurovirulence when injected into the host. The antibody epitopes appeared to be on the surface hemagglutinin protein. Amino acid substitutions in measles hemagglutinin appear to alter both antigenicity and neurovirulence.

Measles virus also appears to change its binding affinity for different cellular receptors during adaptation to cell culture (Nielsen et al. 2001). The amino acid changes associated with receptor affinity occur in the surface hemagglutinin protein. Further experimental evolution studies of this system will provide more information on how viruses modulate receptor binding and cell tropism during adaptation to different kinds of host cells.

The life cycle of arthropod-borne viruses (arboviruses) typically alternates between vertebrate hosts and blood-feeding arthropod vectors. The viruses replicate in both hosts. Arboviruses have RNA genomes and therefore the potential for high genetic diversity. However, many studies have reported a high degree of antigenic conservation and slow rates of molecular evolution (reviewed by Cooper and Scott 2001). Scott et al. (1994) and Weaver et al. (1999) suggested that alternating hosts impose a constraint on molecular change.

Cooper and Scott (2001) used experimental evolution to study how alternating hosts potentially constrain adaptive change. They passaged viral lineages in cell culture through either mosquito cells only, avian cells only, or alternating between mosquito and avian cells. They then measured various characteristics of infectivity and growth on insect, avian, or mammalian host cells.

The different passage histories produced significant differences in infectivity and growth between the lineages. The lineages that alternated between the two host types expressed intermediate phenotypes relative to those lineages passaged only in one cell type. Alternation apparently favored compromise between changing selective regimes. Further experimental evolution studies in vivo may provide more insight into how multiple selective pressures constrain the rate of evolutionary change.

Moya et al. (2000) review experimental evolution studies of vesicular stomatitis virus, an RNA virus. They particularly emphasize that high mutation rates and large population sizes of RNA viruses affect evolutionary potential by maintaining a large diversity of variant genotypes. Those variants provide material for a rapid response to new or changing selective pressures. The consequences of varying population size on the rate of adaptation have been analyzed under controlled experimental conditions.

A few bacterial studies analyzed escape mutants in response to controlled antibody pressure (e.g., Jensen et al. 1995; Solé et al. 1998). Other scattered studies of experimental evolution have been done on nonviral pathogens, but none approaches the scope of the viral experiments.

13.6 Problems for Future Research

1. Decoy antigenic variation. The first infection of a host initially stimulates the naive IgM antibody repertoire, which has relatively low affinity and broad specificity. The mature, high-affinity antibody response develops by various processes, including competition between antibodies based on binding affinity.

A pathogen gains if its most highly antigenic sites have low rates of neutralization or high rates of antigenic change. Highly antigenic decoy sites can draw antibody pressure away from sites more sensitive to neutralization or more strongly constrained against change because of essential function.

Laeeq et al. (1997) showed that IgM antibody pressure selects variants in the receptor binding site, whereas mature, high-affinity antibodies select variants in the major antigenic sites outside of the binding pocket. The immunodominant sites draw the maturing repertoire away from the binding pocket.

To what extent have immunodominant sites evolved to draw antibody pressure away from more sensitive sites? This is a difficult question, because immunodominant sites may happen to be away from receptor binding pockets or other functional sites for a variety of reasons.

No experimental systems developed so far provide a clear way to address this problem. One needs experimental control of initial antibody pressure and a feedback mechanism that enhances antibody pressure on epitopes with stronger antibody binding. Feedback favors epitopes with relatively lower rates of neutralization to evolve relatively stronger antibody binding. Such decoy sites might additionally be favored if they could tolerate a broad array of amino acid escape mutants.

This sort of experimental evolution would provide clues about the forces that have shaped immunodominance. Mathematical models of immunodominance such as those developed by Nowak and May (2000) would aid in designing experiments and clarifying evolutionary process.

2. Genetic background. Experimental evolution studies of avian and human H3 showed that a single amino acid change at position 226 of HA1 determines avian $\alpha(2,3)$-tropic or human $\alpha(2,6)$-tropic binding for sialic acid (Rogers et al. 1983, 1989). An open question concerns the role of the genetic background in conditioning the effects of a particular substitution. These experiments could be repeated, starting with genotypes that have different amino acid substitutions at varying distances from site 226.

3. Kinetics of pleiotropy. Several escape mutants have been generated by application of MAbs. It would be interesting to know the pleiotropic consequences of antibody escape mutants for other components of fitness, such as binding to host receptors, growth rate, and virulence. These fitness components depend on various kinetic processes within the host. A study that matched amino acid substitutions to kinetic processes would illuminate the mechanistic basis of fitness and provide insight into the microevolutionary patterns of change in proteins.

Most work on influenza has emphasized human isolates of influenza A. Those isolates can be grown in vivo in mice and other hosts, but the change in hosts compromises interpretations of kinetics and fitness. It would be interesting to develop an experimental model of influenza A in aquatic birds, the ancestral host for this virus. This would allow study of natural variation in avian isolates coupled with in vivo experimental analysis of fitness components.

4. Balancing selection of receptor binding. Influenza binding affinity for host receptors appears to be balanced at an intermediate level. Some substitutions raise affinity, and other substitutions lower affinity. Cell culture studies of FMDV and other pathogens show that binding affinity and receptor tropism evolve readily in experimental settings. It would be interesting to learn more about the selective pressures that modulate such affinities. The fitness effects no doubt depend on kinetic rates of cellular binding and entry balanced against rates of aggregation on inappropriate surfaces and in places hidden from or exposed to immune effectors. Substitutions that modulate these rate processes may also affect antibody binding. Study of these processes depends on a good in vivo system in which selective pressures can be varied and fitness components can be measured.

5. Kinetic consequences of neutralization mechanisms. Preliminary studies of neutralization kinetics provide some clues about how antibody binding affects fitness. Different mechanistic models of neutralization could be transformed into a family of mathematical models for neutralization kinetics. Those models would clarify predicted response to experimental manipulation under different assumptions, allowing better tests of the mechanistic assumptions. In addition, models would suggest how changes in different aspects of neutralization would affect viral fitness. The more sensitive steps in neutralization would be under more intense selective pressure for change, suggesting a testable prediction for which amino acid sites would be most likely to respond during experimental evolution. These studies would link molecular mechanisms, kinetic consequences, and evolutionary forces.

14 Experimental Evolution: CTL Escape

CTL pressure favors amino acid substitutions in pathogen epitopes that escape recognition. Escape substitutions may avoid peptide processing and transport, reduce binding to MHC molecules, or lower affinity for the T cell receptor (Borrow and Shaw 1998). In this chapter, I discuss experimental evolution studies of CTL escape. I also discuss nonevolutionary studies that provide background or suggest promising experimental systems.

The first section reviews mechanisms of escape during peptide cleavage and transport. Two studies of murine leukemia virus describe single amino acid substitutions that changed patterns of peptide cleavage in cellular proteasomes. One substitution added a cleavage site within an epitope. Before the substitution, a significant amount of that epitope was transported to the endoplasmic reticulum, bound to MHC molecules, and presented to CTLs at the cell surface. The new cleavage site greatly reduced the abundance of the epitope available for MHC binding. A different substitution abrogated cleavage at the carboxyl terminus of an epitope, preventing transport of the peptide from the proteasome to the endoplasmic reticulum.

The second section describes escape from binding to MHC molecules during experimental evolution. Studies of influenza and lymphocytic choriomeningitis virus used a transgenic mouse with almost all of its CTLs specific for a single epitope, creating intense selective pressure for escape. Structural analyses of the peptide-MHC complex illuminate the biochemical mechanisms by which escape variants reduce binding to MHC. Experiments with simian immunodeficiency virus compared the spread of amino acid substitutions in several epitopes when in different host MHC genotypes. If the host had an MHC molecule that could present a particular epitope, that epitope was much more likely to evolve escape substitutions during infection.

The third section summarizes escape from binding to the T cell receptor (TCR). The experimental evolution studies of influenza and lymphocytic choriomeningitis with transgenic, monoclonal T cells yielded some TCR escape substitutions. Structural studies of peptide-MHC complexes and binding affinity studies of the complexes with TCRs clarified the biochemical mechanisms by which escape occurs.

The fourth section considers how the function of pathogen proteins may be altered by CTL escape substitutions. The Tax protein of human T cell leukemia virus type 1 provides a major target for CTL attack. Intense immune pressure selects for escape substitutions in naturally occurring infections. Tax plays a key role in many viral and cellular processes that affect viral fitness. Functional studies of Tax mutants suggest that substitutions reduce Tax performance. In HIV, amino acid substitutions in response to drugs sometimes increase binding to MHC molecules. It may be that the wild-type sequence reflects a balance between protein function and avoidance of MHC binding. Drugs or other experimental perturbations may upset that balance, exposing the mechanisms that mediate balancing selection.

The fifth section lists kinetic processes that determine the success or failure of escape variants. Kinetic processes connect the biochemical mechanisms of molecular interaction to the ultimate fitness consequences that shape observed patterns of antigenic variation. No experimental evolutionary studies have focused on these kinetic processes.

The final section highlights some topics for future research.

14.1 Cleavage and Transport of Peptides

Cellular proteasomes continuously chop up proteins into smaller peptides. Proteasomal cleavage patterns of proteins determine which peptides will be transported into the endoplasmic reticulum by transporter (TAP) molecules and made available for binding and presentation by the MHC system.

Single amino acid substitutions can affect proteasomal cleavage patterns (references in Beekman et al. 2000). Ossendorp et al. (1996) compared an eight-residue CTL epitope in two different murine leukemia viruses. Those epitopes differ by a K→R substitution in the first position. The R residue adds an additional, strong cleavage site within the epitope, causing a large reduction in the abundance of the R-containing epitope available for MHC presentation.

Cleavage does not occur instantaneously for all proteins. Instead, varying sites affect rates of cleavage and consequently relative abundances of different peptides. Ossendorp et al. (1996) present kinetic data for the accumulation of the K- and R-containing epitopes, and show that a large difference in abundance arises early in digestion, on the order of one hour.

Beekman et al. (2000) studied a different epitope in the same pair of murine leukemia viruses. In this case, an amino acid substitution at the residue flanking the C-terminus of the epitope affected both cleavage and transport. An aspartic acid residue at this position prevented cleavage precisely at the C-terminal site of the epitope and prevented transport by TAP. Thus, the epitope remained intact, but the peptide was not carried to the site of MHC binding.

These studies demonstrate that cleavage and transport can affect CTL response. But no data show how commonly amino acid substitutions abrogate efficient cleavage and transport. Experimental evolution studies could manipulate immunodominance and kinetic aspects of within-host infections to measure the frequency of the escape mechanism under different conditions.

14.2 MHC Binding

Amino acid substitutions can reduce affinity of epitopes for binding to MHC molecules. This may prevent MHC from transporting bound epitopes to the cell surface. Alternatively, peptide-MHC complexes may be presented on the cell surface, but higher off-rates of the peptide reduce the opportunity for interaction with T cell receptors (TCRs). Several experimental evolution studies report mutations that reduce peptide-MHC binding.

LCMV

Mice infected with lymphocytic choriomeningitis virus (LCMV) form the best-studied experimental system (Pircher et al. 1990; Weidt et al. 1995; Moskophidis and Zinkernagel 1995). LCMV is a noncytopathic RNA virus that naturally infects mice. The infection can be controlled or eliminated by a strong CTL response of the host. In H2-b mice, the MHC molecule D^b presents the viral glycoprotein epitope GP33–43 and the MHC molecule K^b presents the overlapping GP34–43 epitope (Puglielli et al. 2001).

Genetically modified (transgenic) mouse lines have been developed that express a TCR specific for GP33–43 presented by MHC D^b. Most (75–

90%) of the CTLs in these mice express the TCR for GP33–43 (Pircher et al. 1990). These CTLs clear low doses of LCMV. High doses produce an initial viremia and subsequent decline under CTL pressure, followed by the appearance of CTL escape variants (Pircher et al. 1990). The rather extreme immunodominance of this experimental system provides a good model for studying molecular details of escape variants.

Puglielli et al. (2001) used this system to study amino acid substitutions in response to CTL pressure against D^b-restricted GP33–43. They infected transgenic mice with high doses of LCMV virus. After the initial viremia and subsequent decline in titers in response to CTL pressure, viral titers increased. They isolated viruses from this later period to determine if escape variants had evolved and, if so, by what mechanism. These late viruses had a V→A substitution at the third position (site 35) of GP33–43 that nearly abolished binding to MHC D^b.

Binding affinity of a peptide to MHC class I molecules typically depends on a small number of anchor residues in the peptide (Janeway et al. 1999). For example, an MHC molecule may have two anchor positions such that the fifth and ninth amino acids from the amino terminus (lower-numbered end) of the peptide determine the main portion of binding affinity. Structurally, such anchors may be pockets in the MHC molecule into which side chains from amino acids can fit. An amino acid with a side chain that fits well into the MHC pocket will bind with high affinity. A substitution in the peptide at an anchor position to a different amino acid with significantly altered shape or charge often diminishes or abolishes effective binding of the peptide-MHC complex. Substitutions at nonanchor residues usually have much smaller effects on binding affinity.

The third binding position of MHC D^b is neither the primary nor auxiliary anchor residue according to previous studies (Rammensee et al. 1995). However, Tissot et al. (2000) solved the structure of D^b bound to the LCMV wild-type epitope at GP33–43 (fig. 14.1). They found that the peptide residue at position three had its side chain buried in the D^b binding cleft and, apparently, certain substitutions such as V→A at this location can disrupt binding in the manner of an anchor position (Puglielli et al. 2001).

Moskophidis and Zinkernagel (1995) studied the same system with H2-b mice and LCMV virus. Evolution within experimentally infected mice produced substitutions in immunodominant CTL epitopes. The

(a)

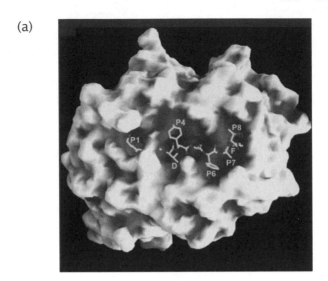

(b)

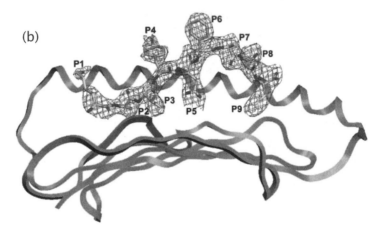

Figure 14.1   Binding of LCMV epitope GP33-41 to the H-2 mouse MHC molecule D^b. The nine amino acids of the epitope in positions 33–41 of the protein are labeled as P1-P9. (a) The epitope fits into the MHC binding groove. The bound epitope exposes P4 and P6-P8; the groove shelters the other residues. (b) Side-view diagram shows the buried and exposed residues. Rammensee et al. (1995) list P5 and P9 as anchor residues; P2 and P3 also occur deep in the groove. From Tissot et al. (2000).

substitutions N→D and N→S at position 280 of epitope GP275-289 abolished presentation by MHC molecule D^b. This position forms an anchor residue for binding to D^b.

Moskophidis and Zinkernagel (1995) also studied the V→L substitution at position 35 of GP32–42 originally obtained in the experimental evolution studies of Pircher et al. (1990). Both D^b and K^b can present this epitope. The V→L change, which occurred in a nonanchor residue for both MHC molecules, did not significantly reduce binding to either MHC molecule. The substitution did significantly reduce CTLs directed against this epitope when presented by D^b.

From these studies, two different substitutions at GP35 were analyzed (position P3 in fig. 14.1). Puglielli et al. (2001) found that a V→A substitution at GP35 abrogated binding to D^b, whereas Moskophidis and Zinkernagel (1995) found that a V→L change did not affect binding to D^b. Although this site was previously considered as a nonanchor residue, the L and A substitutions had significantly different effects on MHC binding. Interestingly, the V→L substitution, which did not affect binding affinity to the MHC molecule, did reduce the affinity of the peptide-MHC complex for a TCR (see section 14.3 below, *TCR Binding*).

SIV

Several authors suggest that HIV escape from CTLs plays an important role in the dynamics and persistence of infection within individual hosts (e.g., McMichael and Phillips 1997; Nowak and May 2000). Many lines of evidence from human hosts support this argument. But human infections cannot be controlled or manipulated experimentally. Several experimental evolution studies of simian immunodeficiency virus (SIV) infections in rhesus macaques have recently been published.

Allen et al. (2000) infected eighteen rhesus macaques with cloned SIV. All ten hosts expressing the MHC class I molecule Mamu-A*01 made CTLs to Tat28–35, the SL8 epitope in the Tat protein. Up to 10% of circulating CTLs recognized this epitope during the acute phase of viremia three to four weeks after infection. However, the frequency of Tat-specific CTLs dropped sharply after the acute phase, suggesting escape from recognition.

Sequencing at eight weeks after infection showed that five of ten Mamu-A*01 positive animals had mutations in the SL8 epitope, with little variation outside of this epitope. By contrast, only one of eight Mamu-A*01 negative hosts had mutations in the SL8 epitope. Four of the amino acid substitutions in SL8 effectively destroyed binding to Mamu-

A∗01. Three of these substitutions occurred at position 8, the primary anchor site, and one substitution occurred at position 2, the secondary anchor site. Two other substitutions reduced binding by less than two orders of magnitude: a substitution at position 1 reduced binding by 67%, and a substitution at position 5 reduced binding by 85%.

Z. W. Chen et al. (2000) observed CTL escape in SIV infections of rhesus macaques mediated by a single T→A substitution in an epitope of the Gag protein. The Mamu-A∗01 MHC molecule presents this Gag181–189 epitope on the cell surface. The substitution did not affect binding affinity of Mamu-A∗01 for Gag181–189. However, the peptide-MHC complexes could stimulate CTL response only when in vitro target cells where experimentally pulsed with high concentrations of the mutated epitope. Z. W. Chen et al. (2000) conclude that the substitution increases the off-rate of binding, causing a high dissociation rate of peptide-MHC complexes on the cell surface. High experimental concentrations of the epitope in vitro may overcome the high dissociation rates and provide enough peptide-MHC complexes on the cell surface to stimulate CTLs.

Many studies of CTL escape either use nearly monoclonal T cells or follow only one viral epitope. This leaves open the problem of whether polyclonal CTL responses to multiple epitopes favor escape in the same way as CTL responses to a single epitope. Evans et al. (1999) addressed this issue by following the within-host evolution of five distinct CTL epitopes of the Env and Nef proteins in five rhesus macaques experimentally infected by SIV. All hosts had the same MHC class II genotype and thus similar presentation of epitopes to helper T cells.

Hosts B and B′ had the same MHC class I genotype and progressed rapidly to disease without making a strong CTL response. The other three hosts made strong initial CTL responses. Hosts A and D progressed slowly to disease, whereas host C progressed at an intermediate rate. The intermediate progressor, host C, differed from the fast progressors by having MHC class I molecules Mamu-A∗11 and Mamu-B∗17. These MHC molecules presented two epitopes, Env497–504 and Nef165–173. One slow progressor, host A, differed from the fast progressors by having MHC class I molecules Mamu-B∗03 and Mamu-B∗04, which present three epitopes, Env575–583, Nef136–146, and Nef62–70. The other slow progressor, host D, had all four class I molecules listed for hosts A and C, and presented all five epitopes.

Evans et al. (1999) sequenced *env* and *nef* genes at various times during the course of infection. For the five epitopes listed above, each host had viral populations dominated by escape mutants only for those epitopes that they could present by their class I MHC molecules. For example, host C viruses were dominated by escape mutants in Env497–504 and Nef165-173 but not in the other three epitopes. This demonstrates selective pressure on multiple epitopes, defined by MHC class I presentation. Some of the escape variants abolished MHC binding to the epitopes, whereas others apparently reduced TCR recognition.

INFLUENZA

Price et al. (2000) infected mice with a human isolate of influenza. These transgenic mice expressed a monoclonal TCR specific for the influenza nucleoprotein epitope NP366–374, leading to a narrow and strong CTL response directed against this epitope. This intense selective pressure favored escape variants in this nine-residue epitope at positions 5, 6, 7, and 9, each escape variant having only one altered position.

Young et al. (1994) described the structure of the MHC D^b molecule bound to this NP epitope. This structural information allowed Price et al. (2000) to interpret the substitutions they observed in response to CTL pressure. Positions 5 and 9 form anchor sites buried in the MHC binding groove. Three different amino acid replacements at position 5 greatly reduced binding affinity for D^b and consequently abrogated CTL stimulation.

A substitution at position 9 reduced affinity for D^b less than 10-fold. In spite of the relatively small change in binding affinity for MHC, this substitution also abolished CTL response. Price et al. (2000) cite data to suggest that peptide processing and transport do not play a role, so the mechanism of escape by this substitution remains unclear.

14.3 TCR Binding

I continue with the influenza study by Price et al. (2000), which ended the previous section. I then return to the LCMV experimental system, which provides the first combined information on structure, binding affinity, and escape mutations with respect to peptide-MHC interactions with the TCR.

INFLUENZA

The structural study of Young et al. (1994) demonstrated that binding between MHC D^b and the NP366–374 epitope exposes positions 6 and 7. These exposed positions could potentially interact with the TCR. Haanen et al. (1999) showed a dominant role for position 7 by tetramer staining of TCR bound to peptide-MHC complexes. These previous structural and binding studies did not implicate position 6 as important for TCR affinity.

Price et al. (2000) observed three substitutions at positions 6 and one at position 7 that bound to D^b with the same affinity as the wild type. These escape variants avoided binding by the transgenic, monoclonal CTL.

Price et al. (2000) compared the ability of the wild type and an M→I substitution at position 6 to stimulate a CTL response in immunocompetent mice with a polyclonal repertoire. The M→I substitution attracted 3-10-fold fewer CTLs than did the wild type. Thus, this substitution at position 6 that escaped the transgenic monoclonal CTLs did not abolish polyclonal CTL stimulation. These observations suggest that the total TCR repertoire includes a set of overlapping specificities with varying affinity, allowing recognition of the altered ligand.

LCMV

In the section above on MHC binding, I described the V→L substitution of LCMV at GP35 (P3) that provided escape from transgenic CTLs in experimental infections of mice (Moskophidis and Zinkernagel 1995). This substitution did not significantly reduce binding affinity of the GP33–41 epitope for the MHC molecule D^b. Moskophidis and Zinkernagel (1995) concluded that this substitution interfered with stimulation of CTLs by the peptide-MHC complex.

Tissot et al. (2000) analyzed the structure and affinity of the peptide-MHC complex bound to the same TCR used by Moskophidis and Zinkernagel (1995). The V→L substitution at P3 reduced binding affinity to the TCR by a factor of 50, even though P3 is buried in the peptide-MHC binding groove (fig. 14.1). Tissot et al. (2000) suggest that the relatively bulky leucine reside caused shifting of the structure and a slight movement in residues P2 and P4. The residue at P4 is exposed and had the strongest effect on binding affinity to the TCR, so movement of P4 could be responsible for the change in affinity. Escape variants with a Y→F substitution at P4 obtained during experimental evolution in vivo cause a 100-fold decline in affinity for the TCR.

14.4 Functional Consequences of Escape

Escape substitutions change amino acids in pathogen proteins. Those changed proteins may have altered performance, affecting pathogen fitness in ways other than CTL escape. Ideally, experimental studies of escape would provide information about changed functional characteristics of pathogen proteins and the associated fitness consequences. I am not aware of any such analyses for CTL escape in experimentally controlled systems. Two uncontrolled studies provide some clues.

First, Niewiesk et al. (1995) analyzed CTL escape variants of human T cell leukemia virus (HTLV-1) in naturally infected human hosts. They focused on the Tax protein, a major target of CTLs. Individuals with MHC type HLA-A2 simultaneously recognize at least five epitopes of Tax (Parker et al. 1994). Niewiesk et al. (1995) found that in HLA-A2 subjects, 24 of 179 isolates had substitutions in epitopes presented by HLA-A2. By contrast, in subjects without HLA-A2, only one of 116 of these epitopes had a substitution. CTLs appear to be imposing strong selective pressure that favors escape. Nine different substitutions occurred across the five Tax epitopes. Each substitution abolished CTL attack of the associated epitope.

HTLV-1 is a retrovirus that integrates itself into the host genome. The Tax protein is a trans-acting transcriptional regulator that modulates expression of several viral and cellular genes (Yoshida 2001). Because HTLV-1 typically occurs as an integrated provirus in host cells, viral replication occurs by transmission within the lineages of host cells and by transmission between cells. Tax appears to affect several aspects of the cell cycle, potentially enhancing cell division and reducing cell death.

Niewiesk et al. (1995) tested the nine observed Tax substitutions for potency as activators of one viral and two cellular promoters of transcription. Potencies were compared with activation by a consensus sequence. Three substitutions had lowered ability to activate the viral promoter, and all nine substitutions caused lowered or no activation of two cellular promoters. The fitness consequences of these substitutions could not be measured directly. In vitro studies introduced mutations into the Tax protein and demonstrated that most mutations abolished Tax function (Smith and Greene 1990; Semmes and Jeang 1992). Thus, Tax appears to be highly constrained, suggesting that substitutions accumulate only under very strong CTL pressure.

A second study analyzed the selective pressure imposed by a drug (Samri et al. 2000). This study of human patients with HIV compared the viral reverse transcriptase (RT) protein before and after application of nucleoside inhibitors of RT. Substitutions in RT that escape drug pressure also reduce viral fitness (Coffin 1995; Back et al. 1996; Harrigan et al. 1998; Sharma and Crumpacker 1999). Samri et al. (2000) showed that, on average, drug escape mutants increased CTL recognition, most likely by enhanced binding to common MHC molecules.

Samri et al.'s (2000) preliminary study raises some interesting problems. Amino acid sequences of viral proteins may be shaped by two opposing pressures: contribution to viral function and escape from immune recognition. Thus, amino acid substitutions in response to a third force, such as a drug, may be likely to reduce protein performance or enhance recognition by the host immune system. In the case of RT, both reduced performance and enhanced MHC recognition may have occurred.

A particular viral sequence reflects the balance between functional performance and avoidance of CTL recognition via MHC presentation. Experimentally applied selective pressures such as drugs may provide information about the functional and immune selective pressures that shaped the wild-type sequence.

14.5 Kinetics of Escape

Experimental evolutionary studies have not focused on the kinetics by which escape variants arise and spread within hosts or within populations. I briefly list six issues.

IMMUNODOMINANCE

The first experimentally controlled studies of escape from CTLs used extreme immunodominance (Pircher et al. 1990). In that system, genetically constructed mice produced the identical TCR on 75–90% of circulating T cells. That extreme, monoclonal TCR distribution creates powerful selection favoring escape mutants for epitopes recognized by the dominant TCR.

More realistic polyclonal distributions of TCRs may not favor escape so easily (Borrow and Shaw 1998; Haanen et al. 1999). A single viral mutation can abrogate recognition of a particular epitope, but the virus carrying the mutant will likely express other epitopes recognized by different CTLs. By this argument, partial escape means partial recognition and death.

The degree of immunodominance plays an important role. For some pathogens and hosts, a typical response may primarily target a single epitope, with fewer CTLs focusing on subdominant epitopes. In this case, the pressure on the lead epitope favors escape. Other infections may have a broader and more even CTL response against several epitopes. Escape at one epitope does not alleviate recognition at several other epitopes. However, escape at multiple epitopes may be observed within individual hosts (Evans et al. 1999). The role of immunodominance in escape depends on the rate of killing by CTLs relative to the rate of viral transmission between cells (McMichael and Phillips 1997; Nowak and May 2000).

RATE OF KILLING VERSUS RATE OF TRANSMISSION

Consider a cytopathic virus—one that bursts its host cell when liberating progeny virions. A CTL escape mutant gains if it enhances the probability of cellular burst before CTL-mediated death. This probability depends on the race between the CTLs to kill infected cells and the viruses to liberate progeny. Escape at a dominant epitope provides benefit if the aggregate rate of killing via subdominant epitopes allows a higher probability of burst before death.

Noncytopathic viruses leak progeny virions from intact host cells. Here the race occurs between, on the one hand, CTL-induced death and, on the other hand, the time before the first viral progeny release and then the subsequent rate of progeny production. CTL escape has no benefit if pressure on other epitopes still kills before initial progeny production. If some infected cells survive to produce new virions, the benefit of escape at one epitope depends on the expected increase in cellular longevity during the productive phase of virion release and the probability that released viruses transmit to new host cells.

The roles of these different rate processes could be combined into a mathematical model by extending the approach of Nowak and May (2000). Experimental control over TCR diversity, CTL intensity, and comparison of cytopathic and noncytopathic viruses could provide tests of the mechanistic processes contained in the mathematical formulation.

MULTIPLICITY OF INFECTION

Higher multiplicity of infection may reduce the rate at which escape mutants spread (McMichael and Phillips 1997). Suppose two viruses infect a host cell. One virus expresses an escape mutant that avoids recognition by the dominant CTLs, whereas the other virus expresses the common epitope recognized by the dominant CTLs. This dually infected cell presents the common epitope on its surface, making it susceptible to recognition by CTLs. The escape mutant benefits only to the extent that fewer recognized peptides occur on the cell surface—lower density may reduce the rate of killing, and that reduction may in turn allow more of the escape variant's progeny to be transmitted.

DOSAGE AND POPULATION SIZE WITHIN HOSTS

In experimental studies, escape mutants arise more often as infecting dose increases (Pircher et al. 1990). At low doses, the host clears infection before escape mutants spread. Higher dose most likely produces larger population size during the initial viremia, increasing the time and the number of pathogens available to make a particular mutant.

Experimental manipulations could test the contributions of dosage, pathogen population size within the host, and time to clearance. Waiting time for an escape mutant also depends on the mutation rate, which could perhaps be varied by comparing genotypes that differed in mutation rate.

RATE OF CLEARANCE AND TRANSMISSION BETWEEN HOSTS

Rapidly cleared infections provide little opportunity for the transmission of escape variants. Such variants spread within hosts only after intense CTL pressure begins. If the infection clears rapidly, then the potential escape variants do not increase sufficiently within the host to contribute significantly to transmission to other hosts.

MHC Polymorphism and Transmission between Hosts

CTL escape may depend on reduced binding to an MHC molecule or on changed affinity between TCRs and the peptide-MHC complex. Hosts vary in the highly polymorphic MHC alleles. Escape from one host's MHC binding does not provide protection if most other hosts carry different MHC alleles. Long-term spread of an MHC escape variant depends on the frequency at which viruses encounter the particular MHC molecule and the intensity of forces against the escape variant. Such countering forces include creation of new sequences that bind well to different MHC molecules and functional attributes that affect the performance of the viral protein.

Further insight may be gained by multiple passage experiments. Viruses could be passed through a sequence of hosts with either the same or varying MHC genotypes. The changing frequencies of amino acid substitutions could be tracked under different regimes of fluctuating selection.

14.6 Problems for Future Research

1. Immunodominance and timing of epitope expression. Infected cells express different pathogen proteins at different times. Proteins expressed relatively early may be more likely to attract a dominant CTL response because they occur on the cell surface for longer periods of time. The role of timing could be studied in the following experimental evolution design.

Create a host with a biclonal TCR repertoire focused on two different pathogen epitopes, one expressed early and the other expressed late. Also create two different hosts with monoclonal TCRs, one focused on the early epitope and the other focused on the late epitope. Finally, create a host immunodeficient in CTL response. Infect the four different host types with cloned genotypes of a pathogen. If early expressed epitopes attract stronger CTL responses, then the biclonal host should induce fewer escape substitutions in the late expressed epitope than the monoclonal host focused on the late epitope. The relative escape rates in the monoclonal hosts focused on early and late epitopes calibrate escape rates in the absence of competition between epitopes.

A similar design may be accomplished by using different host MHC genotypes to turn on or off the pressure on epitopes expressed at different times.

2. Immunodominance and probability of escape. Pressure from a single kind of MAb often gives rise to antibody escape mutants. By contrast, simultaneous pressure from two or more MAbs can prevent spread of escape substitutions because a pathogen needs to escape simultaneously from multiple killing agents. A similar experiment can be developed for CTLs by using different MHC host genotypes. In experimental evolution studies, hosts that can effectively present a broader variety of epitopes should restrict the spread of escape substitutions relative to hosts with narrower presentation.

3. Performance versus avoiding MHC recognition. Substitutions that avoid MHC recognition may reduce other components of fitness. This hypothesis can be tested by evolving pathogens in different regimes of MHC-mediated selection and then competing the evolved pathogens to determine relative fitness. In this design, one starts with a cloned pathogen genotype. Some lineages can be passaged in a sequence of hosts with the same MHC genotype, others in hosts with varying MHC genotypes, and controls in hosts immunodeficient for CTL response. Competition between various pairs of evolved pathogens can be used to estimate the fitness costs of substitutions that avoid MHC recognition.

Some sites may have the potential to abrogate MHC recognition but fail to acquire escape substitutions during experimental evolution. Nonvarying sites may identify key functional residues. This can be tested by site-directed mutagenesis.

4. Spread of TCR escape substitutions between hosts. Klenerman and Zinkernagel (1998) demonstrated original antigenic sin of TCR escape mutants in LCMV. To simplify a bit, suppose epitope B is a TCR escape variant derived from epitope A. If a host is first exposed to epitope A, subsequent exposure to epitope B tends to reinforce the response against epitope A. Similarly, hosts initially exposed to B, then challenged with A, enhance their response to the first epitope, B. Thus, memory tends to recall TCRs to previous, cross-reacting epitopes.

This memory effect may influence the spread of TCR escape substitutions within a population. To study the evolutionary consequences, an experimental evolution design could follow the fate of particular substitutions through serial passage in hosts with various histories of prior exposure. For example, what sort of evolutionary response would occur in a series of hosts each previously exposed to epitope A? Each previously exposed to epitope B? What about a sequence of hosts with varying exposure histories?

5. Altered peptide ligands. The affinity and kinetics of TCR binding to peptide-MHC ligands influences regulatory control of CTL clones (Davis et al. 1998; Germain and Štefanová 1999). Variant epitopes present altered peptide ligands (APLs) to the TCR. It may be that APLs can interfere with CTL attack by preventing expansion of CTLs with matching TCR specificities. Experimental evolution may favor APLs that interfere with CTL attack. APL variants could be measured for binding properties to TCRs (Tissot et al. 2000) and tendency to spread under various experimental conditions.

6. Dependence of TCR escape on TCR germline genes. Germline genes recombine to make diverse TCRs. The role of the germline genotype in the TCR repertoire could be studied by selecting for TCR escape mutants in hosts with different TCR germline genotypes.

7. Laboratory adaptation. Experimental evolution creates adaptations to the particular in vitro or in vivo laboratory conditions. These conditions only partially reflect selection in the wild. Laboratory studies provide an opportunity to relate biochemical mechanism to kinetics, and kinetics to fitness. Mathematical models aid the controlled, experimental dissection of these relations (Nowak and May 2000). Controlled analysis must be complemented by study of variation and adaptation in natural isolates. The next chapter discusses aspects of natural variation.

15

Measuring Selection with Population Samples

Experimental evolution provides insight into kinetic and mechanistic aspects of parasite escape from host immunity. Such experimental studies clarify selective forces that influence change at certain amino acid sites. But experimental studies provide only a hint of what actually occurs in natural populations, in which selective pressures and evolutionary dynamics differ significantly from those in controlled laboratory studies. It is important to combine experimental insights with analyses of variation in natural populations. In this chapter, I discuss how population samples of nucleotide sequences provide information about natural selection of antigenic variation.

I focus on themes directly related to the goal of this book—the synthesis between different kinds of biological analyses. In particular, I show how analysis of population samples complements studies of molecular structure and experimental evolution. Several books and articles review the methods to analyze population samples and the many different types of applications (Kimura 1983; Nei 1987; Nee et al. 1995; Hillis et al. 1996; Li 1997; Page and Holmes 1998; Crandall 1999; Hughes 1999; Nei and Kumar 2000; Otto 2000; Rodrigo and Learn 2000; Yang and Bielawski 2000; Bush 2001; Overbaugh and Bangham 2001).

The first section describes how different kinds of natural selection cause different patterns of nucleotide substitutions. Thus, the pattern of nucleotide substitutions observed in a population sample of sequences can sometimes be used to infer the kind of selection. The simplest pattern concerns the number of nucleotide changes that cause an amino acid substitution (nonsynonymous) relative to the number of nucleotide changes that do not cause an amino acid substitution (synonymous). If natural selection does not affect the relative success of amino acid variants, then nonsynonymous and synonymous nucleotide substitutions occur at the same rate. An excess of nonsynonymous substitutions suggests that natural selection favored those changes, providing evidence for positive selection of amino acid replacements.

The second section presents two examples of positive selection on parasite antigens. The surface antigen Tams1 of the protozoan *Theileria annulata* induces a strong antibody response in cattle, its primary host. A sample of nucleotide sequences showed that strong positive selection occurred in a few small regions of the Tams1 antigen, suggesting that those regions have been under strong selection for escape from host immunity. The group A streptococci cause sporadic epidemics of "strep throat." Streptococcal inhibitor of complement (Sic) is the most variable protein of these bacteria. In a sample of 892 nucleotide sequences, 77 of 86 nucleotide changes caused amino acid substitutions, a large excess of nonsynonymous substitutions. Very strong natural selection by host antibodies apparently drives rapid change in Sic.

The third section continues with more examples of positive selection on parasite antigens. These examples improve on earlier studies by estimating the rates of synonymous and nonsynonymous nucleotide changes for each individual amino acid. This is important because an epitope often requires only one or two amino acid changes to escape from binding by a specific antibody or T cell. Identification of particular amino acid sites under strong selection can confirm predictions for the location of epitopes based on structural data and experimental analysis of escape mutants. Positively selected sites can also suggest the location of new epitopes not found by other methods and provide clues about which amino acid variants should be included in multicomponent vaccines.

The fourth section turns to recent studies of influenza A that correlate amino acid changes at positively selected sites with the subsequent success of the lineage. This correlation between substitutions and fitness provides an opportunity to predict future evolution—new variants arising at positively selected sites are predicted to be the progenitors of future lineages. Yearly influenza A isolates from 1983 to 1997 provided sequences on which to test this prediction method retrospectively. In nine of eleven years, the changes at positively selected sites predicted which lineage would give rise to the future influenza population.

The final section highlights some topics for future research.

15.1 Kinds of Natural Selection

Different kinds of natural selection leave different patterns of nucleotide substitutions. These patterns can be observed in a sample of sequences isolated from a population, allowing one to infer the type of selection.

SYNONYMOUS AND NONSYNONYMOUS NUCLEOTIDE SUBSTITUTIONS

The genetic code maps three sequential nucleotides (a codon) to a single amino acid or to a stop signal. The four different nucleotides combine to make $4^3 = 64$ different codons. The 64 codons specify 20 different amino acids plus a stop signal, leading to an average of $64/21 \approx 3$ different codons for each amino acid or stop signal. This degenerate aspect of the code means that some nucleotide substitutions do not change the encoded amino acid or stop signal.

Nucleotide substitutions that do not cause an amino acid change are called *synonymous;* those that do change the encoded amino acid are called *nonsynonymous.* Synonymous substitutions do not affect the amino acid sequence and therefore should not be affected by natural selection of phenotype. By contrast, nonsynonymous substitutions can be affected by selection because they do change the encoded protein. If there is no selection on proteins, then the same forces of mutation and random sampling influence all nucleotide changes, causing the rate of nonsynonymous substitutions, d_N, to equal the rate of synonymous substitutions, d_S (Nei 1987; Li 1997; Page and Holmes 1998).

POSITIVE AND NEGATIVE SELECTION

When natural selection favors change in amino acids, the nonsynonymous substitution rate d_N rises. Thus, $d_N > d_S$ measured in a sample of sequences implies that natural selection has favored evolutionary change. This contribution of selection to the rate of amino acid change above the background measured by d_S is called *positive selection.* Parasite epitopes often show signs of positive selection as they change to escape recognition by host immunity (Yang and Bielawski 2000).

By contrast, negative selection removes amino acid changes, preserving the amino acid sequence against the spread of mutations. Negative selection reduces the nonsynonymous substitution rate, causing $d_N < d_S$.

The great majority of sequences show negative selection, suggesting that most amino acid replacements are deleterious and are removed by natural selection. In cases where positive selection does occur, the nonsynonymous replacements often cluster on protein surfaces involved in some sort of specific recognition. In these positively selected proteins, amino acid sites structurally hidden from external recognition often show the typical signs of negative selection (see references in the introduction to this chapter).

FREQUENCY-DEPENDENT SELECTION

A rare antigenic variant has an advantage because it avoids immune memory in hosts induced by more common variants. This is an example in which the success of an allele depends on its frequency, a kind of frequency-dependent selection (Conway 1997).

Selection favoring rare types can cause two different patterns of evolutionary change. First, transient polymorphisms may arise, in which novel variants increase when rare and eventually dominate the population, driving out the previous variants. This reduces genetic variation at all nucleotide sites linked to the favored substitution.

Second, balanced polymorphisms may occur, in which rare variants increase but then are held in check as they rise in frequency. This protects genetic variants from extinction because they rise when rare but decline when common. Nucleotide sites linked to those sites under selection also enjoy protection against extinction because they receive a selective boost whenever they become rare. This increases genetic variation at all nucleotide sites linked to the site under selection. Thus, transient polymorphisms decrease genetic variation in sequences linked to a favored site, and balanced polymorphisms increase genetic variation in sequences linked to a favored site.

15.2 Positive Selection to Avoid Host Recognition

Many examples of positive selection come from genes involved in host-parasite recognition (Endo et al. 1996; Hughes 1999; Yang and Bielawski 2000). These sequence analyses provide information about how selection has shaped the structure and function of proteins. For example, one may combine analysis of positive selection with structural data to determine which sites are exposed to antibody pressure. In the absence of structural data, sequences can be used to predict which sites are structurally exposed and can change and which sites are either not exposed or functionally constrained. I briefly summarize a few cases in this section.

THEILERIA ANNULATA

The tick-borne protozoan *Theileria annulata* causes disease in cattle (Gubbels et al. 2000). The surface antigen Tams1 induces a strong antibody response and has been considered a candidate for developing a vaccine. However, Tams1 varies antigenically; thus studies have focused on the molecular nature of the variability to gain further insight. The structure and function of Tams1 have not been determined.

Recently, Gubbels et al. (2000) analyzed a population sample of nucleotide sequences to predict which domains of Tams1 change in response to host immunity and which domains do not vary because of structural or functional constraints. They found seven domains with elevated rates of nonsynonymous substitutions compared with synonymous substitutions (fig. 15.1), suggesting that these regions may be exposed to antibody pressure. Some domains had relatively little nonsynonymous change, indicating that structural or functional constraints preserve amino acid sequence. These inferences provide guidance in vaccine design and point to testable hypotheses about antigenicity and structure.

GROUP A STREPTOCOCCI

Group A streptococci (GAS) infect the upper respiratory tract of humans, causing "strep throat." GAS epidemics develop quickly and typically last one to three years (Martin and Single 1993; Muotiala et al. 1997). Streptococcal inhibitor of complement (Sic) is the most variable protein of GAS (Hoe et al. 1999). This extracellular protein interferes with the host's complement system of immunity, a key defense against invading bacteria.

Hoe et al. (1999) sequenced the *sic* gene in 892 GAS isolates. These sequences had insertions, deletions, and nonsynonymous substitutions that encode 158 variant Sic proteins. Of the single nucleotide changes, 77 of 86 caused amino acid substitutions (nonsynonymous), demonstrating strong positive selection.

Figure 15.2 shows the phylogenetic relationship between sequences from Ontario, Canada, in 1996. Most variants could be linked to each

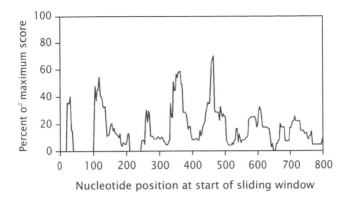

Figure 15.1   The seven peaks identify the major regions of positive selection in the Tams1 protein. The eighteen sequences analyzed in this figure have about 870 nucleotides. The analysis focused on a sliding window (Endo et al. 1996) of 60 nucleotides (20 amino acids). For each window shown on the x axis, the numbers of nonsynonymous and synonymous nucleotide substitutions were calculated by comparing the eighteen sequences. The y axis shows the strength of positive selection measured as follows. For each window of 60 nucleotides, each pair of sequences was compared. Each paired comparison was scored for the statistical significance of positive selection based on the numbers of nonsynonymous and synonymous changes between the pair, with a score of zero for nonsignificant, a score of one for significant, and a score of two for highly significant. The maximum score is twice the number of comparisons; the actual score is the sum of significance values for each comparison; and the percentage of the maximum is the actual divided by the maximum multiplied by 100. From Gubbels et al. (2000), with permission of Elsevier Science.

other by a small number of changes, as shown in the figure. The starlike shape of the phylogeny suggests that the isolates diverged rapidly from a common ancestor during the course of the local epidemic. This rapid divergence implies very strong selection for change, most likely caused by escape from host antibodies (Hoe et al. 1999).

15.3 Phylogenetic Analysis of Nucleotide Substitutions

Initial studies of selection often used small numbers of sequences, typically fewer than one hundred. Small sample sizes required aggregating observations across all nucleotide sites to gain sufficient statistical power. Conclusions focused on whether selection was positive, negative, or neutral when averaged over all sites. With slightly larger samples, one could do a sliding window analysis as in figure 15.1 to in-

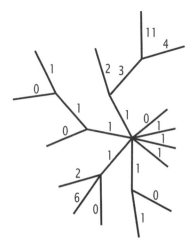

Figure 15.2 Phylogeny for Group A streptococcal *sic* alleles from a local epidemic in Ontario, Canada. Each tip corresponds to one isolate. The numbers on each branch indicate the number of molecular differences between each node. From Hoe et al. (1999), with permission of *Nature Medicine*.

fer the kind of selection averaged over sets of amino acids that occur contiguously in the two-dimensional sequence (Endo et al. 1996).

We have seen throughout this book that major changes in binding and antigenicity often require only one or a few amino acid changes. The analytical methods that aggregate over whole sequences or sliding windows often fail to detect selection at the scale of single-site substitutions, which appears to be the proper scale for understanding antigenic evolution.

Recently, larger samples of sequences have provided the opportunity to study the rates of synonymous and nonsynonymous substitutions at individual nucleotide sites. Each individual substitution occurs within a lineal history of descent, that is, a change occurs between parent and offspring. To study each substitution directly, one must first arrange a sample of sequences into lineal relationships by building a phylogenetic tree. From the tree, one can infer the nucleotide sequence of ancestors, and therefore trace the history of each nucleotide change through time.

Each nucleotide change can be classified as synonymous or nonsynonymous. For each amino acid site, one can sum up the numbers of synonymous and nonsynonymous nucleotide changes across the entire phylogeny and derive the associated rates of change. With appropriate statistics, one determines for each amino acid site whether nonsynonymous changes occur significantly more or less often than synonymous changes (Hasegawa et al. 1993; Wakely 1993; Bush et al. 1999; Meyer et al. 1999; Suzuki and Gojobori 1999; Yang and Bielawski 2000; Bush 2001).

The concepts of measuring positive and negative selection remain the same. However, for the first time, the statistical power has been raised to the point where analysis of population samples provides significant insight into the evolution of antigens. The power derives from studying the relative success of alternate amino acids at a single site. Important selective forces include the amino acids at other sites as well as binding properties to host immune molecules and other host receptors.

HIV

Yamaguchi-Kabata and Gojobori (2000) analyzed selection on individual amino acid sites in gp120, the major exposed glycoprotein on the HIV-1 envelope. gp120 contains the primary host-cell receptor that binds to the host's CD4 molecules on the surfaces of various immune cells. gp120 also has the secondary host-cell receptor that binds either the host's CCR5 or CXCR4 molecules—the viral binding specificity for these second receptors determines the kinds of host immune cells infected by the virus. gp120 carries major antibody epitopes as well as CTL epitopes.

Yamaguchi-Kabata and Gojobori (2000) studied amino acid variations at 422 sites in 186 sequences of HIV-1 subtype B. Significant positive selection occurred at 33 sites, and significant negative selection occurred at 63 sites. As with most proteins, negative selection or no apparent selection dominated over the whole sequence, with positive selection limited to a minority of sites.

Previous work had split the linear amino acid sequence into five variable and five constant domains based on the inferred tendency for genetic variation in each region (Modrow et al. 1987). The variable domains mostly occur in exposed loops, whereas the constant regions mostly occur in a core that may be partly protected.

Yamaguchi-Kabata and Gojobori (2000) found that, when analyzing selection on individual amino acids, sites in the variable domains did have a relatively greater tendency to be positively rather than negatively selected. By contrast, those sites in the constant domains had a relatively greater tendency to be negatively rather than positively selected. However, many positively selected sites occurred in the constant domains.

Yamaguchi-Kabata and Gojobori (2000) focused on individual sites with regard to location on the three-dimensional structure and in relation to potential selective pressures. For example, fifteen of the thirty-three positively selected sites clustered on the face of the gp120 core opposite the CD4 binding site. Seven of these sites occurred in positions 335–347, which form an α-helix that is alternately exposed on the surface and hidden in the core. The positively selected sites occurred at exposed positions, whereas three of the interior sites were highly conserved although they lacked elevated ratios of synonymous to nonsynonymous substitutions.

The other positively selected sites in this region also occurred on the exposed surface near the 335–347 α-helix. These other sites had dispersed sequence locations ranging from positions 291 to 446 that are brought together in the three-dimensional structure. Yamaguchi-Kabata and Gojobori (2000) propose that this cluster of fifteen positively selected sites may form discontinuous epitopes. Previously, this partially recessed region was not considered a key location for antibody binding.

Foot-and-Mouth Disease Virus

Haydon et al. (2001) analyzed selection on individual amino acid sites of foot-and-mouth disease virus. Most sites showed mild to strong negative selection, as usually occurs. At seventeen sites they found evidence of significant positive selection. Twelve of these positively selected sites occurred at positions that had previously been observed to develop escape mutants in experimental evolution studies that imposed pressure by monoclonal antibodies. The other five sites indicate candidates for further experimental analysis.

Haydon et al.'s (2001) study of natural isolates gives further evidence that a small number of amino acid sites determines a large fraction of antigenic evolution to escape antibody recognition. The combination of analyses on structure, experimental evolution, and natural variation provide an opportunity to study how complex evolutionary forces together determine the evolutionary dynamics of particular amino acids.

15.4 Predicting Evolution

The studies on positive selection in the previous section could not correlate amino acid substitutions with the actual success of the viruses. In each case, selection was inferred strictly from the patterns of nucleotide substitutions in a sample of sequences.

Bush et al.'s (1999) study of influenza takes the next step by associating particular amino acid substitutions with the success or failure of descendants that carry the substitutions. Influenza allows such studies because sequences have been collected each year over the past several decades, providing a history of which substitutions have led to success over time.

The influenza data can be used to predict future evolution by two steps. First, previous patterns of substitutions and the successes of associated lineages suggest which amino acid sites contain variants that enhance fitness. Second, new variants arising at those key sites are predicted to be the progenitors of future lineages.

THE SHAPE OF PHYLOGENIES

Predicting evolution based on amino acid substitutions requires a correlation between substitutions and the success of lineages. Many parasites do not have such broad-scale correlations. For example, figure 15.2 shows a star-shaped phylogeny for streptococcal divergence. This kind of phylogeny retains multiple, diverging lineages along several branches. Although selection may guide the relative success of different substitutions within a lineage, the lineages along different branches apparently do not compete. Thus, one cannot use particular substitutions to predict which lineages will eventually dominate the future population.

HIV-1 also has multiple diverging lineages that create star-shaped phylogenies (fig. 15.3). This makes sense because HIV-1 currently forms an expanding population with little competition between lineages. Many different lineages continue to spread to naive hosts that have no prior immune memory of infection. Thus, at the population level, immune pressure does not favor one lineage over another by amino acid substitutions that escape widely dispersed immune memory in hosts.

In the HIV-1 phylogeny, the different subtypes coalesce to a common ancestor that probably occurred near the origin of the HIV-1 epidemic

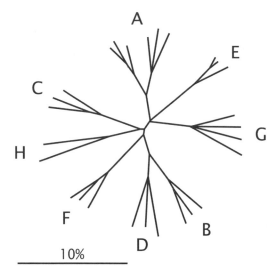

Figure 15.3   The phylogeny of the HIV-1 subtypes based on the *env* gene, which includes the coding for the gp120 protein. The letters name the different subtypes. The bar shows the length along branches corresponding to 10% divergence in sequence. From McCutchan (1999), with permission from Johns Hopkins University Press.

in humans. Various studies estimate that the ancestor occurred during the first half of the twentieth century (Korber et al. 2000; Yusim et al. 2001).

Comparison of HIV-1 subtypes may not be the appropriate scale at which to study the correlation between amino acid substitutions and fitness. The subtypes are to some extent separated geographically and may not compete directly. Even within regions, HIV-1 continues to spread to naive hosts, so escape from immune memory at a few key antibody epitopes would not dominate the relative success of lineages. It would be interesting to see the shapes of HIV-1 phylogenies based on samples collected over several years from a single region.

Figure 15.4 shows the kinds of phylogenetic shapes that may occur. Only the extreme case in figure 15.4d provides enough differential success (fitness) between lineages to correlate amino acid substitutions with fitness. In the other shapes, the signal of differential success would usually not be strong enough to associate particular substitutions with the survival of a lineage. However, the dominance of a single lineage as in figure 15.4d does not guarantee an association between success and any

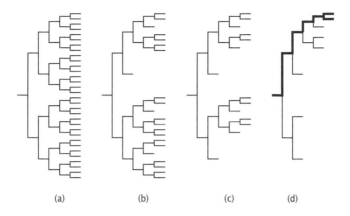

Figure 15.4   Differences in success between lineages in a phylogeny influence the shape of the tree. All trees shown with their ancestral node on the left. Time increases from left to right. (a) Shape when all lineages survive. This corresponds to a star phylogeny when drawn as in fig. 15.3 with lineages radiating out from the ancestor in the center of the phylogeny. (b) Tips that stop in the middle of the tree represent lineages that have gone extinct. Some extinctions occur in this case, but many different lineages have survived to the present. (c) Greater differential success between lineages; however, no single winner emerges in any time period. (d) Only a single lineage survives over time, shown in bold. In each time period, a single lineage gives rise to all survivors a few generations into the future.

particular characteristic of the parasite. Powerful epidemics that start from just a few individuals also give rise to skewed phylogenetic trees, but the progenitors of those epidemics may simply have been lucky and may show no tendency to carry particular traits.

INFLUENZA

Influenza A phylogenies have just the sort of shape that could allow correlation between particular substitutions and fitness. The trees in figure 15.5 show a single successful lineage continuing through time, with many branches diverging and dying off over short periods of time.

Bush et al. (1999) used trees such as those in figure 15.5 to analyze amino acid substitutions in the hemagglutinin HA1 domain. They assigned each variable amino acid site to zero or more of four different sets: 18 sites were positively selected with d_N significantly greater than d_S, 16 sites were associated with the receptor binding site of the HA1

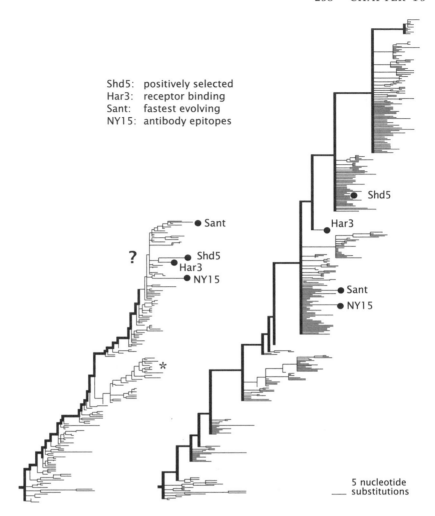

Shd5: positively selected
Har3: receptor binding
Sant: fastest evolving
NY15: antibody epitopes

Figure 15.5 Phylogeny of influenza A hemagglutinin HA1 domain. The tree on the left shows evolutionary relationships between isolates from subtype H3 from 1983 to 1994. The horizontal axis measures the number of nucleotide substitutions between isolates, which correlates closely with time. Thus, the lower isolates come from earlier seasons, with time increasing up and to the right. The bold line shows the single lineage that succeeded through time. The asterisk shows another lineage that succeeded for about five years after its divergence from the main line, but eventually died out. See the text for a description of the labeled isolates (filled circles) and how the left tree was used to predict evolution in the upper part of the right tree, which contains the data from 1983 to 1994 plus three additional years from 1994 to 1997. From Bush et al. (1999), with permission from the American Association for the Advancement of Science.

surface, 20 sites evolved relatively faster than the other sites, and 41 sites were in or near the well-known antibody epitope domains A and B.

Suppose amino acid changes in one of the four sets consistently correlated with the ultimate success of a lineage. Then, at any time, one could predict which of the currently circulating isolates would be most closely related to the progenitor of future lineages. In particular, those lineages with the most amino acids that had recently changed at the key sites would be most likely to succeed. In influenza, success probably occurs by escaping the host's immunological antibody memory caused by recent epidemics.

Variant sites near key antibody epitopes would be good candidates to produce antibody escape. However, Bush et al. (1999) found that the variant amino acids at positively selected sites provided the best information about future success. In other words, those sites with amino acid replacements favored by selection in the past also provided the best information about which amino acid changes would lead to success in the future.

Bush et al. (1999) did not truly predict future evolution. Instead, they used data from 1983 to 1997 to form eleven retrospective tests. A retrospective test analyzed data from 1983 to year x and predicted subsequent evolution in the years following x, where x varied between 1986 and 1997.

Figure 15.5 shows the structure of one retrospective comparison. The left tree contains data from 1983 to 1994. The bold line along the left marks the single dominant "trunk" lineage. At the question mark, just before 1994, the data can no longer resolve the trunk lineage because several variants cocirculated at that time and the trunk can be resolved only after one knows which of those lineages succeeded.

The filled circles show four isolates from 1994 that represented the four classifications for variable amino acids. Shd5 (A/Shangdong/5/94) represented the lineage with the greatest number of recent amino acid changes at sites that had been positively selected in the past, as inferred from the 1983–1997 data. The Har3 (A/Harbin/3/94) lineage had variant amino acids near the receptor binding site. The Sant (A/Santiago/7198/94) lineage had variant amino acids at those sites that had evolved rapidly in the past. The NY15 (A/New York/15/94) lineage had variant sites in or near antibody epitopes A and B.

The right tree includes additional data from 1994 to 1997. Those data show which of the 1994 lineages succeeded and which died out. Successful prediction means choosing the isolate closest on the tree (most alike genetically) with the lineage that continues along the trunk and gives rise to the future population. It turned out that Shd5 was closest to the successful trunk lineage among the candidates. In other words, the most changes in previously positively selected sites predicted which lineage succeeded in subsequent years.

Bush et al. (1999) reported a systematic analysis of retrospective tests in eleven years. In nine of those eleven years, the lineage that contained the most changes relative to its ancestor at the eighteen positively selected sites identified the section of the tree from which the future trunk emerged. The sites in the antibody epitopes only identified seven of eleven trunk lineages, and the other amino acid sets did worse. Thus, positive selection provided the best signal for which amino acid changes correlated most closely with fitness.

Foot-and-Mouth Disease Virus

Feigelstock et al. (1996) sequenced foot-and-mouth disease virus isolates from a 1993–94 epidemic in Argentina. The epidemic strains contained amino acid replacements at a small number of sites that had previously been identified as crucial for escape from monoclonal antibodies. Feigelstock et al. (1996) suggested a prediction method similar to the one used by Bush et al. (1999): identify those few key amino acid sites that correlate with fitness, then predict that lineages with changes at those sites will be likely candidates to spread in the future.

Feigelstock et al. (1996) chose sites by previous reports of escape from monoclonal antibodies in experimental evolution. Bush et al. (1999) chose sites by analysis of positive selection from population samples. It would be interesting to compare these two methods in a single study of the same evolving parasite population.

15.5 Problems for Future Research

1. Episodic selection. Bush et al. (1999) found eighteen amino acid sites under positive selection in subtype H3 of influenza A. Substitutions at these positively selected sites correlated with the future success of

MEASURING SELECTION · 261

lineages during the years of sampling, 1983–1997. In the future, will these eighteen sites continue to be the primary target of selection?

On the one hand, the eighteen sites may indeed be the most important for escape from protective antibodies. If so, future samples will continue to find positive selection focused on these sites. On the other hand, different sites may dominate in the future, with little future selective change in the currently positively selected sites. A changing focus of selection may arise from evolving structural features of the viral surface that expose or hide different sites or from a changed distribution in the immune memory profiles of hosts.

If episodic selection frequently occurs, then the time scale over which one studies substitution patterns plays a critical role in inference. Simply measuring aggregate rates of synonymous and nonsynonymous substitutions may turn out to be a rather crude tool that misses a large proportion of the changes brought about by natural selection. As more data accumulate, it will become important to match statistical methods with explicit hypotheses about the biological processes of selection and the temporal scale over which selection varies.

2. Kinds of selection detectable from standard analyses of population samples. Influenza has certain characters that make it a particularly good model for simple analysis of positive selection. Epidemic strains often have wide distribution; thus, there is relatively less spatial variation in the exposure of hosts to different strains than for many other parasites. The wide and relatively uniform distribution of epidemics creates relatively uniform selective pressure on the virus. In addition, infections do not persist within hosts, so most selective pressure on the surface hemagglutinin glycoprotein arises by escape from antibody recognition during transmission between hosts. The uniformity of selective pressure means that aggregate samples can provide clear signals.

By contrast, other parasites may face multiple selective pressures that vary over relatively small spatial and temporal scales. For example, Rouzine and Coffin (1999) analyzed 213 *pro* sequences of HIV-1 from eleven infected individuals. This sampling scheme allowed them to analyze the different patterns of selection within hosts and between hosts. This may be particularly important in HIV, which causes long, persistent infections within hosts. HIV probably faces relatively little pressure from immune memory during transmission between hosts, but does experience different MHC genotypes between hosts and different selective pressures on T cell epitopes.

Rouzine and Coffin (1999) found evidence only for negative selection within hosts. They propose various models of selection within and between hosts that could be tested by further sampling and analysis. The point here is that a simple aggregation of sequences over the entire population may not be informative given the different kinds of selection that act over various temporal and spatial scales.

3. Sampling methods to collect sequences. I mentioned in the *Problems for Future Research* section of chapter 11 that most population samples have been collected for reasons other than phylogenetic analysis. For example, each year epidemic surveillance teams collect thousands of influenza isolates from across the world. Sequencing labs choose only a small fraction of the isolates for analysis. They typically use antigenic screening to pick isolates that differ significantly from the common, recently circulating strains. This biased sampling supports vaccine design but may affect analyses of selection and other population-level processes. Recent calls for wider and better-designed sampling should lead to great opportunities for population studies (Layne et al. 2001).

Nonlinear processes of transmission and stochastic effects of small effective population sizes in epidemics strongly influence the patterns of evolutionary change. Random sampling may not be the best design for studying the population consequences of nonlinear transmission and stochastic fluctuations. New theoretical work on sampling and inference would help to guide the advanced screening and analysis technologies that will be put in place in the coming years.

4. Selection on archival variants. Several parasites such as *Trypanosoma brucei* and *Borrelia hermsii* store archival libraries of antigenic variants. They express only one variant at a time. Strong positive selection probably favored diversification of the archival variants during the initial evolution of antigenic switching. However, once a genome contains a large library of diverged variants, negative selection may act primarily to retain the existing antigenic differences between the variants.

I found only one analysis of archival variants. Rich et al. (2001) studied one sequence from each of eleven different loci that contain antigenic variants of the variable short protein (Vsp) of *Borrelia hermsii*. This sample showed significant recombination between the loci, suggesting that divergence between antigenic variants may arise by intragenomic mixing of protein domains. Their sampling did not provide multiple alleles at individual loci, so they did not report on the selective pressures recently acting on each individual locus. An extended study that analyzed variation within and between loci would be interesting.

5. Inferring selection from the spatial distribution of allele frequencies. Rare antigenic variants often have an advantage because they encounter specific immune memory less often than common antigens. Conway (1997) suggested that this rare-type advantage promotes a balanced distribution of allele frequencies among antigenic variants. By this theory, such balancing selection reduces the fluctuations in allele frequencies when compared with loci experiencing little or no selection. The neutral loci would have allele frequencies drifting over time and space, whereas the balanced antigenic loci would face a continual pressure to raise any allele frequency that temporarily dropped to a low level.

Conway (1997) suggested that one could infer which loci experienced strong immune selection by examining the spatial distribution of allele frequencies. Balancing selection may cause immune-selected loci to have a more even, less variable distribution of allele frequencies across space than other loci.

Conway et al. (2000) tested this idea by examining the spatial distribution of allele frequencies for Msp1, a dominant surface protein of *Plasmodium falciparum*. They divided the long (5 kb) *msp1* gene into domains and measured the allele frequencies for each domain over six African and two Southeast Asian populations. Recombination occurs frequently within the gene, causing low linkage disequilibrium between domains. One domain, *block 2*, had very even distributions of its three allelic types over the different populations within each continent. The other domains all had significant variations in allele frequency over the populations. Conway et al. (2000) also showed that hosts with IgG antibodies against block 2 enjoyed some protection against malaria. From these data, Conway et al. (2000) concluded that *block 2* is an important antigenic site.

Conway et al.'s (2000) spatial analysis of allele frequencies provides an interesting approach to identifying key antigenic sites. However, the theoretical prediction of relatively stable allele frequencies over space requires further study.

Frequency dependence with an advantage for rare types commonly occurs in models of host-parasite interactions (Anderson and May 1991). In the typical model, frequency dependence causes strong fluctuations in allele frequencies rather than stable allele frequencies. The fluctuations arise because of feedbacks between host and parasite types. A rare parasite type, x, increases because most hosts do not recognize the rare type. As x increases in frequency, this favors an increase in the frequency of the hosts that recognize x, causing in turn a decline in the frequency of x. The decline in x favors a loss of host recognition for x. Low frequencies of x and of host recognition start the cycle again.

Conway (1997) suggested that frequency dependence stabilizes allele frequencies rather than causes enhanced fluctuations. This may be true for the particular dynamics that follow from *Plasmodium* demography and the time course of host immune memory. However, this should be studied with theoretical models that analyze fluctuations over space in antigenic allele frequencies and host memory profiles.

16

Recap of Some Interesting Problems

My *Problems for Future Research* span many different technical and conceptual challenges for understanding antigenic variation. These fifty-six problems arise from my synthesis of the molecular processes of recognition, the dynamics of infections within hosts, the variability of populations, and the methods for studying evolution.

There is no point in covering once again so many diverse topics. Instead, I have chosen to recap four examples, to highlight the kinds of problems that integrate different levels of analysis. I summarize each example briefly, as a reminder of the potential for integrating structure, function, biochemical kinetics, population dynamics, and evolution.

16.1 Population-Level Explanation for Low Molecular Variability

Immune memory against the measles virus provides lifelong protection because the measles virus does not evolve widespread escape variants. Measles can vary its dominant surface antigen, hemagglutinin, and limited variation does occur (Griffin 2001). So it is an interesting puzzle why antigenic variants do not spread as in many other viruses.

Perhaps the very high infectiousness of measles causes the common strain to spread so widely in the host population that little heterogeneity occurs among hosts in immune memory profiles. If memory responds against a few different epitopes, then no single-step mutational change allows a measles variant to spread between previously infected hosts. The only "nearby" susceptible class of hosts arises from the influx of naive newborns, which depends on the birthrate of the host population. Naive hosts do not impose selective pressure for antigenic change.

This explanation for the lack of antigenic variation suggests that the epidemiological properties of the parasite and the demographic structure of the hosts affect the patterns of molecular variation in antigens. These population processes do not control the possible types of variation or the molecular recognition between host and parasite, but instead shape the actual distribution of variants.

A population-level explanation for the measles virus's lack of widespread antigenic variation may be wrong. The lack of variation may simply reflect conservation of some essential viral function in a dominant antigen, such as binding to host receptors. My point here is that the lack of molecular variation does not necessarily mean that the explanation resides at the molecular level. Population processes can strongly influence the distribution of molecular variants.

16.2 Molecular-Level Explanation for Population Dynamics

The causal chain can move in the other direction, from the molecular nature of host-parasite recognition to the dynamics of populations. For example, five or so amino acids determine most of the binding energy between an antibody and an antigen. Often a single amino acid substitution in the antigen can abolish the defensive capability of a particular antibody specificity for a matching epitope. This type of recognition is qualitative, in which a single change determines whether or not recognition occurs.

Binding reactions may change in a qualitative way between molecular variants. But the dynamics of an infection within a host depend on all of the parasite's epitopes and all of the specific B and T cell lineages that recognize different epitopes. The interactions within the host between the population of parasites and the populations of different immune cells determine immunodominance, the number of different epitopes that stimulate a strong immune response.

Immunodominance sets the number of amino acid substitutions needed to avoid host recognition. This aggregate recognition at the level of individual hosts controls the spread of antigenic variants through a population of previously exposed hosts. Thus, molecular interactions affect immunodominance, and immunodominance sets the pace of evolutionary change and the distribution of variants in parasite populations.

16.3 Binding Kinetics and the Dynamics of Immunodominance

The control of immunodominance remains poorly understood. Rao's (1999) analyses suggest the kinds of studies that may generate new insight. Rao showed that initial stimulation of B cells depended on an affinity window for binding between antibodies and epitopes. Low-affinity binding did not stimulate division of B cell lineages, whereas high-affinity antibodies bound the antigen so effectively that the B cell receptors received little stimulation. Intermediate affinity provided the strongest stimulation for initial expansion of B cell clones.

After initial stimulation and production of IgM, the next phase of B cell competition occurs during affinity maturation and the shift to IgG production. The B cell receptors with the highest on-rates of binding for antigen tended to win the race to pass through affinity maturation. The limiting step may be competition for stimulation by helper T cells. This competition for T cell help apparently depends on the rate at which B cells acquire antigens rather than on the equilibrium affinity of binding to antigens.

Equilibrium affinity is the ratio of the rate at which bonds form (on-rate) to the rate at which bonds break (off-rate). The contrast between the early selection of equilibrium affinity (on:off ratio) and the later selection of on-rate may provide insight into the structural features of binding that separately control on-rates and off-rates. This is a superb opportunity to relate structure to function via the kinetic processes that regulate the immune response.

16.4 Diversity and Regulation of Archival Repertoires

Some parasites store archival libraries of antigenic variants in their genomes. Switching expression between variants may allow the parasite to escape recognition by immune responses directed at previously expressed variants. Alternatively, a sequence of variants may exploit the mechanisms of immune recognition and regulation to interfere with the ability of the host to mount new responses to variants expressed later in the sequence. Variants can potentially interfere with new host responses by exploiting original antigenic sin—the tendency of the host to enhance a cross-reactive response to a previously encountered antigen instead of generating a new and more focused response to a novel variant.

The interesting problem concerns the evolution of the archival repertoire. How do the different molecular mechanisms of escape and immune interference shape the diversity and cross-reactivity of variants stored within each parasite's genome?

The type of immune recognition may influence the pattern of diversification between antigenic variants. For example, IgM antibodies with relatively low affinity and high cross-reactivity control *Borrelia hermsii*, a spirochete with an archival library of variants (Barbour and Bundoc 2001). By contrast, many parasites face control by the more highly specific IgA and IgG antibodies. It would be interesting to know if *B. hermsii* requires a relatively greater molecular distance between variants to escape IgM cross-reactivity than parasites controlled by IgG antibodies. If so, then *B. hermsii's* variants may have diverged under a different pattern of specificity and cross-reactivity from that influencing the divergence of variants in other parasites.

Parasites with archival variants have particularly interesting dynamics within hosts. If the variants are produced too quickly, the host develops specific immunity against all types early in the infection, and the infection cannot persist for long. If the variants arise too slowly, the parasite risks clearance before switching to a novel type. Thus, the pacing of molecular switches in the parasite must be tuned to the dynamics of the host's immune response. This system of contained dynamics within individual hosts may be particularly amenable to experimental study, providing insight into the interactions between host immunity, antigenic escape variants, the shaping of antigenic repertoires, and the evolution of the molecular control systems that regulate antigenic switching.

16.5 Final Note

The technical advances in molecular biology have greatly accelerated the pace of discovery in immunology and parasite biology. When reviewing various topics, I found that many key articles had been published in the past eighteen months.

This book's synthesis may soon be outdated with regard to the latest details for each particular subject. But, for the first time, it has been possible to see the subject as a whole, to discuss in an informed way the interactions between different processes and different ways of study. The problems that I raised for future study will continue to provide key challenges for many years to come.

References

Abraham, J. M., Freitag, C. S., Clements, J. R., and Eisenstein, B. I. 1985. An invertible element of DNA controls phase variation of type 1 fimbriae of *Escherichia coli*. *Proceedings of the National Academy of Sciences* 82:5724-5727.

Abrams, S. I., and Schlom, J. 2000. Rational antigen modification as a strategy to upregulate or downregulate antigen recognition. *Current Opinion in Immunology* 12:85-91.

Ada, G. 1999. The immunology of vaccination. In Plotkin, S. A., and Orenstein, W. A., eds., *Vaccines*, 3d ed., pp. 28-39. W. B. Saunders, Philadelphia.

Agarwal, A., Nayak, B. P., and Rao, K. V. S. 1998. B cell responses to a peptide epitope. VII. Antigen-dependent modulation of the germinal center reaction. *Journal of Immunology* 161:5832-5841.

Agarwal, A., and Rao, K. V. S. 1997. B cell responses to a peptide epitope. III. Differential T helper thresholds in recruitment of B cell fine specificities. *Journal of Immunology* 159:1077-1085.

Agarwal, A., Sarkar, S., Nazbal, C., Balasundaram, G., and Rao, K. V. S. 1996. B cell responses to a peptide epitope. I. The cellular basis for restricted recognition. *Journal of Immunology* 157:2779-2788.

Agarwal, P., Oldenburg, M. C., Czarneski, J. E., Morse, R. M., Hameed, M. R., Cohen, S., and Fernandes, H. 2000. Comparison study for identifying promoter allelic polymorphism in interleukin 10 and tumor necrosis factor alpha genes. *Diagnostic Molecular Pathology* 9:158-164.

Agur, Z. 1992. Mathematical models for African trypanosomiasis. *Parasitology Today* 8:128-129.

Agur, Z., Abiri, D., and van der Ploeg, L. H. T. 1989. Ordered appearance of antigenic variants of African trypanosomes explained in a mathematical model based on a stochastic switch process and immune-selection against putative switch intermediates. *Proceedings of the National Academy of Sciences USA* 86:9626-9630.

Ahmed, R., and Gray, D. 1996. Immunological memory and protective immunity: understanding their relation. *Science* 272:54-60.

Alamgir, A. S. M., Matsuzaki, Y., Hongo, S., Tsuchiya, E., Sugawara, K., Muraki, Y., and Nakamura, K. 2000. Phylogenetic analysis of influenza C virus nonstructural (NS) protein genes and identification of the NS2 protein. *Journal of General Virology* 81:1933-1940.

Albrecht, P., Ennis, F. A., Saltzmann, E. J., and Krugman, S. 1977. Persistence of maternal antibody in infants beyond 12 months. mechanisms of measles vaccine failure. *Journal of Hygiene* 86:291-304.

Alcami, A., and Koszinowski, U. H. 2000. Viral mechanisms of immune evasion. *Trends in Microbiology* 8:410-418.

Allen, T. M., O'Connor, D. H., Jing, P., Dzuris, J. L., Mothé, B. R., Vogel, T. U., Dunphy, E., Liebl, M. E., Emerson, C., Wilson, N., Kunstman, K. J., Wang, X., Allison, D. B., Hughes, A. L., Desrosiers, R. C., Altman, J. D., Wolinsky, S. M., Sette, A., and Watkins, D. I. 2000. Tat-specific cytotoxic T lymphocytes select for SIV escape variants during resolution of primary viraemia. *Nature* 407:386–390.

Almarri, A., and Batchelor, J. R. 1994. HLA and hepatitis B infection. *Lancet* 344:1194–1195.

Altman, J. D., Moss, P. A. H., Goulder, P. J. R., Barouch, D. H., McHeyzer-Williams, M. G., Bell, J. I., McMichael, A. J., and Davis, M. M. 1996. Phenotypic analysis of antigen-specific T lymphocytes. *Science* 274:94–96.

Anderson, R. M., and May, R. M. 1991. *Infectious Diseases of Humans: Dynamics and Control.* Oxford University Press, Oxford.

Anderson, T. J. C., Haubold, B., Williams, J. T., Estrada-Franco, J. G., Richardson, L., Mollinedo, R., Bockarie, M., Mikili, J., Mharakurwa, S., French, N., Whitworth, J., Velez, I. D., Brockman, A. H., Nosten, F., Ferreira, M. U., and Day, K. P. 2000. Microsatellite markers reveal a spectrum of population structures in the malaria parasite *Plasmodium falciparum. Molecular Biology and Evolution* 17:1467–1482.

Andreasen, V., Lin, J., and Levin, S. A. 1997. The dynamics of cocirculating influenza strains conferring partial cross-immunity. *Journal of Mathematical Biology* 35:825–842.

Aslam, N., and Turner, C. M. R. 1992. The relationship of variable antigen expression and population growth rates in *Trypanosoma brucei. Parasitology Research* 78:661–664.

Avrameas, S. 1991. Natural autoantibodies: from horror autotoxicus to gnothi seauton. *Immunology Today* 12:154–159.

Awad-El-Kariem, F. M. 1999. Does *Cryptosporidium parvum* have a clonal population structure? *Parasitology Today* 15:502–504.

Ayala, F. J. 1995. The myth of Eve: molecular biology and human origins. *Science* 270:1930–1936.

Babiker, H. A., and Walliker, D. 1997. Current views on the population structure of *Plasmodium falciparum:* implications for control. *Parasitology Today* 13:262–267.

Back, N. K., Nijhuis, M., Keulen, W., Boucher, C. A., Oude Essink, B. O., van Kuilenburg, A. B., van Gennip, A. H., and Berkout, B. 1996. Reduced replication of 3TC-resistant HIV-1 variants in primary cells due to a processivity defect of the reverse transcriptase enzyme. *EMBO Journal* 15:4040–4049.

Badovinac, V. P., Tvinnereim, A. R., and Harty, J. T. 2000. Regulation of antigen-specific CD8$^+$ T cell homeostasis by perforin and interferon-γ. *Science* 290: 1354–1357.

Banchereau, J., Briere, F., Caux, C., Davoust, J., Lebecque, S., Liu, Y.-J., Pulendran, B., and Palucka, K. 2000. Immunobiology of dendritic cells. *Annual Review of Immunology* 18:767–811.

Baranowski, E., Ruiz-Jarabo, C. M., Sevilla, N., Andreu, D., Beck, E., and Domingo,

E. 2000. Cell recognition by foot-and-mouth disease virus that lacks the RGD integrin-binding motif: flexibility in aphthovirus receptor usage. *Journal of Virology* 74:1641–1647.

Barbet, A. F., and Kamper, S. M. 1993. The importance of mosaic genes to trypanosome survival. *Parasitology Today* 9:63–66.

Barbour, A. G. 1987. Immunobiology of relapsing fever. *Contributions to Microbiology and Immunology* 8:125–137.

Barbour, A. G. 1993. Linear DNA of *Borrelia* species and antigenic variation. *Trends in Microbiology* 1:236–239.

Barbour, A. G., and Bundoc, V. 2001. In vitro and in vivo neutralization of the relapsing fever agent *Borrelia hermsii* with serotype-specific immunoglobulin M antibodies. *Infection and Immunity* 69:1009–1015.

Barbour, A. G., Burman, N., Carter, C. J., Kitten, T., and Bergstrom, S. 1991. Variable antigen genes of the relapsing fever agent *Borrelia hermsii* are activated by promoter addition. *Molecular Microbiology* 5:489–493.

Barbour, A. G., and Hayes, S. F. 1986. Biology of *Borrelia* species. *Microbiological Reviews* 50:381–400.

Barbour, A. G., and Stoenner, H. G. 1985. Antigenic variation of *Borrelia hermsii*. In Herskowitz, I., and Simon, M. I., eds., *Genome Rearrangement*. UCLA Symposium on Molecular and Cellular Biology, New Series, Vol. 20. Alan Liss, Inc., New York.

Barnabé, C., Brisse, S., and Tibayrenc, M. 2000. Population structure and genetic typing of *Trypanosoma cruzi*, the agent of Chagas disease: a multilocus enzyme electrophoretic approach. *Parasitology* 120:513–526.

Barnwell, J. W. 1999. Malaria: a new escape and evasion tactic. *Nature* 398:562–563.

Barragan, A., Kremsner, P. G., Weiss, W., Wahlgren, M., and Carlson, J. 1998. Age-related buildup of humoral immunity against epitopes for rosette formation and agglutination in African areas of malaria endemicity. *Infection and Immunity* 66:4783–4787.

Barry, J. D. 1986. Antigenic variation during *Trypanosoma vivax* infections of different host species. *Parasitology* 92:51–65.

Barry, J. D. 1997. The relative significance of mechanisms of antigenic variation in African trypanosomes. *Parasitology Today* 13:212–218.

Barry, J. D., Peeling, R. W., and Brunham, R. C. 1999. Analysis of the original antigenic sin antibody response to the major outer membrane protein of *Chlamydia trachomatis*. *Journal of Infectious Diseases* 179:180–186.

Barry, J. D., and Turner, C. M. R. 1991. The dynamics of antigenic variation and growth of African trypanosomes. *Parasitology Today* 7:207–211.

Barry, J. D., and Turner, C. M. R. 1992. Mathematical models for African trypanosomiasis—reply. *Parasitology Today* 8:129.

Barton, N. H., and Turelli, M. 1987. Adaptive landscapes, genetic distance and the evolution of quantitative characters. *Genetical Research* 49:157–173.

Beaumont, T., van Nuenen, A., Broersen, S., Blattner, W. A., Lukashov, V. V., and

Schuitemaker, H. 2001. Reversal of human immunodeficiency virus type 1 IIIB to a neutralization-resistant phenotype in an accidentally infected laboratory worker with a progressive clinical course. *Journal of Virology* 75:2246–2252.

Bednarek, M. A., Sauma, S. Y., Gammon, M. C., Porter, G., Tamhankar, S., Williamson, A. R., and Zweerink, H. J. 1991. The minimum peptide epitope from the influenza virus matrix protein: extra and intracellular loading of HLA-A2. *Journal of Immunology* 147:4047–4053.

Beekman, N. J., van Veelen, P. A., van Hall, T., Neisig, A., Sijts, A., Camps, M., Kloetzel, P.-M., Neefjes, J. J., Melief, C. J., and Ossendorp, F. 2000. Abrogation of CTL epitope processing by single amino acid substitution flanking the C-terminal proteasome cleavage site. *Journal of Immunology* 164:1898–1905.

Belz, G. T., Xie, W., Altman, J. D., and Doherty, P. C. 2000. A previously unrecognized H-2D^b-restricted peptide prominent in the primary influenza A virus-specific CD8$^+$ T-cell response is much less apparent following secondary challenge. *Journal of Virology* 74:3486–3493.

Benjamin, D. C., Berzofsky, J. A., East, I. J., Gurd, F. R. N., Hannum, C., Leach, S. J., Margoliash, E., Michael, J. G., Miller, A., Prager, E. M., Reichlin, M., Sercarz, E. E., Smith-Gill, S. J., Todd, P. E., and Wilson, A. C. 1984. The antigenic structure of proteins: a reappraisal. *Annual Review of Immunology* 2:67–101.

Benjamin, D. C., and Perdue, S. S. 1996. Site-directed mutagenesis in epitope mapping. *Methods in Enzymology* 9:508–515.

Bennett, A. F., and Lenski, R. E. 1999. Experimental evolution and its role in evolutionary physiology. *American Zoologist* 39:346–362.

Bennink, J. R., and Doherty, P. C. 1981. The response to H-2-different virus-infected cells is mediated by long-lived T lymphocytes and is diminished by prior virus priming in a syngeneic environment. *Cellular Immunology* 61:220–224.

Berinstein, A., Roivainen, M., Hovi, T., Mason, P. W., and Baxt, B. 1995. Antibodies to the vitronectin receptor (integrin $\alpha_v\beta_3$) inhibit binding and infection of foot-and-mouth disease virus to cultured cells. *Journal of Virology* 69:2664–2666.

Bernard, K. A., Klimstra, W. B., and Johnston, R. E. 2000. Mutations in the E2 glycoprotein of Venezuelan equine encephalitis virus confer heparan sulfate interaction, low morbidity, and rapid clearance from blood of mice. *Virology* 276:93–103.

Bertoletti, A., Sette, A., Chisari, F. V., Penna, A., Levrero, M., De Carli, M., Fiaccadori, F., and Ferrari, C. 1994. Natural variants of cytotoxic epitopes are T-cell receptor antagonists for antiviral cytotoxic T cells. *Nature* 369:407–410.

Bhattacharjee, A. K., and Glaudemans, C. P. J. 1978. Dual binding specificities in MOPC 384 and 870 murine myeloma immunoglobulins. *Journal of Immunology* 120:411–413.

Biozzi, G., Cabrera, W. H., Mouton, D., and Ibanez, D. M. 1982. Restricted and general polygenic regulation of antibody responsiveness. In Benacerraf, B., ed., *Immunogenetics and Immune Regulation*, p. 31. Masson Italia Editori, Milan.

Bizebard, T., Gigant, B., Rigolet, P., Rasmussen, B., Diat, O., Bösecke, P., Wharton, S. A., Skehel, J. J., and Knossow, M. 1995. Structure of influenza virus haemagglutinin complexed with a neutralizing antibody. *Nature* 376:92–94.

Bobkov, A., Cheingsong-Popov, R., Salminen, M., McCutchan, F., Louwagie, J., Ariyoshi, K., Whittle, H., and Weber, J. 1996. Complex mosaic structure of the partial envelope sequence from a Gambian HIV type 1 isolate. *AIDS Research and Human Retroviruses* 12:169–171.

Borre, M. B., Owen, C. A., Keen, J. K., Sinha, K. A., and Holder, A. A. 1995. Multiple genes code for high-molecular-mass rhoptry proteins of *Plasmodium yoelii*. *Molecular and Biochemical Parasitology* 70:149–155.

Borrow, P., and Shaw, G. M. 1998. Cytotoxic T-lymphocyte escape viral variants: how important are they in viral evasion of immune clearance in vivo? *Immunological Reviews* 164:37–51.

Borst, P., Rudenko, G., Blundell, P. A., van Leeuwen, F., Cross, M. A., McCulloch, R., Gerrits, H., and Chaves, I. M. F. 1997. Mechanisms of antigenic variation in African trypanosomes. *Behring Institute Mitteilungen* 99:1–15.

Bousso, P., Levraud, J.-P., Kourilsky, P., and Abasado, J.-P. 1999. The composition of a primary T cell response is largely determined by the timing of recruitment of individual T cell clones. *Journal of Experimental Medicine* 189:1591–1600.

Brannan, L. R., Turner, C. M. R., and Phillips, R. S. 1994. Malaria parasites undergo antigenic variation at high rates in vivo. *Proceedings of the Royal Society of London Series B Biological Sciences* 256:71–75.

Brisse, S., Barnabé, C., and Tibayrenc, M. 2000a. Identification of six *Trypanosoma cruzi* phylogenetic lineages by random amplified polymorphic DNA and multilocus enzyme electrophoresis. *International Journal for Parasitology* 30:35–44.

Brisse, S., Dujardin, J.-C., and Tibayrenc, M. 2000b. Identification of six *Trypanosoma cruzi* lineages by sequence-characterised amplified region markers. *Molecular and Biochemical Parasitology* 111:95–105.

Brown, I. H., Ludwig, S., Olsen, C. W., Hannoun, C., Scholtissek, C., Hinshaw, V. S., Harris, P. A., McCauley, J. W., and Strong, I. 1997. Antigenic and genetic analyses of H1N1 influenza A viruses from European pigs. *Journal of General Virology* 78:553–562.

Bruyere, A., Wantroba, M., Flasinski, S., Dzianott, A., and Bujarski, J. J. 2000. Frequent homologous recombination events between molecules of one RNA component in a multipartite RNA virus. *Journal of Virology* 74:4214–4219.

Buonagurio, D. A., Nakada, S., Desselberger, U., Krystal, M., and Palese, P. 1985. Noncumulative sequence changes in the hemagglutinin genes of influenza C virus isolates. *Virology* 146:221–232.

Burch, C. L., and Chao, L. 1999. Evolution by small steps and rugged landscapes in the RNA virus variant ϕ6. *Genetics* 151:921–927.

Burkhart, C., Freer, G., Castro, R., Adorini, L., Wiesmuller, K. H., Zinkernagel, R. M., and Hengartner, H. 1994. Characterization of T helper epitopes of the glycoprotein of vesicular stomatitis virus. *Journal of Virology* 68:1573–1580.

Burrows, S. R., Khanna, R., Burrows, J. M., and Moss, D. J. 1994. An alloresponse in humans is dominated by cytotoxic T lymphocytes (CTL) cross-reactive with a single Epstein-Barr virus CTL epitope: implications for graft-versus-host disease. *Journal of Experimental Medicine* 179:1155–1161.

Burrows, S. R., Silins, S. L., Moss, D. J., Khanna, R., Misko, I. S., and Argaet, V. P. 1995. T cell receptor repertoire for a viral epitope in humans is diversified by tolerance to a background major histocompatibility complex antigen. *Journal of Experimental Medicine* 182:1703–1715.

Busch, D. H., Pilip, I. M., Vijh, S., and Pamer, E. G. 1998. Coordinate regulation of complex T cell populations responding to bacterial infection. *Immunity* 8:353–362.

Bush, R. M. 2001. Predicting adaptive evolution. *Nature Reviews Genetics* 2:387–392.

Bush, R. M., Bender, C. A., Subbarao, K., Cox, N. J., and Fitch, W. M. 1999. Predicting the evolution of influenza A. *Science* 286:1921–1925.

Buss, L. W. 1987. *The Evolution of Individuality.* Princeton University Press, Princeton, New Jersey.

Butz, E. A., and Bevan, M. J. 1998. Massive expansion of antigen-specific CD8+ T cells during an acute virus infection. *Immunity* 8:167–175.

Buus, S. 1999. Description and prediction of peptide-MHC binding: the 'human MHC project.' *Current Opinion in Immunology* 11:209–213.

Byers, V. S., and Sercarz, E. E. 1968. The x-y-z scheme of immunocyte maturation. *Journal of Experimental Medicine* 128:715–728.

Byrnes, A. P., and Griffin, D. E. 2000. Large-plaque mutants of Sindbis virus show reduced binding to heparan sulfate, heightened viremia, and slower clearance from the circulation. *Journal of Virology* 74:644–651.

Cadavid, D., Pachner, A. R., Estanislao, L., Patalapati, R., and Barbour, A. G. 2001. Isogenic serotypes of *Borrelia turnicatae* show different localization in the brain and skin of mice. *Infection and Immunity* 69:3389–3397.

Calisher, C. H., Karabatsos, N., Dalrymple, J. M., Shope, R. E., Porterfield, J. S., Westaway, E. G., and Brandt, W. E. 1989. Antigenic relationships between flaviviruses as determined by cross-neutralization tests with polyclonal antisera. *Journal of General Virology* 70:37–43.

Callan, M. F. C., Tan, L., Annels, N., Ogg, G. S., Wilson, J. D. K., O'Callaghan, C. A., Steven, N., McMichael, A. J., and Rickinson, A. B. 1998. Direct visualization of antigen-specific CD8+ T cells during the primary immune response to Epstein-Barr virus in vivo. *Journal of Experimental Medicine* 187:1395–1402.

Caporale, L. H. 1999. Chance favors the prepared genome. *Annals of the New York Academy of Sciences* 870:1–21.

Carrillo, C., Borca, M., Moore, D. M., Morgan, D. O., and Sobrino, F. 1998. In vivo analysis of the stability and fitness of variants recovered from foot-and-mouth disease virus quasispecies. *Journal of General Virology* 79:1699–1706.

Caton, A. J., Brownlee, G. G., Yewdell, J. W., and Gerhard, W. 1982. The antigenic structure of the influenza virus A/PR/8/34 hemagglutinin (H1 subtype). *Cell* 31:417–427.

Chackerian, B., Rudensey, L. M., and Overbaugh, J. 1997. Specific N-linked and O-linked glycosylation modifications in the envelope V1 domain of simian immunodeficiency virus variants that evolve in the host after recognition by neutralizing antibodies. *Journal of Virology* 71:7719–7727.

Chao, L., and Cox, E. C. 1983. Competition between high and low mutating strains of *Escherichia coli*. *Evolution* 37:125–134.

Chapman, B. A., Burt, M. J., Frampton, C. M., Collett, J. A., Yeo, K. H., Wilkinson, I. D., Cook, H. B., Barclay, M. J., Ross, A. G., and George, P. M. 2000. The prevalence of viral hepatitis (HAV, HBC and HCV) in the Christchurch community. *New Zealand Medical Journal* 113:394–396.

Charlesworth, B., Sniegowski, P., and Stephan, W. 1994. The evolutionary dynamics of repetitive DNA in eukaryotes. *Nature* 371:215–220.

Chen, Q., Fernandez, V., Sundström, A., Schlichtherle, M., Datta, S., Hagblom, P., and Wahlgren, M. 1998. Developmental selection of *var* gene expression in *Plasmodium falciparum*. *Nature* 394:392–395.

Chen, W., Antón, L. C., Bennink, J. R., and Yewdell, J. W. 2000. Dissecting the multifactorial causes of immunodominance in class I–restricted T cell responses to viruses. *Immunity* 12:83–93.

Chen, W., Khilko, S., Fecondo, J., Margulies, D. H., and McLuskey, J. 1994. Determinant selection of major histocompatibility complex class I–restricted antigenic peptides is explained by class I–peptide affinity and is strongly influenced by nondominant anchor residues. *Journal of Experimental Medicine* 180:1471–1483.

Chen, Z. J., Wheeler, C. J., Shi, W., Wu, A. J., Yarboro, C. H., Gallagher, M., and Notkins, A. L. 1998. Polyreactive antigen-binding B cells are the predominant cell type in the newborn B cell repertoire. *European Journal of Immunology* 28:989–994.

Chen, Z. W., Craiu, A., Shen, L., Kuroda, M. J., Iroku, U. C., Watkins, D. I., Voss, G., and Letvin, N. L. 2000. Simian immunodeficiency virus evades a dominant epitope-specific cytotoxic T lymphocyte response through mutation resulting in the accelerated dissociation of viral peptide and MHC class I. *Journal of Immunology* 164:6474–6479.

Chisari, F. V. 1995. Hepatitis B virus immunopathogenesis. *Annual Review of Immunology* 13.29–60.

Ciurea, A., Klenerman, P., Hunziker, L., Horvath, E., Senn, B. M., Ochsenbein, A. F., Hengartner, H., and Zinkernagel, R. M. 2000. Viral persistence in vivo through selection of neutralizing antibody-escape variants. *Proceedings of the National Academy of Sciences USA* 97:2749–2754.

Cleghorn, F. R., Jack, N., Carr, J. K., Edwards, J., Mahabir, B., Sill, A., McDanal, C. B., Connolly, S. M., Goodman, D., Bennetts, R. Q., O'Brien, T. R., Weinhold, K. J., Bartholomew, C., Blattner, W. A., and Greenberg, M. L. 2000. A distinctive clade B HIV type 1 is heterosexually transmitted in Trinidad and Tobago. *Proceedings of the National Academy of Sciences USA* 97:10532-10537.

Cleveland, S. M., Taylor, H. P., and Dimmock, N. J. 1997. Selection of neutralizing antibody escape mutants with type A influenza virus HA-specific polyclonal antisera: possible significance for antigenic drift. *Epidemiology and Infection* 118:149-154.

Coffin, J. M. 1995. HIV population dynamics in vivo: implications for genetic variation, pathogenesis, and therapy. *Science* 267:483-489.

Coffin, J. M. 1996. Retroviridae: the viruses and their replication. In Fields, B. N., Knipe, D. M., and Howley, P. M., eds., *Fields Virology*, 3d ed., pp. 763-843. Lippincott-Raven, Philadelphia.

Coffman, R. L., and Beebe, A. M. 1998. Genetic control of the T cell response to *Leishmania major* infection. In Gupta, S., Sher, A., and Ahmed, R., eds., *Mechanisms of Lymphocyte Activitation and Immune Regulation VII: Molecular Determinants of Microbial Immunity*, pp. 61-66. Plenum Press, New York.

Cohen, S., and Lambert, P. H. 1982. Malaria. In Cohen, S., and Warren, D., eds., *Immunology of Parasitic Infections*, 2d ed., pp. 422-438. Blackwell, London.

Cole, G. A., Hogg, T. L., Coppola, M. A., and Woodland, D. L. 1997. Efficient priming of CD8+ memory T cells specific for a subdominant epitope following Sendai virus infection. *Journal of Immunology* 158:4301-4309.

Colman, P. M. 1998. Structure and function of the neuraminidase. In Nicholson, K. G., Webster, R. G., and Hay, A. J., eds., *Textbook of Influenza*, pp. 65-73. Blackwell Science, Oxford.

Connor, R. I., Sheridan, K. E., Ceradini, D., Choe, S., and Landau, N. R. 1997. Change in coreceptor use correlates with disease progression in HIV-1-infected individuals. *Journal of Experimental Medicine* 185:621-628.

Connor, R. J., Kawaoka, Y., Webster, R. G., and Paulson, J. C. 1994. Receptor specificity in human, avian, and equine H2 and H3 influenza virus isolates. *Virology* 205:17-23.

Constant, S. L., and Bottomly, K. 1997. Induction of Th1 and Th2 CD4+ T cell responses: the alternative approaches. *Annual Review of Immunology* 15:297-322.

Conway, D. J. 1997. Natural selection on polymorphic malaria antigens and the search for a vaccine. *Parasitology Today* 13:26-29.

Conway, D. J., Cavanagh, D. R., Tanabe, K., Roper, C., Mikes, Z. S., Sakihama, N., Bojang, K. A., Oduola, A. M. J., Kremsner, P. G., Arnot, D. E., Greenwood, B. M., and McBride, J. S. 2000. A principal target of human immunity to malaria identified by molecular population genetic and immunological analyses. *Nature Medicine* 6:689-692.

Conway, D. J., Roper, C., Oduola, A. M. J., Arnot, D. E., Kremsner, P. G., Grobusch,

M. P., Curtis, C. F., and Greenwood, B. M. 1999. High recombination rate in natural populations of *Plasmodium falciparum*. *Proceedings of the National Academy of Sciences USA* 96:4506–4511.

Cooper, L. A., and Scott, T. W. 2001. Differential evolution of eastern equine encephalitis virus populations in response to host cell type. *Genetics* 157:1403–1412.

Cornelissen, M., Kampinga, G., Zorgdrager, F., and Goudsmit, J. 1996. Human Immunodeficiency virus type 1 subtypes defined by *env* show high frequency of recombinant *gag* genes. *Journal of Virology* 70:8209–8212.

Couceiro, J. N., Paulson, J. C., and Baum, L. G. 1993. Influenza virus strains selectively recognize sialyloligosaccharides on human respiratory epithelium: the role of the host cell in selection of hemagglutinin receptor specificity. *Virus Research* 29:155–165.

Cowell, L., Kepler, T. B., Janitz, M., Lauster, R., and Mitchison, N. A. 1998. The distribution of variation in regulatory gene segments as present in MHC class II promoters. *Genome Research* 8:124–134.

Cox, N. J., and Bender, C. A. 1995. The molecular epidemiology of influenza viruses. *Seminars in Virology* 6:359–370.

Cox, N. J., and Subbarao, K. 2000. Global epidemiology of influenza: past and present. *Annual Review of Medicine* 51:407–421.

Crandall, K. A., ed. 1999. *The Evolution of HIV*. Johns Hopkins University Press, Baltimore, Maryland.

Crill, W. D., Wichman, H. A., and Bull, J. J. 2000. Evolutionary reversals during viral adaptation to alternating hosts. *Genetics* 154:27–37.

Croft, M., and Swain, S. L. 1992. Analysis of CD4$^+$ T cells that provide contact-dependent bystander help to B cells. *Journal of Immunology* 149:3157–3165.

Crow, J. F., and Kimura, M. 1970. *An Introduction to Population Genetics Theory*. Burgess, Minneapolis, Minnesota.

Daser, A., Mitchison, H., Mitchison, A., and Müller, B. 1996. Non-classical-MHC genetics of immunological disease in man and mouse. The key role of pro-inflammatory cytokine genes. *Cytokine* 8:593–597.

Davis, M. M., Boniface, J. J., Reich, Z., Lyons, D., Hampl, J., Arden, B., and Chien, Y. 1998. Ligand recognition by $\alpha\beta$ T cell receptors. *Annual Review of Immunology* 16:523–544.

de Lana, M., da Silveira, A., Bastrenta, B., Barnabé, C., Noël, S., and Tibayrenc, M. 2000. *Trypanosoma cruzi*: infectivity of clonal genotype infections in acute and chronic phases in mice. *Experimental Parasitology* 96:61–66.

Deitsch, K. W., Moxon, E. R., and Wellems, T. E. 1997. Shared themes of antigenic variation and virulence in bacterial, protozoal, and fungal infections. *Microbiology and Molecular Biology Reviews* 61:281–293.

Deitsch, K. W., and Wellems, T. E. 1996. Membrane modifications in erythrocytes parasitized by *Plasmodium falciparum*. *Molecular and Biochemical Parasitology* 76:1–10.

del Portillo, H. A., Fernandez-Becerra, C., Bowman, S., Oliver, K., Preuss, M., Sanchez, C. P., Schneider, N. K., Villalobos, J. M., Rajandream, M.-A., Harris, D., Perera da Silva, L. H., Barrell, B., and Lanzer, M. 2001. A superfamily of variant genes encoded in the subtelomeric region of *Plasmodium vivax. Nature* 410:839–842.

Deng, Y., Yewdell, J. W., Eisenlohr, L. C., and Bennink, J. R. 1997. MHC affinity, peptide liberation, T cell repertoire, and immunodominance all contribute to the paucity of MHC class I–restricted peptides recognized by antiviral CTL. *Journal of Immunology* 158:1507–1515.

Dick, L. R., Aldrich, C., Jameson, S. C., Moomaw, C. R., Pramanik, B. C., Doyle, C. K., Demartino, G. N., Bevan, M. J., Forman, J. M., and Slaughter, C. A. 1994. Proteolytic processing of ovalbumin and beta-galactosidase by the proteasome to yield antigenic peptides. *Journal of Immunology* 152:3884–3894.

Dimmock, N. J. 1993. Neutralization of animal viruses. *Current Topics in Microbiology and Immunology* 183:1–149.

Dimmock, N. J. 1995. Update on the neutralization of animal viruses. *Reviews in Medical Virology* 5:165–179.

Doherty, P. C., Biddison, W. E., Bennink, J. R., and Knowles, B. B. 1978. Cytotoxic T-cell responses in mice infected with influenza and vaccinia viruses vary in magnitude with H-2 genotype. *Journal of Experimental Medicine* 148:534–543.

Doherty, P. C., and Christensen, J. P. 2000. Accessing complexity: the dynamics of virus-specific T cell responses. *Annual Review of Immunology* 18:561–592.

Dougan, D. A., Malby, R. L., Gruen, L. C., Kortt, A. A., and Hudson, P. J. 1998. Effects of substitutions in the binding surface of an antibody on antigen affinity. *Protein Engineering* 11:65–74.

Dowdle, W. R. 1999. Influenza A virus recycling revisited. *Bulletin of the World Health Organization* 77:820–828.

Drake, J. W., Charlesworth, B., Charlesworth, D., and Crow, J. F. 1998. Rates of spontaneous mutation. *Genetics* 148:1667–1686.

Drake, J. W., and Holland, J. J. 1999. Mutation rates among RNA viruses. *Proceedings of the National Academy of Sciences USA* 96:13910–13913.

Drescher, J., and Aron, R. 1999. Influence of the amino acid differences between the hemagglutinin HA1 domains of influenza virus H1N1 strains on their reaction with antibody. *Journal of Medical Virology* 57:397–404.

Dutton, R. W., Bradley, L. M., and Swain, S. L. 1998. T cell memory. *Annual Review of Immunology* 16:201–223.

Earn, D. J. D., Rohani, P., Bolker, B. M., and Grenfell, B. T. 2000. A simple model for complex dynamical transitions in epidemics. *Science* 287:667–670.

Edfors-Lilja, I., Wattrang, E., Marklund, L., Moller, M., Andersson-Eklund, L., Andersson, L., and Fossum, C. 1998. Mapping quantitative trait loci for immune capacity in the pig. *Journal of Immunology* 161:829–835.

Edwards, M. J., and Dimmock, N. J. 2000. Two influenza A virus-specific Fabs neutralize by inhibiting virus attachment to target cells, while neutralization by their IgGs is complex and occurs simultaneously through fusion inhibition and attachment inhibition. *Virology* 278:423-435.

El-Omar, E. M., Carrington, M., Chow, W.-H., McColl, K. E. L., Bream, J. H., Young, H. A., Herrera, J., Lissowska, J., Yuan, C.-C., Rothman, N., Lanyon, G., Martin, M., Fraumeni, Jr., J. F., and Rabkin, C. S. 2000. Interleukin-1 polymorphisms associated with increased risk of gastric cancer. *Nature* 404:398-402.

Endo, T., Ikeo, K., and Gojobori, T. 1996. Large-scale search for genes on which positive selection may operate. *Molecular Biology and Evolution* 13:685-690.

Engelhard, V. H., Lacy, E., and Ridge, J. P. 1991. Influenza A-specific, HLA-A2.1-restricted cytotoxic T lymphocytes from HLA-A2.1 transgenic mice recognize fragments of the M1 protein. *Journal of Immunology* 146:1226-1232.

Enright, M. C., and Spratt, B. G. 1999. Multilocus sequence typing. *Trends in Microbiology* 7:482-487.

Evans, D. T., O'Connor, D. H., Jing, P., Dzuris, J. L., Sidney, J., da Silva, J., Allen, T. M., Horton, H., Venham, J. E., Rudersdorf, R. A., Vogel, T., Pauza, C. D., Bontrop, R. E., DeMars, R., Sette, A., Hughes, A. L., and Watkins, D. I. 1999. Virus-specific cytotoxic T-lymphocyte responses select for amino-acid variation in simian immunodeficiency virus Env and Nef. *Nature Medicine* 5:1270-1276.

Farber, D. L. 2000. T cell memory: heterogeneity and mechanisms. *Clinical Immunology* 95:173-181.

Farci, P., Shimoda, A., Coiana, A., Diaz, G., Peddis, G., Melpolder, J. C., Strazzera, A., Chien, D. Y., Munoz, S. J., Balestrieri, A., Purcell, R. H., and Alter, H. J. 2000. The outcome of acute hepatitis C predicted by the evolution of viral quasispecies. *Science* 288:339-344.

Fazekas de St. Groth, S., and Webster, R. G. 1966a. Disquisitions on original antigenic sin. I. Evidence in man. *Journal of Experimental Medicine* 124:331-345.

Fazekas de St. Groth, S., and Webster, R. G. 1966b. Disquisitions on original antigenic sin. II. Proof in lower creatures. *Journal of Experimental Medicine* 124:347-361.

Feavers, I. M., Fox, A. J., Gray, S., Jones, D. M., and Maiden, M. C. J. 1996. Antigenic diversity of meningococcal outer membrane protein PorA has implications for epidemiological analysis and vaccine design. *Clinical and Diagnostic Laboratory Immunology* 3:444-450.

Feigelstock, D. A., Mateu, M. G., Valero, M. L., Andreu, D., Domingo, E., and Palma, E. L. 1996. Emerging foot-and-mouth disease virus variants with antigenically critical amino acid substitutions predicted by model studies using reference viruses. *Vaccine* 14:97-102.

Ferguson, N., Anderson, R., and Gupta, S. 1999. The effect of antibody dependent enhancement on the transmission dynamics and persistence of multiple-strain pathogens. *Proceedings of the National Academy of Sciences USA* 96:790-794.

Fischetti, V. A. 1991. Streptococcal M protein. *Scientific American* 264(6):32-39.

Fish, S., Zenowich, E., Fleming, M., and Manser, T. 1989. Molecular analysis of original antigenic sin. I. Clonal selection, somatic mutation, and isotype switching during a memory B cell response. *Journal of Experimental Medicine* 170:1191-1209.

Fleury, D., Barrère, B., Bizebard, T., Daniels, R. S., Skehel, J. J., and Knossow, M. 1999. A complex of influenza hemagglutinin with a neutralizing antibody that binds outside the virus receptor binding site. *Nature Structural Biology* 6:530-534.

Fleury, D., Wharton, S. A., Skehel, J. J., Knossow, M., and Bizebard, T. 1998. Antigen distortion allows influenza virus to escape neutralization. *Nature Structural Biology* 5:119-123.

Forsyth, K. P., Philip, G., Smith, T., Kum, E., Southwell, B., and Brown, G. V. 1989. Diversity of antigens expressed on the surface of the erythrocytes infected with mature *Plasmodium falciparum* parasites in Papua New Guinea. *American Journal of Tropical Medicine and Hygiene* 41:259-265.

Foster, C. B., Lehrnbecher, T., Samuels, S., Stein, S., Mol, F., Metcalf, J. A., Wyvill, K., Steinberg, S. M., Kovacs, J., Blauvelt, A., Yarchoan, R., and Chanock, S. J. 2000. An IL6 promoter polymorphism is associated with a lifetime risk of development of Kaposi sarcoma in men infected with human immunodeficiency virus. *Blood* 96:2562-2567.

Fox, G., Parry, N. R., Barnett, P. V., McGinn, B., Rowlands, D. J., and Brown, F. 1989. The cell attachment site on foot-and-mouth disease virus includes the amino acid sequence RGD (arginine-glycine-aspartic acid). *Journal of General Virology* 70:625-637.

Francis, T. 1953. The newe acquayantance. *Annals of Internal Medicine* 39:203-212.

Franco, A., Ferrari, C., Sette, A., and Chisari, F. V. 1995. Viral mutations, TCR antagonism and escape from the immune response. *Current Opinion in Immunology* 7:524-531.

Frank, S. A. 1993. Coevolutionary genetics of plants and pathogens. *Evolutionary Ecology* 7:45-75.

Frank, S. A. 1994. Recognition and polymorphism in host-parasite genetics. *Philosophical Transactions of the Royal Society of London B* 346:283-293.

Frank, S. A. 1996. Models of parasite virulence. *Quarterly Review of Biology* 71:37-78.

Frank, S. A. 1999. A model for the sequential dominance of antigenic variants in African trypanosome infections. *Proceedings of the Royal Society of London B* 266:1397-1401.

Frank, S. A. 2001. Multiplicity of infection and the evolution of hybrid incompatibility in segmented viruses. *Heredity* 87:522-529.

Fry, E. E., Lea, S. M., Jackson, T., Newman, J. W. I., Ellard, F. M., Blakemore, W. E., Abu-Ghazaleh, R., Samuel, A., King, A. M. Q., and Stuart, D. I. 1999. The structure and function of foot-and-mouth disease virus-oligosaccharide receptor complex. *EMBO Journal* 18:543–554.

Fujita, K., Maeda, K., Yokoyama, N., Miyazawa, T., Kai, C., and Mikami, T. 1998. In vitro recombination of feline herpesvirus type 1. *Archives of Virology* 143:25–34.

Fussenegger, M. 1997. Different lifestyles of human pathogenic procaryotes and their strategies for phase and antigenic variation. *Symbiosis* 22:85–153.

Fussenegger, M., Rudel, T., Barten, R., Ryll, R., and Meyer, T. F. 1997. Transformation competence and type-1 pilus biogenesis in *Neisseria gonorrhoeae:* a review. *Gene* 192:125–134.

Gao, P., Robertson, D. L., Carruthers, C. D., Li, Y., Bailes, E., Kosrikis, L. G., Salminen, M. O., Bibollet-Ruche, F., Peeters, M., Ho, D. D., Shaw, G. M., Sharp, P. M., and Hahn, B. H. 1998. An isolate of human immunodeficiency virus type 1 originally classified as subtype I represents a complex mosaic comprising three different group M subtypes (A, G, and I). *Journal of Virology* 72:10234–10241.

Germain, R. N., and Štefanová, I. 1999. The dynamics of T cell receptor signaling: complex orchestration and the key roles of tempo and cooperation. *Annual Review of Immunology* 17:467–522.

Ghany, M. G., Ayola, B., Villamil, F. G., Gish, R. G., Rojter, S., Vierling, J. M., and Lok, A. S. F. 1998. Hepatitis B virus S mutants in liver transplant recipients who were reinfected despite hepatitis B immune globulin prophylaxis. *Hepatology* 27:213–222.

Gianfrani, C., Oseroff, C., Sidney, J., Chesnut, R. W., and Sette, A. 2000. Human memory CTL response specific for influenza A virus is broad and multispecific. *Human Immunology* 61:438–452.

Gilbert, S. C., Plebanski, M., Gupta, S., Morris, J., Cox, M., Aidoo, M., Kwiatkowski, D., Greenwood, B. M., Whittle, H. C., and Hill, A. V. S. 1998. Association of malaria parasite population structure, HLA, and immunological antagonism. *Science* 279:1173–1177.

Golub, E. S., and Green, D. R. 1991. *Immunology: A Synthesis,* 2d ed. Sinauer Associates, Sunderland, Massachusetts.

Good, M. F., Zevering, Y., Currier, J., and Bilsborough, J. 1993. Original antigenic sin, T cell memory, and malaria sporozoite immunity: an hypothesis for immune evasion. *Parasite Immunology* 15:187–193.

Goulder, P. J. R., Brander, C., Tang, Y., Tremblay, C., Colbert, R. A., Addo, M. M., Rosenberg, E. S., Nguyen, T., Allen, R., Trocha, A., Altfeld, M., He, S., Bunce, M., Funkhouser, R., Pelton, S. I., Burchett, S. K., McIntosh, K., Korber, B. T. M., and Walker, B. D. 2001. Evolution and transmission of stable CTL escape mutations in HIV infection. *Nature* 412:334–338.

Gow, P. J., and Mutimer, D. 2000. Mechanisms of hepatitis B virus escape after immunoglobulin therapy. *Current Opinion in Infectious Disease* 13:643–646.

Gras-Masse, H., Georges, B., Estaquier, J., Tranchand-Bunel, D., Tartar, A., Druilhe, P., and Auriault, C. 1999. Convergent peptide libraries, or mixotopes, to elicit or to identify specific immune responses. *Current Opinion in Immunology* 11:223–228.

Gravenor, M. B., and Lloyd, A. L. 1998. Reply to: models for the in-host dynamics of malaria revisited: errors in some basic models lead to large over-estimates of growth rates. *Parasitology* 117:409–410.

Gravenor, M. B., McLean, A. R., and Kwiatkowski, D. 1995. The regulation of malaria parasitaemia: parameter estimates for a population model. *Parasitology* 110:115–122.

Gray, A. R. 1965. Antigenic variation in a strain of *Trypanosoma brucei* transmitted by *Glossina morsitans* and *G. palpalis*. *Journal of General Microbiology* 41:195–214.

Gray, D. 2000. Thanks for the memory. *Nature Immunology* 1:11–12.

Gray-Owen, S. D., Lorenzen, D. R., Haude, A., Meyer, T. F., and Dehio, C. 1997. Differential Opa specificities for CD66 receptors influence tissue interactions and cellular response to *Neisseria gonorrhoeae*. *Molecular Microbiology* 26:971–980.

Griffin, D. E. 2001. Measles virus. In Knipe, D. M., and Howley, P. M., eds., *Fields Virology,* 4th ed., pp. 1401–1441. Lippincott-Raven, Philadelphia.

Gross, M. D., and Siegel, E. C. 1981. Incidence of mutator strains in *Escherichia coli* and coliforms in nature. *Mutation Research* 91:107–110.

Guardiola, J., Maffei, A., Lauster, R., Mitchison, N. A., Accolla, R. S., and Sartoris, S. 1996. Functional significance of polymorphism among MHC class II gene promoters. *Tissue Antigens* 48:615–625.

Gubbels, M.-J., Katzer, F., Hide, G., Jongejan, F., and Shiels, B. R. 2000. Generation of a mosaic pattern of diversity in the major merozoite-piroplasm surface antigen of *Theileria annulata*. *Molecular and Biochemical Parasitology* 110:23–32.

Guillot, S., Caro, V., Cuervo, N., Korotkova, E., Combiescu, M., Persu, A., Aubert-Combiescu, A., Delpeyroux, F., and Crainic, R. 2000. Natural genetic exchanges between vaccine and wild poliovirus strains in humans. *Journal of Virology* 74:8434–8443.

Gupta, S., and Day, K. P. 1994. A strain theory of malaria transmission. *Parasitology Today* 10:476–481.

Gupta, S., Ferguson, N., and Anderson, R. 1998. Chaos, persistence, and evolution of strain structure in antigenically diverse infectious agents. *Science* 280:912–915.

Gupta, S., Maiden, M. C. J., and Anderson, R. M. 1999. Population structure of pathogens: the role of immune selection. *Parasitology Today* 15:497–501.

Gupta, S., Maiden, M. C. J., Feavers, I. M., Nee, S., May, R. M., and Anderson, R. M. 1996. The maintenance of strain structure in populations of recombining infectious agents. *Nature Medicine* 2:437–442.

Gupta, S. C., Hengartner, H., and Zinkernagel, R. M. 1986. Primary antibody responses to a well-defined and unique antigen are not enhanced by preimmunization with carrier: analysis in a viral model. *Proceedings of the National Academy of Sciences USA* 83:2604–2608.

Gutjahr, T. S., O'Rourke, M., Ison, C. A., and Spratt, B. G. 1997. Arginine-, hypoxanthine-, uracil-requiring isolates of *Neisseria gonorrhoeae* are a clonal lineage within a non-clonal population. *Microbiology* 143:633–640.

Guttman, D. S. 1997. Recombination and clonality in natural populations of *Escherichia coli. Trends in Ecology and Evolution* 12:16–22.

Haanen, J. B. A. G., Wolkers, M. C., Kruisbeek, A. M., and Schumacher, T. N. M. 1999. Selective expansion of cross-reactive CD8+ memory T cells by viral variants. *Journal of Experimental Medicine* 190:1319–1328.

Hackstadt, T. 1999. Cell biology. In Stephens, R. S., ed., *Chlamydia: Intracellular Biology, Pathogenesis, and Immunity*, pp. 101–138. American Society for Microbiology, Washington, D.C.

Hajós, J. P., Pijnenburg, J., Usmany, M., Zuidema, D., Závadszky, P., and Vlak, J. M. 2000. High frequency recombination between homologous baculoviruses in cell culture. *Archives of Virology* 145:159–164.

Harindranath, N., Ikematsu, H., Notkins, A. L., and Casali, P. 1993. Structure of the VH and VL segments of polyreactive and monoreactive human natural antibodies to HIV-1 and *Escherichia coli* β-galactosidase. *International Immunology* 5:1523–1533.

Harrigan, P. R., Bloor, S., and Larder, B. A. 1998. Relative replicative fitness of zidovudine-resistant human immunodeficiency virus type 1 isolates in vitro. *Journal of Virology* 72:3773–3778.

Harrison, S. C. 1989. Picornaviruses: finding the receptors. *Nature* 338:205–206.

Hartl, D. L., and Clark, A. G. 1997. *Principles of Population Genetics,* 3d ed. Sinauer Associates, Sunderland, Massachusetts.

Hartl, D. L., and Taubes, C. H. 1996. Compensatory nearly neutral mutations: selection without adaptation. *Journal of Theoretical Biology* 182:303–309.

Hasegawa, M., Di Rienzo, A., Kocher, T. D., and Wilson, A. C. 1993. Toward a more accurate time scale for the human mitochondrial DNA tree. *Journal of Molecular Evolution* 37:347–354.

Hastings, I. M., and Wedgwood-Oppenheim, B. 1997. Sex, strains and virulence. *Parasitology Today* 13:375–383.

Hauser, S. L. 1995. T-cell receptor genes. *Annals of the New York Academy of Sciences* 756:233–240.

Haydon, D. T., Bastos, A. D., Knowles, N. J., and Samuel, A. R. 2001. Evidence for positive selection in foot-and-mouth disease virus capsid genes from field isolates. *Genetics* 157:7–15.

Haydon, D. T., and Woolhouse, M. E. J. 1998. Immune avoidance strategies in RNA viruses: fitness continuums arising from trade-offs between immunogenicity and antigenic variability. *Journal of Theoretical Biology* 193:601–612.

Haywood, A. M. 1994. Virus receptors: binding, adhesion strengthening, and changes in viral structure. *Journal of Virology* 68:1–5.

Hedrick, P. W. 2000. *Genetics of Populations,* 2d ed. Jones and Bartlett, Boston.

Hetzel, C., and Anderson, R. M. 1996. The within-host cellular dynamics of bloodstage malaria: theoretical and experimental studies. *Parasitology* 113: 25–38.

Hide, G., Welburn, S. C., Tait, A., and Maudlin, I. 1994. Epidemiological relationships of *Trypanosoma brucei* stocks from south east Uganda: evidence for different population structures in human infective and non-human infective isolates. *Parasitology* 109:95–111.

Hill, A. V. S. 1998. The immunogenetics of human infectious diseases. *Annual Review of Immunology* 16:593–617.

Hillis, D. M., Moritz, C., and Mable, B. K., eds. 1996. *Molecular Systematics.* Sinauer Associates, Sunderland, Massachusetts.

Hiromoto, Y., Saito, T., Lindstrom, S. E., Li, Y., Nerome, R., Sugita, S., Shinjoh, M., and Nerome, K. 2000. Phylogenetic analysis of the three polymerase genes (PB1, PB2 and PA) of the influenza B virus. *Journal of General Virology* 81:929–937.

Hoe, N. P., Nakashima, K., Lukomski, S., Grigsby, D., Liu, M., Kordari, P., Dou, S.-J., Pan, X., Vuopio-Varkila, J., Salmelinna, S., McGeer, A., Low, D. E., Schwartz, B., Schuchat, A., Naidich, S., de Lorenzo, D., Fu, Y.-X., and Musser, J. M. 1999. Rapid selection of complement-inhibiting protein variants in group A streptococcus epidemic waves. *Nature Medicine* 5:924–929.

Hohler, T., Gerken, G., Notghi, A., Lubjuhn, R., Taheri, H., Protzer, U., Lohr, H. F., Schneider, P. M., Meyer zum Buschenfelde, K. H., and Rittner, C. 1997. HLA-DRB1*1301 and *1302 protect against chronic hepatitis B. *Journal of Hepatology* 26:503–507.

Holland, J. J., ed. 1992. *Genetic Diversity of RNA Viruses.* Springer-Verlag, New York.

Hollingshead, S. K., Fischetti, V. A., and Scott, J. R. 1986. Complete nucleotide sequence of type 6 M protein of the group A streptococcus: repetitive structure and membrane anchor. *Journal of Biological Chemistry* 261:1677–1686.

Hollingshead, S. K., Fischetti, V. A., and Scott, J. R. 1987. Size variation in group A streptococcal protein is generated by homologous recombination between intragenic repeats. *Molecular and General Genetics* 207:196–203.

Holmes, E. C., Zhang, L. Q., Simmonds, P., Ludlam, C. A., and Leigh Brown, A. J. 1992. Convergent and divergent sequence evolution in the surface envelope glycoprotein of human immunodeficiency virus type 1 within a single infected patient. *Proceedings of the National Academy of Sciences* 89:4835–4839.

Housworth, W. J., and Spoon, M. M. 1971. The age distribution of excess mortality during A2 Hong Kong influenza outbreaks. *American Journal of Epidemiology* 94:348–350.

Hughes, A. L. 1992. Positive selection and interallelic recombination at the merozoite surface antigen-1 (MSA-1) locus of *Plasmodium falciparum*. *Molecular Biology and Evolution* 9:381–393.

Hughes, A. L. 1999. *Adaptive Evolution of Genes and Genomes*. Oxford University Press, Oxford.

Hughes, A. L., and Verra, F. 2001. Very large long-term effective population size in the virulent human malaria parasite *Plasmodium falciparum*. *Proceedings of the Royal Society of London Series B Biological Sciences* 268:1855–1860.

Hughes, M. K., and Hughes, A. L. 1995. Natural selection on *Plasmodium* surface proteins. *Molecular and Biochemical Parasitology* 71:99–113.

Hulst, M. M., van Gennip, H. G. P., and Moormann, R. J. M. 2000. Passage of classical swine fever virus in cultured swine kidney cells selects virus variants that bind to heparan sulfate due to a single amino acid change in envelope protein E^{rns}. *Virology* 276:93–103.

Hurwitz, J. L., Heber-Katz, E., Hackett, C. J., and Gerhard, W. 1984. Characterization of the murine TH response to influenza virus hemagglutinin: evidence for three major specificities. *Journal of Immunology* 133:3371–3377.

Hynes, R. O. 1992. Integrins: versatility, modulation, and signaling in cell adhesion. *Cell* 69:11–25.

Icenogle, J. C., Shiwen, H., Duke, G., Gilbert, S., Rueckert, R., and Anderegg, J. 1983. Neutralization of poliovirus by a monoclonal antibody: kinetics and stoichiometry. *Virology* 127:412–425.

Iida, S., Meyer, J., Kennedy, K. E., and Arber, W. 1982. A site-specific, conservative recombination system carried by bacteriophage P1: mapping the recombinase gene *cin* and the crossover sites *cix* for the inversion of the C-segment. *EMBO Journal* 1:1445–1453.

Iqbal, J., Perlmann, P., and Berzins, K. 1993. Serologic diversity of antigens expressed on the surface of *Plasmodium falciparum* infected erythrocytes in Punjab (Pakistan). *Transactions of the Royal Society of Tropical Medicine and Hygiene* 87:583–588.

Jackson, T., Blakemore, W., Newman, J. W. I., Knowles, N. J., Mould, A. P., Humphries, M. J., and King, A. M. Q. 2000. Foot-and-mouth disease virus is a ligand for the high-affinity binding conformation of integrin $\alpha5\beta1$: influence of the leucine residue within the RGDL motif on selectivity of integrin binding. *Journal of General Virology* 81:1383–1391.

Jackson, T., Ellard, F. M., Abu-Ghazaleh, R., Brookes, S. M., Blakemore, W. E., Corteyn, A. H., Stuart, D. I., Newman, J. W. I., and King, A. M. Q. 1996. Efficient infection of cells in culture by type O foot-and-mouth disease virus requires binding to cell surface heparan sulfate. *Journal of Virology* 70:5282–5287.

Jackson, T., Sheppard, D., Denyer, M., Blakemore, W. E., and King, A. M. Q. 2000. The epithelial integrin $\alpha v\beta6$ is a receptor for foot-and-mouth disease virus. *Journal of Virology* 74:4949–4956.

Jameson, S. C., and Bevan, M. J. 1995. T cell receptor antagonists and partial agonists. *Immunity* 2:1–11.

Jamieson, B. D., and Ahmed, R. 1989. T cell memory: long-term persistence of virus-specific cytotoxic T cells. *Journal of Experimental Medicine* 169:1993–2005.

Janeway, Jr., C. A. 1993. How the immune system recognizes invaders. *Scientific American* 269(3):73–79.

Janeway, Jr., C. A., Travers, P., Capra, J. D., and Walport, M. J. 1999. *Immunobiology: The Immune System in Health and Disease.* Garland Publishers, New York.

Jaulin, C., Casanova, J.-L., Romero, P., Luescher, I., Cordey, A.-S., Maryanski, J. L., and Kourilsky, P. 1992. Highly diverse T cell recognition of a single *Plasmodium berghei* peptide presented by a series of mutant H-2 K^d molecules. *Immunity* 4:47–55.

Jenni, L., Marti, S., Schweizer, J., Betschart, B., Le Page, R. W. F., Wells, J. M., Tait, A., Paindavoine, P., Pays, E., and Steinert, M. 1986. Hybrid formation between trypanosomes during cyclical transmission. *Nature* 322:173–175.

Jensen, L. T., Laderoged, S., Birkelund, S., and Christiansen, G. 1995. Selection of *Mycoplasma hominis* PG21 deletion mutants by cultivation in the presence of monoclonal antibody 552. *Infection and Immunity* 63:3336–3347.

Jetzt, A. E., Yu, H., Klarmann, G. J., Ron, Y., Preston, B. D., and Dougherty, J. P. 2000. High rate of recombination throughout the human immunodeficiency virus type 1 genome. *Journal of Virology* 74:1234–1240.

Jung, H. C., Kim, J. M., Song, I. S., and Kim, C. Y. 1997. *Heliobacter pylori* induces an array of pro-inflammatory cytokines in human gastric epithelial cells: quantification of mRNA for interleukin-8, -1 α/β, granulocyte-macrophage colony-stimulating factor, monocyte chemoattractant protein-1 and tumour necrosis factor-alpha. *Journal of Gastroenterology and Hepatology* 12:473–480.

Jyssum, K. 1960. Observations on two types of genetic instability in *Escherichia coli. Acta Pathologica et Microbiologica Scandinavica* 48:113–120.

Kamp, D., Kahmann, R., Zipser, D., Broker, T. R., and Chow, L. T. 1978. Inversion of the G DNA segment of phage Mu controls phage infectivity. *Nature* 271:577–580.

Kaverin, N. V., Smirnov, Y. A., Govorkova, E. A., Rudneva, I. A., Gitelman, A. K., Lipatov, A. S., Varich, N. L., Yamnikova, S. S., Makarova, N. V., Webster, R. G., and Lvov, D. K. 2000. Cross-protection and reassortment studies with avian H2 influenza viruses. *Archives of Virology* 145:1059–1066.

Kawaoka, Y., Krauss, S., and Webster, R. G. 1989. Avian-to-human tranmission of the PB1 gene of influenza A viruses in the 1957 and 1968 pandemics. *Journal of Virology* 63:4603–4608.

Keitel, T., Kramer, A., Wessner, H., Scholz, C., Schneider-Mergener, J., and Höhne, W. 1997. Crystallographic analysis of anti-p24 (HIV-1) monoclonal antibody cross-reactivity and polyspecificity. *Cell* 91:811–820.

Kilbourne, E. D., Laver, W. G., Schulman, J. L., and Webster, R. G. 1968. Antiviral activity of antiserum specific for an influenza virus neuraminidase. *Journal of Virology* 2:281–288.

Kimata, J. T., Kuller, L., Anderson, D. B., Dailey, P., and Overbaugh, J. 1999. Emerging cytopathic and antigenic simian immunodeficiency virus variants influence AIDS progression. *Nature Medicine* 5:535–541.

Kimura, M. 1983. *The Neutral Theory of Molecular Evolution.* Cambridge University Press, Cambridge.

Klenerman, P., Rowland-Jones, S., McAdam, S., Edwards, J., Daenke, S., Lalloo, D., Koppe, B., Rosenberg, W., Boyd, D., and Edwards, A. 1994. Cytotoxic T-cell activity antagonized by naturally occurring HIV-1 Gag variants. *Nature* 369:403–407.

Klenerman, P., and Zinkernagel, R. M. 1998. Original antigenic sin impairs cytotoxic T lymphocyte responses to viruses bearing variant epitopes. *Nature* 394:482–485.

Klimstra, W. B., Ryman, K. D., and Johnston, R. E. 1998. Adaptation of Sindbis virus to BHK cells selects for use of heparan sulfate as an attachment receptor. *Journal of Virology* 72:7357–7366.

Knipe, D. M., and Howley, P. M., eds. 2001. *Fields Virology,* 4th ed. Lippincott-Raven, Philadelphia.

Kollmann, T. R., Pettoello-Mantovani, M., Katopodis, N. F., Hachamvitch, M., Rubinstein, A., Kim, A., and Goldstein, H. 1996. Inhibition of acute in vivo human immunodeficiency virus infection by human interleukin 10 treatment of SCID mice implanted with human fetal thymus and liver. *Proceedings of the National Academy of Sciences USA* 93:3126–3131.

Korber, B., Muldoon, M., Theiler, J., Gao, F., Gupta, R., Lapedes, A., Hahn, B. H., Wolinsky, S., and Bhattacharya, T. 2000. Timing the ancestor of the HIV-1 pandemic strains. *Science* 288:1789–1796.

Kosinski, R. J. 1980. Antigenic variation in trypanosomes: a computer analysis of variant order. *Parasitology* 80:343–357.

Kostolanský, F., Varečková, E., Betáková, T., Mucha, V., Russ, G., and Wharton, S. A. 2000. The strong positive correlation between effective affinity and infectivity neutralization of highly cross-reactive monoclonal antibody IIB4, which recognizes antigenic site B on influenza A virus haemagglutinin. *Journal of General Virology* 81:1727–1735.

Kramer, A., Keitel, T., Winkler, K., Stöcklein, W., Höhne, W., and Schneider-Mergener, J. 1997. Molecular basis for the binding promiscuity of an anti-p24 (HIV-1) monoclonal antibody. *Cell* 91:799–809.

Kropshofer, H., Hämmerling, G. J., and Vogt, A. B. 1999. The impact of the non-classical MHC proteins HLA-DM and HLA-DO on loading of MHC class II molecules. *Immunological Reviews* 172:267–278.

Kumar, V., Bansal, V. J., Rao, K. V. S., and Jameel, S. 1992. Hepatitis B virus envelope epitopes: gene assembly and expression in *Escherichia coli* of an immunologically reactive novel multiple-epitope polypeptide 1 (MEP-1). *Gene* 110:137–144.

Kuno, G., Chang, G.-J., Tsuchiya, K. R., Karabatsos, N., and Cropp, C. B. 1998. Phylogeny of the genus *Flavivirus*. *Journal of Virology* 72:73–83.

Laeeq, S., Smith, C. A., Wagner, S. D., and Thomas, D. B. 1997. Preferential selection of receptor-binding variants of influenza virus hemagglutinin by the neutralizing antibody repertoire of transgenic mice expressing a human immunoglobulin μ minigene. *Journal of Virology* 71:2600–2605.

Lamb, R. A., and Krug, R. M. 2001. *Orthomyxoviridae:* the viruses and their replication. In Knipe, D. M., and Howley, P. M., eds., *Fields Virology*, 4th ed., pp. 1487–1531. Lippincott-Raven, Philadelphia.

Lambkin, R., and Dimmock, N. J. 1996. Longitudinal study of an epitope-biased serum haemagglutinin-inhibition antibody response in rabbits immunized with type A influenza virions. *Vaccine* 14:212–218.

Lambkin, R., McLain, L., Jones, S. E., Aldridge, S. L., and Dimmock, N. J. 1994. Neutralization escape mutants of type A influenza virus are readily selected by antisera from mice immunized with whole virus: a possible mechanism for antigenic drift. *Journal of General Virology* 75:3493–3502.

Lancefield, R. C. 1962. Current knowledge of type-specific M antigens of group A streptococci. *Journal of Immunology* 89:307–313.

Landweber, L. F. 1999. Experimental RNA evolution. *Trends in Ecology and Evolution* 14:353–358.

Larsen, O., Andersson, S., da Silva, Z., Hedegaard, K., Sandstrom, A., Naucler, A., Dias, F., Melbye, M., and Aaby, P. 2000. Prevalences of HTLV-1 infection and associated risk determinants in an urban population in Guinea–Bissau, West Africa. *Journal of Acquired Immune Deficiency Syndrome* 25:157–163.

Latek, R. R., and Unanue, E. R. 1999. Mechanisms and consequences of peptide selection by the I-A^k class II molecule. *Immunological Reviews* 172:209–228.

Latham, J. L., and Burgess, A. E. 1977. *Elementary Reaction Kinetics,* 3d ed. Butterworths, London.

Laukkanen, T., Carr, J. K., Janssens, W., Liitsola, K., Gotte, D., McCutchan, F. E., de Coul, E. O., Cornelissen, M., Heyndrickx, L., and van der Groen, G. 2000. Virtually full-length subtype F and F/D recombinant HIV-1 from Africa and South America. *Virology* 269:95–104.

Lavoie, T. B., Mohan, S., Lipschultz, C. A., Grivel, J.-C., Li, Y., Mainhart, C. R., Kam-Morgan, L. N. W., Drohan, W. N., and Smith-Gill, S. J. 1999. Structural differences among monoclonal antibodies with distinct fine specificities and kinetic properties. *Molecular Immunology* 36:1189–1205.

Layne, S. P., Beugelsdijk, T. J., Patel, C. K., Taubenberger, J. K., Cox, N. J., Gust, I. D., Hay, A. J., Tashiro, M., and Lavanchy, D. 2001. A global lab against influenza. *Science* 293:1729.

LeClerc, J. E., Li, B., Payne, W. L., and Cebula, T. A. 1996. High mutation frequencies among *Escherichia coli* and *Salmonella* pathogens. *Science* 274:1208–1211.

Leigh, E. G. 1970. Natural selection and mutability. *American Naturalist* 104: 301–305.

Lescar, J., Pellegrini, M., Souchon, H., Tello, D., Poljak, R. J., Peterson, N., Greene, M., and Alzari, P. M. 1995. Crystal structure of a cross-reaction complex between Fab F9.13.7 and guinea fowl lysozyme. *Journal of Biological Chemistry* 270:18067–18076.

Levin, B. R., and Bull, J. J. 1994. Short-sighted evolution and the virulence of pathogenic microorganisms. *Trends in Microbiology* 2:76–81.

Levinson, G., and Gutman, G. A. 1987. Slipped-strand mispairing: a major mechanism for DNA sequence evolution. *Molecular Biology and Evolution* 4:203–221.

Li, C. C. 1976. *First Course in Population Genetics*. Boxwood Press, Pacific Grove, California.

Li, W.-H. 1997. *Molecular Evolution*. Sinauer Associates, Sunderland, Massachusetts.

Liang, S., Mozdzanowska, K., Palladino, G., and Gerhard, W. 1994. Heterosubtypic immunity to influenza type A virus in mice. *Journal of Immunology* 152:1653–1661.

Liebert, U. G., Flanagan, S. G., Loffler, S., Baczko, K., ter Meulen, V., and Rima, B. K. 1994. Antigenic determinants of measles virus hemagglutinin associated with neurovirulence. *Journal of Virology* 68:1486–1493.

Lin, J., Andreasen, V., and Levin, S. A. 1999. Dynamics of influenza A drift: the linear three-strain model. *Mathematical Biosciences* 162:33–51.

Lindstrom, S. E., Hiromoto, Y., Nerome, R., Omoe, K., Sugita, S., Yamazaki, Y., Takahashi, T., and Nerome, K. 1998. Phylogenetic analysis of the entire genome of influenza A (H3N2) viruses from Japan: evidence for genetic reassortment of the six internal genes. *Journal of Virology* 72:8021–8031.

Lindstrom, S. E., Hiromoto, Y., Nishimura, H., Saito, T., Nerome, R., and Nerome, K. 1999. Comparative analysis of evolutionary mechanisms of the hemagglutinin and three internal protein genes of inflenza B virus: multiple cocirculating lineages and frequent reassortment of the NP, M, and NS genes. *Journal of Virology* 73:4413–4426.

Llorente, M., Sánchez-Palomino, S., Mañes, S., Luca, P., Kremer, L., de Alborán, I. M., Torán, J. L., Alcamí, J., del Real, G., and Martínez-A., C. 1999. Natural human antibodies retrieved by phage display libraries from healthy donors: polyreactivity and recognition of human immunodeficiency virus type 1 gp120 epitopes. *Scandinavian Journal of Immunology* 50:270–279.

Lord, C. C., Barnard, B., Day, K., Hargrove, J. W., McNamara, J. J., Paul, R. E. L., Trenholme, K., and Woolhouse, M. E. J. 1999. Aggregation and distribution of strains in microparasites. *Philosophical Transactions of the Royal Society of London B* 354:799–807.

Louis, P., Eliaou, J.-F., Kerlan-Candon, S., Pinet, V., Vincent, R., and Clot, J. 1993. Polymorphism in the regulatory region of *HLA-DRB* genes correlating with haplotype evolution. *Immunogenetics* 38:21–26.

Louis, P., Vincent, R., Cavadore, P., Clot, J., and Eliaou, J.-F. 1994. Differential transcriptional activities of *HLA-DR* genes in the various haplotypes. *Journal of Immunology* 153:5059–5067.

MacLeod, A., Turner, C. M. R., and Tait, A. 1999. A high level of mixed *T. brucei* infections in tsetse flies detected by three hypervariable minisatellites. *Molecular and Biochemical Parasitology* 102:237–248.

MacLeod, A., Tweedie, A., Welburn, S. C., Maudlin, I., Turner, C. M. R., and Tait, A. 2000. Minisatellite marker analysis of *Trypanosoma brucei:* reconciliation of clonal, panmictic, and epidemic population genetic structures. *Proceedings of the National Academy of Sciences USA* 97:13442–13447.

Madrenas, J. 1999. Differential signalling by variant ligands of the T cell receptor and the kinetic model of T cell activation. *Life Sciences* 64:717–731.

Malorny, B., Morelli, G., Kusecek, B., Kolberg, J., and Achtman, M. 1998. Sequence diversity, predicted two-dimensional protein structure, and epitope mapping of neisserial Opa proteins. *Journal of Bacteriology* 180:1323–1330.

Man, S., Newberg, M. H., Crotzer, V. L., Luckey, C. J., Williams, N. S., Chen, Y., Huczko, E. L., Ridge, J. P., and Engelhard, V. H. 1995. Definition of a human T cell epitope from influenza A non-structural protein 1 using HLA-A2.1 transgenic mice. *International Immunology* 7:597–605.

Man, S., Ridge, J. P., and Engelhard, V. H. 1994. Diversity and dominance among TCR recognizing HLA-A2.1(+) influenza matrix peptide in human MHC class I transgenic mice. *Journal of Immunology* 153:4458–4467.

Manz, R. A., Löhning, M., Cassese, G., Theil, A., and Radbruch, A. 1998. Survival of long-lived plasma cells is independent of antigen. *International Immunology* 10:1703–1711.

Mao, E. F., Lane, L., Lee, J., and Miller, J. H. 1997. Proliferation of mutators in a cell population. *Journal of Bacteriology* 179:417–422.

Marrs, C. F., Reuhl, W. W., Schoolnik, G. K., and Falkow, S. 1988. Pilin gene phase variation of *Moraxella bovis* is caused by an inversion of the pilin gene. *Journal of Bacteriology* 170:3032–3039.

Marsh, K., and Howard, R. J. 1986. Antigens induced on erythrocytes by *P. falciparum:* expression of diverse and conserved determinants. *Science* 231:150–153.

Marsh, S. G. E., Parham, P., and Barber, L. D. 2000. *The HLA FactsBook.* Academic Press, San Diego.

Marshall, D., Sealy, R., Sangster, M., and Coleclough, C. 1999. T_H cells primed during influenza virus infection provide help for qualitatively distinct antibody responses to subsequent immunization. *Journal of Immunology* 163:4673–4682.

Martin, D. R., and Single, L. A. 1993. Molecular epidemiology of group A streptococcus-M type-1 infections. *Journal of Infectious Diseases* 167:1112–1117.

Martin, D. W., and Weber, P. C. 1997. DNA replication promotes high-frequency homologous recombination during *Autograha californica* multiple nuclear polyhedrosis virus infection. *Virology* 232:300–309.

Martín, J., Wharton, S. A., Lin, Y. P., Takemoto, D. K., Skehel, J. J., Wiley, D. C., and Steinhauer, D. A. 1998. Studies of the binding properties of influenza hemagglutinin receptor-site mutants. *Virology* 241:101–111.

Martínez, M. A., Verdaguer, N., Mateu, M. G., and Domingo, E. 1997. Evolution subverting essentiality: dispensability of the cell attachment Arg-Gly-Asp motif in multiply passaged foot-and-mouth disease virus. *Proceedings of the National Academy of Sciences USA* 94.6798–6802.

Martinson, J. J., Chapman, N. H., Rees, D. C., Liu, Y.-T., and Clegg, J. B. 1997. Global distribution of the CCR5 gene 32-basepair deletion. *Nature Genetics* 16:100–103.

Maryanski, J. L., Attuil, V., Bucher, P., and Walker, P. R. 1999. A quantitative, single-cell PCR analysis of an antigen-specific TCR repertoire selected during an in vivo CD8 response: direct evidence for a wide range of clone sizes with uniform tissue distribution. *Molecular Immunology* 36:745–753.

Maryanski, J. L., Casanova, J.-L., Falk, K., Gournier, H., Jaulin, C., Kourilsky, P., Lemonier, F. A., Luthy, R., Rammensee, H. G., Rotzschke, O., Servis, C., and Lopez, J. A. 1997. The diversity of antigen-specific TCR repertoires reflects the relative complexity of epitopes recognized. *Human Immunology* 54:117–128.

Maryanski, J. L., Jongeneel, C. V., Bucher, P., Casanova, J.-L., and Walker, P. R. 1996. Single-cell PCR analysis of TCR repertoires selected by antigen in vivo: a high magnitude CD8 response is comprised of very few clones. *Immunity* 4:47–55.

Mason, D. 1999. A very high level of crossreactivity is an essential feature of the T-cell receptor. *Immunology Today* 19:395–404.

Masurel, N. 1969. Serological characteristics of a 'new' serotype of influenza A virus: the Hong Kong strain. *Bulletin of the World Health Organization* 41:461–468.

Masurel, N. 1976. Swine influenza virus and the recycling of influenza A viruses in man. *Lancet* 22:244–247.

Mateu, M. G. 1995. Antibody recognition of picornaviruses and escape from neutralization: a structural view. *Virus Research* 38:1–24.

Mateu, M. G., Escarmís, C., and Domingo, E. 1998. Mutational analysis of discontinuous epitopes of foot-and-mouth disease virus using an unprocessed capsid promoter precursor. *Virus Research* 53:27–37.

Mateu, M. G., Hernández, J., Martínez, M. A., Feigelstock, D., Lea, S., Peréz, J. J., Giralt, E., Stuart, D., Palma, E. L., and Domingo, E. 1994. Antigenic heterogeneity of a foot-and-mouth disease virus serotype in the field is mediated by very limited sequence variation at several antigenic sites. *Journal of Virology* 68:1407–1417.

Mateu, M. G., Silva, D. A., Rocha, E., De Brum, D. L., Alonso, A., Enjuanes, L., Domingo, E., and Barahona, H. 1988. Extensive antigenic heterogeneity of foot-and-mouth disease virus of serotype C. *Virology* 167:113–124.

Matrosovich, M., Gao, P., and Kawaoka, Y. 1998. Molecular mechanisms of serum resistance of human influenza H3N2 virus and their involvement in virus adaptation in a new host. *Journal of Virology* 72:6373-6380.

Matrosovich, M., Zhou, N., Kawaoka, Y., and Webster, R. 1999. The surface glycoproteins of H5 influenza viruses isolated from humans, chickens, and wild aquatic birds have distinguishable properties. *Journal of Virology* 73:1146-1155.

Matrosovich, M. N., Gambaryan, A. S., Teneberg, S., Piskarev, V. E., Yamnikova, S. S., Lvov, D. K., Robertson, J. S., and Karlsson, K.-A. 1997. Avian influenza A viruses differ from human viruses by recognition of sialyloligosaccharides and gangliosides and by a higher conservation of the HA receptor-binding site. *Virology* 233:224-234.

Maynard Smith, J., Smith, N. H., O'Rourke, M., and Spratt, B. G. 1993. How clonal are bacteria? *Proceedings of the National Academy of Sciences USA* 90:4384-4388.

McCutchan, F. E. 1999. Global diversity in HIV. In Crandall, K. A., ed., *The Evolution of HIV*, pp. 41-101. Johns Hopkins University Press, Baltimore, Maryland.

McLain, L., and Dimmock, N. J. 1994. Single- and multi-hit kinetics of immunoglobulin G neutralization of human immunodeficiency virus type 1 by monoclonal antibodies. *Journal of General Virology* 75:1457-1460.

McMichael, A. J., and Doherty, P. C. 2000. Introduction. *Philosophical Transactions of the Royal Society of London B* 355:315-316.

McMichael, A. J., Gotch, F. M., Dongworth, D. W., Clark, A., and Potter, C. W. 1983a. Declining T-cell immunity to influenza, 1977-1982. *Lancet* 2:762-764.

McMichael, A. J., Gotch, F. M., Noble, G. R., and Beare, P. S. 1983b. Cytotoxic T-cell immunity to influenza. *New England Journal of Medicine* 309:13-17.

McMichael, A. J., and Phillips, R. E. 1997. Escape of human immunodeficiency virus from immune control. *Annual Review of Immunology* 15:271-296.

Menon, J. N., and Bretscher, P. A. 1998. Parasite dose determines the Th1/Th2 nature of the response to *Leishmania major* independently of infection route and strain of host or parasite. *European Journal of Immunology* 28:4020-4028.

Meyer, S., Weiss, G., and von Haeseler, A. 1999. Pattern of nucleotide substitution and rate heterogeneity in the hypervariable regions I and II of human mtDNA. *Genetics* 152:1103-1110.

Meyer, T. F. 1987. Molecular basis of surface antigen variation in *Neisseria*. *Trends in Genetics* 3:319-324.

Michod, R. E. 1997. Cooperation and conflict in the evolution of individuality. I. Multilevel selection of the organism. *American Naturalist* 149:607-645.

Mills, K., Skehel, J., and Thomas, B. 1986. Extensive diversity in the recognition of influenza virus hemagglutinin by murine T helper clones. *Journal of Experimental Medicine* 163:1477-1490.

Mims, C., Nash, A., and Stephen, J. 2001. *Mims Pathogenesis of Infectious Disease*, 5th ed. Academic Press, San Diego.

Mims, C., Playfair, J., Roitt, I., Wakelin, D., and Williams, R. 1998. *Medical Microbiology,* 2d ed. Mosby, London.

Mims, C. A. 1987. *The Pathogenesis of Infectious Disease,* 3d ed. Academic Press, London.

Mims, C. A., Playfair, J. H. L., Roitt, I. M., Wakelin, D., and Williams, R. 1993. *Medical Microbiology.* Mosby, St. Louis, Missouri.

Mitchison, A. 1997. Partitioning of genetic variation between regulatory and coding gene segments: the predominance of software variation in genes encoding introvert proteins. *Immunogenetics* 46:46–52.

Mitchison, N. A., Muller, B., and Segel, R. M. 2000. Natural variation in immune responsiveness, with special reference to immunodeficiency and promoter polymorphism in class II MHC genes. *Human Immunology* 61:177–181.

Modrow, S., Hahn, B. H., Shaw, G. M., Gallo, R. C., Wong-Staal, F., and Wolf, H. 1987. Computer-assisted analysis of envelope protein sequences of seven human immunodeficiency isolates: predictions of antigenic epitopes in conserved and variable regions. *Journal of Virology* 61:570–578.

Moffatt, M. F., Schou, C., Faux, J. A., and Cookson, W. O. C. M. 1997. Germline TCR-A restriction of immunoglobulin E responses to allergen. *Immunogenetics* 46:226–230.

Mohan, K., and Stevenson, M. M. 1998. Acquired immunity to asexual blood stages. In Sherman, I. W., ed., *Malaria: Parasite Biology, Pathogenesis, and Protection,* pp. 467–493. American Society for Microbiology, Washington, D.C.

Montgomery, A. M. P., Reisfeld, R. A., and Cheresh, D. A. 1994. Integrin $\alpha v \beta 3$ rescues melanoma cells from apoptosis in three-dimensional dermal collagen. *Proceedings of the National Academy of Sciences USA* 91:8856–8860.

Moody, A. M., Reyburn, H., Willcox, N., and Newsom-Davis, J. 1998. New polymorphism of the human T-cell receptor AV28S1 gene segment. *Immunogenetics* 48:62–64.

Morrison, J., Elvin, J., Latron, F., Gotch, F., Moots, R., Strominger, J. L., and McMichael, A. 1992. Identification of the nonamer peptide from influenza A matrix protein and the role of pockets of HLA-A2 in its recognition by cytotoxic T lymphocytes. *European Journal of Immunology* 22:903–907.

Moskophidis, D., and Zinkernagel, R. M. 1995. Immunobiology of cytotoxic T-cell escape mutants of lymphocytic choriomeningitis virus. *Journal of Virology* 69:2187–2193.

Mosser, A. G., Leippe, D., and Rueckert, R. R. 1989. Neutralization of picornaviruses: support for the pentamer bridging hypothesis. In Semler, B. L., and Ehrenfeld, E., eds., *Molecular Aspects of Picornavirus Infection and Detection,* pp. 155–167. American Society for Microbiology, Washington, D.C.

Moxon, E. R., Rainey, P. B., Nowak, M. A., and Lenski, R. E. 1994. Adaptive evolution of highly mutable loci in pathogenic bacteria. *Current Biology* 4:24–33.

Moya, A., Elena, S. F., Bracho, A., Miralles, R., and Barrio, E. 2000. The evolution of RNA viruses: a population genetics view. *Proceedings of the National Academy of Sciences USA* 97:6967–6973.

Muñoz-Jordán, J. L., Davies, K. P., and Cross, G. A. M. 1996. Stable expression of mosaic coats of variant surface glycoproteins in *Trypanosoma brucei*. *Science* 272:1795-1797.

Muotiala, A., Seppala, H., Huovinen, P., and Vuopio-Varkila, J. 1997. Molecular comparison of group A streptococci of T1M1 serotype from invasive and noninvasive infections in Finland. *Journal of Infectious Diseases* 175:392-399.

Murali-Krishna, K., Altman, J. D., Suresh, M., Sourdive, D. J. D., Zajac, A. J., Miller, J. D., Slansky, J., and Ahmed, R. 1998. Counting antigen-specific CD8 T cells: a reevaluation of bystander activation during viral infection. *Immunity* 8:177-187.

Mylin, L. M., Bonneau, R. H., Lippolis, J. D., and Tevethia, S. S. 1995. Hierarchy among multiple H-2b-restricted cytotoxic T-lymphocyte epitopes within simian virus 40 T antigen. *Journal of Virology* 69:6665-6677.

Nakagawa, T. Y., and Rudensky, A. Y. 1999. The role of lysosomal proteinases in MHC class II–mediated antigen processing and presentation. *Immunological Reviews* 172:121-129.

Nakajima, S., Nobusawa, E., and Nakajima, K. 2000. Variation in response among individuals to antigenic sites on the HA protein of human influenza virus may be responsible for the emergence of drift strains in the human population. *Virology* 274:220-231.

Nakra, P., Manivel, V., Vishwakarma, R. A., and Rao, K. V. S. 2000. B cell responses to a peptide epitope. X. Epitope selection in a primary response is thermodynamically regulated. *Journal of Immunology* 164:5615-5625.

Nara, P. L., and Garrity, R. 1998. Deceptive imprinting: a cosmopolitan strategy for complicating vaccination. *Vaccine* 16:1780-1787.

Natali, A., Oxford, J. S., and Schild, G. C. 1981. Frequency of naturally occurring antibody to influenza virus antigenic variants selected in vitro with monoclonal antibody. *Journal of Hygiene* 87:185-191.

Natali, A., Pilotti, E., Valcavi, P. P., Chezzi, C., and Oxford, J. S. 1998. Natural and 'in vitro' selected antigenic variants of influenza A virus (H_2N_2). *Journal of Infection* 37:19-23.

Nayak, B. P., Tuteja, R., Manivel, V., Roy, R. P., Vishwakarma, R. A., and Rao, K. V. S. 1998. B cell responses to a peptide epitope. V. Kinetic regulation of repertoire discrimination and antibody optimization for epitope. *Journal of Immunology* 161:3510-3519.

Nee, S., Holmes, E. C., Rambaut, A., and Harvey, P. H. 1995. Inferring population history from molecular phylogenies. *Philosophical Transactions of the Royal Society of London B* 349:25-31.

Neff, S., Sa-Carvalho, D., Rieder, E., Mason, P. W., Blystone, S. D., Brown, E. J., and Baxt, B. 1998. Foot-and-mouth disease virus virulent for cattle utilizes the integrin $\alpha_v\beta_3$ as its receptor. *Journal of Virology* 72:3587-3594.

Nei, M. 1987. *Molecular Evolutionary Genetics*. Columbia University Press, New York.

Nei, M., and Kumar, S. 2000. *Molecular Evolution and Phylogenetics.* Oxford University Press, Oxford.

Neva, F. A. 1977. Looking back for a view of the future: observations of immunity to induce malaria. *American Journal of Tropical Medicine and Hygiene* 26:211–215.

Newman, A. M., Mainhart, C. R., Mallet, C. P., Lavoie, T. B., and Smith-Gill, S. J. 1992. Patterns of antibody specificity during the BALB/c immune response to hen egg white lysozyme. *Journal of Immunology* 149:3260–3272.

Nguyen-Van-Tam, J. S. 1998. Epidemiology of influenza. In Nicholson, K. G., Webster, R. G., and Hay, A. J., eds., *Textbook of Influenza*, pp. 181–206. Blackwell Science, Oxford.

Niedermann, G., Butz, S., Ihlenfeldt, H. G., Grimm, R., Lucchiari, M., Hoschutzky, H., Jung, G., Maier, B., and Eichmann, K. 1995. Contribution of proteasome-mediated proteolysis to the hierarchy of epitopes presented by major histocompatibility complex class I molecules. *Immunity* 2:289–299.

Niedermann, G., Geier, E., Lucchiari-Hartz, M., Hitziger, N., Ramsperger, A., and Eichmann, K. 1999. The specificity of proteasomes: impact on MHC class I processing and presentation of antigens. *Journal of Immunology* 158:1507–1515.

Niedermann, G., King, G., Butz, S., Birsner, U., Grimm, R., Shabanowitz, J., Hunt, D. F., and Eichmann, K. 1996. The proteolytic fragments generated by vertebrate proteasomes: structural relationships to major histocompatibility complex class I binding peptides. *Proceedings of the National Academy of Sciences USA* 93:8572–8577.

Nielsen, L., Blixenkrone-Møller, M., Thylstrup, M., Hansen, N. J. V., and Bolt, G. 2001. Adaptation of wild-type measles virus to CD46 receptor usage. *Archives of Virology* 146:197–208.

Niewiesk, S., Daenke, S., Parker, C. E., Taylor, G., Weber, J., Nightingale, S., and Bangham, C. R. M. 1995. Naturally occurring variants of human T-cell leukemia virus type I Tax protein impair its recognition by cytotoxic T lymphocytes and the transactivation function of Tax. *Journal of Virology* 69:2649–2653.

Nokes, D. J., Anderson, R. M., and Anderson, M. J. 1986. Rubella epidemiology in South East England. *Journal of Hygiene* 86:291–304.

Nowak, M. A., and May, R. M. 2000. *Virus Dynamics: Mathematical Principles of Immunology and Virology.* Oxford University Press, Oxford.

Nowak, M. A., May, R. M., Phillips, R. E., Rowland-Jones, S., Lalloo, D. G., McAdam, S., Klenerman, P., Koppe, B., Sigmund, K., Bangham, C. R. M., et al. 1995. Antigenic oscillations and shifting immunodominance in HIV-1 infections. *Nature* 375:606–611.

Núñez, J. I., Baranowski, E., Molina, N., Ruiz-Jarabo, C. M., Sánchez, C., Domingo, E., and Sobrino, F. 2001. A single amino acid substitution in nonstructural protein 3A can mediate adaptation of foot-and-mouth disease virus to the guinea pig. *Journal of Virology* 75:3077–3083.

Nyambi, P. N., Lewi, P., Peeters, M., Janssens, W., Heyndrickx, L., Fransen, K.,

Andries, K., Vanden Haesevelde, M., Heeney, J., Piot, P., and van der Groen, G. 1997. Study of the dynamics of neutralization escape mutants in a chimpanzee naturally infected with the simian immunodeficiency virus SIVcpz-ant. *Journal of Virology* 71:2320–2330.

Nyambi, P. N., Mbah, H. A., Burda, S., Williams, C., Gorny, M. K., Nádas, A., and Zolla-Pazner, S. 2000a. Conserved and exposed epitopes on intact, native, primary human immunodeficiency virus type 1 virions of group M. *Journal of Virology* 74:7096–7107.

Nyambi, P. N., Nádas, A., Mbah, H. A., Burda, S., Williams, C., Gorny, M. K., and Zolla-Pazner, S. 2000b. Immunoreactivity of intact virions of human immunodeficiency virus type 1 (HIV-1) reveals the existence of fewer HIV-1 immunotypes than genotypes. *Journal of Virology* 74:10670–10680.

Nyambi, P. N., Nkengasong, J., Lewi, P., Andries, K., Janssens, W., Fransen, K., Heyndrickx, L., Piot, P., and van der Groen, G. 1996. Multivariate analysis of human immunodeficiency virus type 1 neutralization data. *Journal of Virology* 70:6235–6243.

O'Brien, S. J., and Dean, M. 1997. In search of AIDS-resistance genes. *Scientific American* 277(3):44–51.

Ochman, H., Lawrence, J. G., and Groisman, E. A. 2000. Lateral gene transfer and the nature of bacterial innovation. *Nature* 405:299–304.

Ochsenbein, A. F., Fehr, T., Lutz, C., Suter, M., Brombacher, F., Hengartner, H., and Zinkernagel, R. M. 1999. Control of early viral and bacterial distribution and disease by natural antibodies. *Science* 286:2156–2159.

Ochsenbein, A. F., Pinschewer, D. D., Sierro, S., Horvath, E., Hengartner, H., and Zinkernagel, R. M. 2000. Protective long-term antibody memory by antigen-driven and T help-dependent differentiation of long-lived memory B cells to short-lived plasma cells independent of secondary lymphoid organs. *Proceedings of the National Academy of Sciences* 97:13263–13268.

O'hUigin, C., Satta, Y., Hausmann, A., Dawkins, R. L., and Klein, J. 2000. The implications of intergenic polymorphism for major histocompatibility complex evolution. *Genetics* 156:867–877.

Oliveira, R. P., Broude, N. E., Macedo, A. M., Cantor, C. R., Smith, C. L., and Pena, S. D. J. 1998. Probing the genetic population structure of *Trypanosoma cruzi* with polymorphic microsatellites. *Proceedings of the National Academy of Sciences USA* 95:3776–3780.

Oliveira, R. P., Melo, A. I. R., Macedo, A. M., Chiari, E., and Pena, S. D. J. 1999. The population structure of *Trypanosoma cruzi:* expanded analysis of 54 strains using eight polymorphic CA-repeat microsatellites. *Memorias do Instituto Oswaldo Cruz, 94 (Suppl. 1)*, 65–70.

Orive, M. E. 1995. Senescence in organisms with clonal reproduction and complex life histories. *American Naturalists* 145:90–108.

Ossendorp, F., Eggers, M., Neisig, A., Ruppert, T., Groettrup, M., Sijts, A., Mengede, E., Kloetzel, P.-M., Neefjes, J., Koszinowski, U., and Melief, C. 1996. A single residue exchange within a viral CTL epitope alters proteasome-mediated degradation resulting in lack of antigen presentation. *Immunity* 5:115-124.

Otto, S. P. 2000. Detecting the form of selection from DNA sequence data. *Trends in Genetics* 16:526-529.

Otto, S. P., and Hastings, I. M. 1998. Mutation and selection within the individual. *Genetica* 102/103:507-524.

Overbaugh, J., and Bangham, C. R. M. 2001. Selection forces and constraints on retroviral sequence variation. *Science* 292:1106-1109.

Oxford, J. S. 2000. Influenza A pandemics of the 20th century with special reference to 1918: virology, pathology and epidemiology. *Reviews in Medical Virology* 10:119-133.

Page, R. D. M., and Holmes, E. C. 1998. *Molecular Evolution: A Phylogenetic Approach.* Blackwell Scientific, Oxford.

Palese, P., and Compans, R. W. 1976. Inhibition of influenza virus replication in tissue culture by 2-deoxy-2,3-dehydro-N-trifluoro-acetyl-neuraminic acid (FANA): mechanism of action. *Journal of General Virology* 33:159-163.

Parker, E. P., Nightingale, S., Taylor, G. P., Weber, J., and Bangham, C. R. M. 1994. Circulating anti-Tax cytotoxic T lymphocytes from human T-cell leukemia virus type I-infected people, with and without tropical spastic paraparesis, recognize multiple epitopes simultaneously. *Journal of Virology* 68:2860-2868.

Paul, R. E. L., and Day, K. P. 1998. Mating patterns of *Plasmodium falciparum*. *Parasitology Today* 14:197-202.

Paul, W. E. 1993. *Fundamental Immunology.* Raven Press, New York.

Paulson, J. C. 1985. Interactions of animal viruses with cell surface receptors. In Conn, M., ed., *The Receptors*, pp. 131-219. Academic Press, New York.

Pays, E. 1985. Gene conversion in trypanosome antigenic variation. *Progress in Nucleic Acid Research and Molecular Biology* 32:1-26.

Pays, E. 1989. Pseudogenes, chimeric genes and the timing of antigen variation in African trypanosomes. *Trends in Genetics* 5:389-391.

Pays, E., Lheureux, M., and Steinert, M. 1981. The expression-linked copy of the surface antigen gene in *Trypanosoma* is probably the one transcribed. *Nature* 292:265-267.

Pays, E., and Nolan, D. 1998. Expression and function of surface proteins in *Trypanosoma brucei. Molecular and Biochemical Parasitology* 91:3-36.

Peng, G., Hongo, S., Kimura, H., Muraki, Y., Sugawara, K., Kitame, F., Numazaki, Y., Suzuki, H., and Nakamura, K. 1996. Frequent occurrence of genetic reassortment between influenza C virus strains in nature. *Journal of General Virology* 77:1489-1492.

Peng, G., Hongo, S., Muraki, Y., Sugawara, K., Nishimura, H., Kitame, F., and Nakamura, K. 1994. Genetic reassortment of influenza C viruses in man. *Journal of General Virology* 75:3619-3622.

Pinilla, C., Martin, R., Gran, B., Appel, J. R., Boggiano, C., Wilson, D. B., and

Houghten, R. A. 1999. Exploring immunological specificity using synthetic peptide combinatorial libraries. *Current Opinion in Immunology* 11:193-202.

Pircher, H., Moskophidis, D., Rohrer, U., Burki, K., Hengartner, H., and Zinkernagel, R. M. 1990. Viral escape by selection of cytotoxic T cell–resistant virus variants in vivo. *Nature* 346:629-633.

Piyasirisilp, S., McCutchan, F. E., Carr, J. K., Sanders-Buell, E., Liu, W., Chen, J., Wagner, R., Wolf, H., Shao, Y., Lai, S., Beyrer, C., and Yu, X.-F. 2000. A recent outbreak of human immunodeficiency virus type 1 infection in southern China was initiated by two highly homogeneous, geographically separated strains, circulating recombinant form AE and a novel BC recombinant. *Journal of Virology* 74:11286-11295.

Plebanski, M., Lee, E. A. M., Hannan, C. M., Flanagan, K. L., Gilbert, S. C., Gravenor, M. B., and Hill, A. V. S. 1999. Altered peptide ligands narrow the repertoire of cellular immune responses by interfering with T-cell priming. *Nature Medicine* 5:565-571.

Plotkin, S. A., and Orenstein, W. A., eds. 1999. *Vaccines,* 3d ed. W. B. Saunders, Philadelphia.

Porcelli, S. A., and Modlin, R. L. 1999. The CD1 system: antigen-presenting molecules for T cell recognition of lipids and glycolipids. *Annual Review of Immunology* 17:297-329.

Porter, P. 1972. Immunoglobulins in bovine mammary secretions: quantitative changes in early lactation and absorption by the neonatal calf. *Immunology* 23:225-237.

Potts, J. R., and Campbell, I. D. 1994. Fibronectin structure and assembly. *Current Opinion in Cell Biology* 6:648-655.

Power, C. A. 2000. Factors that influence T helper cell response to infection. *Current Opinion in Infectious Diseases* 13:209-213.

Prager, E. M. 1993. The sequence-immunology correlation revisited: data for cetacean myoglobins and mammalian lysozymes. *Journal of Molecular Evolution* 37:408-416.

Preiser, P. R., Jarra, W., Capiod, T., and Snounou, G. 1999. A rhoptry-protein-associated mechanism of clonal phenotypic variation in rodent malaria. *Nature* 398:618-622.

Preston, B. D., and Dougherty, J. P. 1996. Mechanisms of retroviral mutation. *Trends in Microbiology* 4:16-21.

Price, D. A., Meier, U.-C., Klenerman, P., Purbhoo, M. A., Phillips, R. E., and Sewell, A. K. 1998. The influence of antigenic variation on cytotoxic T lymphocyte responses in HIV-1 infection. *Journal of Molecular Medicine* 76:699-708.

Price, G. E., Ou, R., Jiang, H., Huang, L., and Moskophidis, D. 2000. Viral escape by selection of cytotoxic T cell–resistant variants in influenza A virus pneumonia. *Journal of Experimental Medicine* 191:1853-1867.

Prigozy, T. I., Naidenko, O., Qasba, P., Elewaut, D., Brossay, L., Khurana, A., Natori, T., Koezuka, Y., Kulkarni, A., and Kronenberg, M. 2001. Glycolipid antigen processing for presentation by CD1d molecules. *Science* 291:664-667.

Puel, A., Groot, P. C., Lathrop, M. G., Demant, P., and Mouton, D. 1995. Mapping of genes controlling quantitative antibody production in Biozzi mice. *Journal of Immunology* 154:5799–5805.

Puglielli, M. T., Zajac, A. J., van der Most, R. G., Dzuris, J. L., Sette, A., Altman, J. D., and Ahmed, R. 2001. In vivo selection of a lymphocytic choriomeningitis virus variant that affects recognition of the GP330043 epitope by H-2D^b but not H-2K^b. *Journal of Virology* 75:5099–5107.

Racaniello, V. R. 2001. *Picornaviridae:* the viruses and their replication. In Knipe, D. M., and Howley, P. M., eds., *Fields Virology,* 4th ed., pp. 685–722. Lippincott-Raven, Philadelphia.

Radman, M. 1999. Enzymes of evolutionary change. *Nature* 401:866–868.

Rammensee, H. G., Friede, T., and Stefanovic, S. 1995. MHC ligand motifs: first listing. *Immunogenetics* 41:178–228.

Rao, K. V. S. 1999. Selection in a T-dependent primary humoral response: new insights from polypeptide models. *APMIS* 107:807–818.

Reeder, J. C., and Brown, G. V. 1996. Antigenic variation and immune evasion in *Plasmodium falciparum* malaria. *Immunology and Cell Biology* 74:546–554.

Rehermann, B., Chang, K. M., McHutchison, J., Kokka, R., Houghton, M., Rice, C. M., and Chisari, F. V. 1996. Differential cytotoxic T-lymphocyte responsiveness to the hepatitis B and C virus in chronically infected patients. *Journal of Virology* 70:7092–7102.

Reichstetter, S., Krellner, P. H., Meenzen, C. M., Kalden, J. R., and Wassmuth, R. 1994. Comparative analysis of sequence variability in the upstream regulatory region of the *HLA-DQB1* gene. *Immunogenetics* 39:207–212.

Reider, E., Baxt, B., and Mason, P. W. 1994. Animal derived antigenic variants of foot-and-mouth disease virus type A$_{12}$ have low affinity for cells in culture. *Journal of Virology* 68:5296–5299.

Reimann, J., and Schirmbeck, R. 1999. Alternative pathways for processing exogenous and endogenous antigens that can generate peptides for MHC class I-restricted presentation. *Immunological Reviews* 172:131–152.

Revollo, S., Oury, B., Laurent, J.-P., Barnabé, C., Quesney, V., Carriere, V., Noël, S., and Tibayrenc, M. 1998. *Trypanosoma cruzi:* impact of clonal evolution of the parasite on its biological and medical properties. *Experimental Parasitology* 89:30–39.

Reyburn, H., Cornélis, F., Russell, V., Harding, R., Moss, P., and Bell, J. 1993. Allelic polymorphism of human T-cell receptor V alpha gene segments. *Immunogenetics* 38:287–291.

Rich, S. M., Ferreira, M. U., and Ayala, F. J. 2000. The origin of antigenic diversity in *Plasmodium falciparum*. *Parasitology Today* 16:390–396.

Rich, S. M., Sawyer, S. A., and Barbour, A. G. 2001. Antien polymorphism in *Borrelia hermsii,* a clonal pathogenic bacterium. *Proceedings of the National Academy of Sciences USA* 98:15038–15043.

Richards, F. F., Konigsberg, W. H., Rosenstein, R. W., and Varga, J. M. 1975. On the specificity of antibodies: biochemical and biophysical evidence indicates the existence of polyfunctional antibody combining regions. *Science* 187:130–137.

Rickinson, A. B., Callan, M. F. C., and Annels, N. E. 2000. T-cell memory: lessons from Epstein-Barr virus infection in man. *Philosophical Transactions of the Royal Society of London B* 355:391–400.

Ripley, L. S. 1999. Predictability of mutant sequences: relationships between mutational mechanisms and mutant specificity. *Annals of the New York Academy of Sciences* 870:159–172.

Robertson, D. L., Anderson, J. P., Bradac, J. A., Carr, J. K., Foley, B., Funkhouser, R. K., Gao, F., Hahn, B. H., Kalish, M. L., Kuiken, C., Learn, G. H., Leitner, T., McCutchan, F., Osmanov, S., Peeters, M., Pieniazek, D., Salminen, M., Sharp, P. M., Wolinsky, S., and Korber, B. 1999. HIV-1 nomenclature proposal: a reference guide to HIV-1 classification. In Kuiken, C. L., Foley, B., Hahn, B., Korber, B., McCutchan, F., Marx, P. A., Mellors, J. W., Mullins, J. I., Sodroski, J., and Wolinksy, S., eds., *Human Retroviruses and AIDS 1999: A Compilation and Analysis of Nucleic Acid and Amino Acid Sequences*, pp. 492–505. Theoretical Biology and Biophysics Group, Los Alamos National Laboratory, Los Alamos, New Mexico.

Robertson, D. L., Hahn, B. H., and Sharp, P. M. 1995. Recombination in AIDS viruses. *Journal of Molecular Evolution* 40:249–259.

Robertson, J. S. 1993. Clinical influenza virus and the embryonated hen's egg. *Reviews in Medical Virology* 3:97–106.

Robertson, J. S. 1999. An overview of host cell selection. In Brown, F., Robertson, J. S., Schild, G. C., and Wood, J. M., eds., *Inactivated Influenza Vaccines Prepared in Cell Culture.* Developments in Biological Standards, vol. 98, pp. 7–11. Karger, Basel.

Robertson, J. S., Cook, P., Attwell, A.-M., and Williams, S. P. 1995. Replicative advantage in tissue culture of egg-adapted influenza virus over tissue-culture derived virus: implications for vaccine manufacture. *Vaccine* 13:1583–1588.

Robinson, J., Malik, A., Parham, P., Bodmer, J. G., and Marsh, S. G. E. 2000. IMGT/HLA database—a sequence database for the human major histocompatibility complex. *Tissue Antigens* 55:280–287.

Rock, K. L., and Goldberg, A. L. 1999. Degradation of cell proteins and the generation of MHC class I–presented peptides. *Annual Review of Immunology* 17:739–779.

Roden, R. B. S., Yutzy, W. H., Fallon, R., Inglis, S., Lowy, D. R., and Schiller, J. T. 2000. Minor capsid protein of human genital papillomaviruses contains subdominant, cross-neutralizing epitopes. *Virology* 270:254–257.

Rodrigo, A. G., and Learn, Jr., G. H., eds. 2000. *Computational and Evolutionary Analysis of HIV Molecular Sequences.* Kluwer Academic, Boston.

Rogers, G. N., Daniels, R. S., Skehel, J. J., Wiley, D. C., Wang, X., Higa, H. H., and Paulson, J. C. 1989. Host-mediated selection of influenza virus receptor variants. *Journal of Biological Chemistry* 260:7362–7367.

Rogers, G. N., and D'Souza, G. L. 1989. Receptor-binding properties of human and animal H1 influenza virus isolates. *Virology* 173:317–322.

Rogers, G. N., Paulson, J. C., Daniels, R. S., Skehel, J. J., Wilson, I. A., and Wiley, D. C. 1983. Single amino acid substitutions in influenza haemagglutinin change receptor binding specificity. *Nature* 304:76–78.

Rohani, P., Earn, D. J. D., and Grenfell, B. T. 1999. Opposite patterns of synchrony in sympatric disease metapopulations. *Science* 286:968–971.

Röhm, C., Zhou, N., Süss, J., MacKenzie, J., and Webster, R. G. 1996. Characterization of a novel influenza hemagglutinin, H15: criteria for determination of influenza A subtypes. *Virology* 217:508–516.

Roost, H. P., Backmann, M. F., Haag, A., Karlinke, U., Pliska, V., Hengartner, H., and Zinkernagel, R. M. 1995. Early high-affinity neutralizing anti-virus IgG responses without further overall improvement of affinity. *Proceedings of the National Academy of Sciences USA* 92:1257–1261.

Roost, H. P., Charan, S., and Zinkernagel, R. M. 1990. Analysis of the kinetics of antiviral memory T help in vivo: characterization of short lived cross-reactive T help. *European Journal of Immunology* 20:2547–2554.

Rose, M. R. 1991. *Evolutionary Biology of Aging*. Oxford University Press, Oxford.

Rostand, K. S., and Esko, J. D. 1997. Microbial adherence to and invasion through proteoglycans. *Infection and Immunity* 65:1–8.

Rottem, S., and Naot, Y. 1998. Subversion and exploitation of host cells by mycoplasmas. *Trends in Microbiology* 6:436–440.

Rouzine, I. M., and Coffin, J. M. 1999. Search for the mechanism of genetic variation in the *pro* gene of human immunodeficiency virus. *Journal of Virology* 73:8167–8178.

Rozsa, W. F., and Marrs, C. F. 1991. Interesting sequence differences between the pilin gene inversion regions of *Moraxella lacunata* ATCC 17956 and *Moraxella bovis* Epp63. *Journal of Bacteriology* 173:4000–4006.

Rudensey, L. M., Kimata, J. T., Long, E. M., Chackerian, B., and Overbaugh, J. 1998. Changes in the extracellular envelope glycoprotein of variants that evolve during the course of simian immunodeficiency virus SIVMne infection affect neutralizing antibody recognition, syncytium formation, and macrophage tropism but not replication, cytopathicity, or CCR-5 coreceptor recognition. *Journal of Virology* 72:209–217.

Rudneva, I. A., Sklyanskaya, E. I., Barulina, O. S., Yamnikova, S. S., Kovaleva, V. P., Tsvetkova, I. V., and Kaverin, N. V. 1996. Phenotypic expression of HA-NA combinations in human-avian influenza A virus reassortants. *Archives of Virology* 141:1091–1099.

Sa-Carvalho, D., Rieder, E., Baxt, B., Rodarte, R., Tanuri, A., and Mason, P. W. 1997. Tissue culture adaptation of foot-and mouth disease virus selects viruses that bind to heparin and are attenuated in cattle. *Journal of Virology* 71:5115–5123.

Saha, K., Zhang, J., Gupta, A., Dave, R., Yimen, M., and Zerhouni, B. 2001. Isolation of primary HIV-1 that target CD8$^+$ T lymphocytes using CD8 as a receptor. *Nature Medicine* 7:65–72.

Salaun, L., Audibert, C., Le Lay, G., Burucoa, C., Fauchere, J. L., and Picard, B. 1998. Panmictic structure of *Helicobacter pylori* demonstrated by the comparative study of six genetic markers. *FEMS Microbiology Letters* 161:231–239.

Salmivirta, M., Lidholt, K., and Linkahl, U. 1996. Heparan sulfate: a piece of information. *FASEB Journal* 10:1270–1279.

Samri, A., Haas, G., Duntze, J., Bouley, J.-M., Calvez, V., Katlama, C., and Autran, B. 2000. Immunogenicity of mutations induced by nucleoside reverse transcriptase inhibitors for human immunodeficiency virus type 1–specific cytotoxic T cells. *Journal of Virology* 74:9306–9312.

Sanna, P. P., Ramiro-Ibañez, F., and De Logu, A. 2000. Synergistic interactions of antibodies in rate of virus neutralization. *Virology* 270:386–396.

Sasisekharan, R., and Venkataraman, G. 2000. Heparin and heparan sulfate: biosynthesis, structure and function. *Current Opinion in Chemical Biology* 4:626–631.

Scherf, A., Hernandez-Rivas, R., Buffet, P., Bottius, E., Benatar, C., Pouvelle, B., Gysin, J., and Lanzer, M. 1998. Antigenic variation in malaria: in situ switching, relaxed and mutually exclusive transcription of *var* genes during intra-erythrocytic development in *Plasmodium falciparum*. *EMBO Journal* 17:5418–5426.

Scherle, P., and Gerhard, W. 1986. Functional analysis of influenza-specific helper T cell clones in vivo: T cells specific for internal viral proteins provide cognate help for B cell responses to hemagglutinin. *Journal of Experimental Medicine* 164:1114–1128.

Schneider-Schaulies, J. 2000. Cellular receptors for viruses: links to tropism and pathogenesis. *Journal of General Virology* 81:1413–1429.

Schofield, D. J., Stephenson, J. R., and Dimmock, N. J. 1997a. High and low efficiency neutralization epitopes on the haemagglutinin of type A influenza virus. *Journal of General Virology* 78:2441–2446.

Schofield, D. J., Stephenson, J. R., and Dimmock, N. J. 1997b. Variations in the neutralizing and haemagglutination-inhibiting activities of five influenza A virus-specific IgGs and their antibody fragments. *Journal of General Virology* 78:2431–2439.

Schols, D., and De Clercq, E. 1996. Human immunodeficiency virus type 1 gp120 induces anergy in human peripheral blood lymphocytes by inducing interleukin-10 production. *Journal of Virology* 70:4953–4960.

Scholtissek, C. 1998. Genetic reassortment of human influenza viruses in nature. In Nicholson, K. G., Webster, R. G., and Hay, A. J., eds., *Textbook of Influenza*, pp. 120–125. Blackwell Science, Oxford.

Schroer, J. A., Bender, T., Feldmann, T., and Kim, K. J. 1983. Mapping epitopes on the insulin molecule using monoclonal antibodies. *European Journal of Immunology* 13:693–700.

Schubert, U., Antón, L. C., Gibbs, J., Norbury, C. C., Yewdell, J. W., and Bennink,

J. R. 2000. Rapid degradation of a large fraction of newly synthesized proteins by proteasomes. *Nature* 404:770-774.

Schumacher, T. N. M. 1999. Immunology: accessory to murder. *Nature* 398:26-27.

Scott, T. W., Weaver, S. C., and Mallampalli, V. L. 1994. Evolution of mosquito-borne viruses. In Morse, S. S., ed., *Evolutionary Biology of Viruses*, pp. 293-324. Raven Press, New York.

Seaman, M. S., Wang, C. R., and Forman, J. 2000. MHC class Ib–restricted CTL provide protection against primary and secondary *Listeria monocytogenes* infection. *Journal of Immunology* 165:5192-5201.

Seder, R. A., and Hill, A. V. S. 2000. Vaccines against intracellular infections requiring cellular immunity. *Nature* 406:793-798.

Seed, J. R. 1978. Competition among serologically different clones of *Trypanosoma brucei gambiense* in vivo. *Journal of Protozoology* 25:526-529.

Semmes, O. J., and Jeang, K.-T. 1992. Mutational analysis of human T-cell leukemia virus type I Tax: regions necessary for function determined with 47 mutant proteins. *Journal of Virology* 66:7183-7192.

Seo, S. H., and Webster, R. G. 2001. Cross-reactive, cell-mediated immunity and protection of chickens from lethal H5N1 influenza virus infection in Hong Kong poultry markets. *Journal of Virology* 75:2516-2525.

Sette, A., Alexander, J., Ruppert, J., Snoke, K., Franco, A., Ishioka, G., and Grey, H. M. 1994. Antigen analog/MHC complexes as specific T cell receptor antagonists. *Annual Review of Immunology* 12:413-431.

Sharma, P. L., and Crumpacker, C. S. 1999. Decreased processivity of human immunodeficiency virus type 1 reverse transcriptase (RT) containing didanosine-selected mutation Leu75Val: a comparative analysis of RT variants Leu-74Val and lamivudine-selected Met184Val. *Journal of Virology* 73:8448-8456.

Shields, P. L., Owsianka, A., Carman, W. F., Boxall, E., Hubscher, S. G., Shaw, J., O'Donnell, K., Elias, E., and Mutimer, D. J. 1999. Selection of hepatitis B surface 'escape' mutants during passive immune prophylaxis following liver transplantion: potential impact of genetic changes on polymerase protein function. *Gut* 45:306-309.

Shin, H. D., Winkler, C., Stephens, J. C., Bream, J., Young, H., Goedert, J. J., O'Brien, T. R., Vlahov, D., Buchbinder, S., Giorgi, J., Rinaldo, C., Donfield, S., Willoughby, A., O'Brien, S. J., and Smith, M. W. 2000. Genetic restriction of HIV-1 pathogenesis to AIDS by promoter alleles of IL10. *Proceedings of the National Academy of Sciences USA* 97:14467-14472.

Shirai, M., Arichi, T., Chen, M., Nishioka, M., Ikeda, K., Takahashi, H., Enomoto, N., Saito, T., Major, M. E., Nakazawa, T., Akatsuka, T., Feinstone, S. M., and Berzofsky, J. A. 1999. T cell recognition of hypervariable region-1 from hepatitis C virus envelope protein with multiple class II MHC molecules in mice and humans: preferential help for induction of antibodies to the hypervariable region. *Journal of Immunology* 162:568-576.

Shirai, M., Arichi, T., Nishioka, M., Nomura, T., Ikeda, K., Kawanishi, K., Engelhard,

V. H., Feinstone, S. M., and Berzofsky, J. A. 1995. CTL responses of HLA-A2.1-transgenic mice specific for hepatitis C viral peptides predict epitopes for CTL of humans carrying HLA-A2.1. *Journal of Immunology* 154:2733-2742.

Sigal, L. J., Crotty, S., Andino, R., and Rock, K. L. 1999. Cytotoxic T-cell immunity to virus-infected non-haematopoietic cells requires presentation of exogenous antigen. *Nature* 398:77-80.

Silverman, M., Zieg, J., Hilmen, M., and Simon, M. 1979. Phase variation in *Salmonella:* genetic analysis of a recombinational switch. *Proceedings of the National Academy of Sciences USA* 76:391-395.

Sim, B. C., Aftahi, N., Reilly, C., Bogen, B., Schwartz, R. H., Gascoigne, N. R., and Lo, D. 1998. Thymic skewing of the CD4/CD8 ratio maps with the T-cell receptor alpha-chain locus. *Current Biology* 8:701-704.

Skehel, J. J., Stevens, D. J., Daniels, R. S., Douglas, A. R., Knossow, M., Wilson, I. A., and Wiley, D. C. 1984. A carbohydrate side chain on hemagglutinins of Hong Kong influenza viruses inhibits recognition by a monoclonal antibody. *Proceedings of the National Academcy of Sciences USA* 81:1779-1783.

Skehel, J. J., and Wiley, D. C. 2000. Receptor binding and membrane fusion in virus entry: the influenza hemagglutinin. *Annual Review of Biochemistry* 69:531-569.

Slatkin, M. 1984. Somatic mutations as an evolutionary force. In Greewood, P. J., Harvey, P. H., and Slatkin, M., eds., *Essays in Honor of John Maynard Smith*, pp. 19-30. Cambridge University Press, Cambridge.

Slifka, M. K., Antia, R., Whitmire, J. K., and Ahmed, R. 1998. Humoral immunity due to long-lived plasma cells. *Immunity* 8:363-372.

Smith, D. J., Forrest, S., Ackley, D. H., and Perelson, A. S. 1999. Variable efficacy of repeated annual influenza vaccination. *Proceedings of the National Academy of Sciences USA* 96:14001-14006.

Smith, J. D., Chitnis, C. E., Craig, A. G., Roberts, D. J., Hudson-Taylor, D. E., Peterson, D. S., Pinches, R., Newbold, C. I., and Miller, L. H. 1995. Switches in expression of *Plasmodium falciparum var* genes correlate with changes in antigenic and cytoadherent phenotypes of infected erythrocytes. *Cell* 82:101-110.

Smith, M. R., and Greene, W. C. 1990. Identification of HTLV-I *tax* trans-activator mutants exhibiting novel transcriptional phenotypes. *Genes and Development* 4:1875-1885.

Smith, M. W., Dean, M., Carrington, M., Winkler, C., Huttley, G. A., Lomb, D. A., Goedert, J. J., O'Brien, T. R., Jacobson, L. P., Kaslow, R., et al. 1997. Contrasting genetic influence of CCR2 and CCR5 variants on HIV-1 infection and disease progression. *Science* 277:959-965.

Smith, V. H., and Holt, R. D. 1996. Resource competition and within-host disease dynamics. *Trends in Ecology and Evolution* 11:386-389.

Sniegowski, P. D., Gerrish, P. J., and Lenski, R. E. 1997. Evolution of high mutation rates in experimental populations of *E. coli. Nature* 387:703-705.

Sobrino, F., Sáiz, M., Jiménez-Clavero, M. A., Núñez, J. I., Rosas, M. F., Baranowski,

E., and Ley, V. 2001. Foot-and-mouth disease virus: a long known virus, but a current threat. *Veterinary Research* 32:1–30.

Solé, M., Bantar, C., Indest, K., Gu, Y., Ramamoorthy, R., Coughlin, R., and Philipp, M. T. 1998. *Borrelia burgdorferi* escape mutants that survive in the presence of antiserum to the OspA vaccine are killed when complement is also present. *Infection and Immunity* 66:2540–2546.

Sompayrac, L. M. 1999. *How the Immune System Works.* Blackwell Science, Malden, Massachusetts.

Sonrier, C., Branger, C., Michel, V., Ruvoen-Clouet, N., Ganiere, J. P., and Andre-Fontaine, G. 2000. Evidence of cross-protection within *Leptospira interrogans* in an experimental model. *Vaccine* 15:86–94.

Soudeyns, H., Paolucci, S., Chappey, C., Daucher, M. B., Graziosi, C., Vaccarezza, M., Cohen, O. J., Fauci, A. S., and Pantaleo, G. 1999. Selective pressure exerted by immunodominant HIV-1-specific cytotoxic T lymophocyte responses during primary infection drives genetic variation restricted to the cognate epitope. *European Journal of Immunology* 29:3629–3635.

Sourdive, D. J. D., Murali-Krishna, K., and Altman, J. D. 1998. Conserved T cell receptor repertoire in primary and memory CD8 T cell responses to an acute viral infection. *Journal of Experimental Medicine* 188:71–82.

Spratt, B. G., Bowler, L. D., Zhang, Q.-Y., Zhou, J., and Maynard Smith, J. 1992. Role of interspecies transfer of chromosomal genes in the evolution of penicillin resistance in pathogenic and commensal *Neisseria* species. *Journal of Molecular Evolution* 34:115–125.

Spratt, B. G., and Maiden, M. C. J. 1999. Bacterial population genetics, evolution and epidemiology. *Philosophical Transactions of the Royal Society of London B* 354:701–710.

Spriggs, M. K. 1996. One step ahead of the game: viral immunomodulatory molecules. *Annual Review of Immunology* 14:101–130.

Springer, T. A. 1990. Adhesion receptors of the immune system. *Nature* 346:425–434.

Stalhammar-Carlemalm, M., Areschoug, T., Larsson, C., and Lindahl, G. 2000. Cross-protection between group A and group B streptococci due to cross-reacting surface proteins. *Journal of Infectious Disease* 182:142–149.

Staudt, L. M., and Gerhard, W. 1983. Generation of antibody diversity in the immune response of BALB/c mice to influenza virus hemagglutinin. I. Significant variation in repertoire expression between individual mice. *Journal of Experimental Medicine* 157:687–704.

Stearns, S. C., Ackermann, M., Doebeli, M., and Kaiser, M. 2000. Experimental evolution of aging, growth, and reproduction in fruitflies. *Proceedings of the National Academy of Sciences USA* 97:3309–3313.

Steinhauer, D. A., and Wharton, S. A. 1998. Structure and function of the haemagglutinin. In Nicholson, K. G., Webster, R. G., and Hay, A. J., eds., *Textbook of Influenza*, pp. 54–64. Blackwell Science, Oxford.

Stern, A., Brown, M., Nickel, P., and Meyer, T. F. 1986. Opacity genes in *Neisseria gonorrhoeae:* control of phase and antigenic variation. *Cell* 47:61-71.

Stern, A., and Meyer, T. F. 1987. Common mechanism controlling phase and antigenic variation in pathogenic neisseriae. *Molecular Microbiology* 1:5-12.

Stevenson, P. G., and Doherty, P. C. 1998. Cell-mediated imune response to influenza virus. In Nicholson, K. G., Webster, R. G., and Hay, A. J., eds., *Textbook of Influenza*, pp. 278-287. Blackwell Science, Oxford.

Stoenner, H. G., Dodd, T., and Larsen, C. 1982. Antigenic variation of *Borrelia hermsii. Journal of Experimental Medicine* 156:1297-1311.

Strauss, E. G., Straus, J. H., and Levine, A. J. 1996. Virus evolution. In Fields, B. N., Knipe, D. M., and Howley, P. M., eds., *Fundamental Virology,* 3d ed., pp. 141-159. Lippincott-Raven, Philadelphia.

Su, C., Jakobsen, I., Gu, X., and Nei, M. 1999. Diversity and evolution of T-cell recpetor variable region genes in mammals and birds. *Immunogenetics* 50:301-308.

Su, C., and Nei, M. 1999. Fifty-million-year-old polymorphism at an immunoglobulin variable region gene locus in the rabbit evolutionary lineage. *Proceedings of the National Academy of Sciences USA* 96:9710-9715.

Su, X., Heatwole, V. M., Wertheimer, S. P., Guinet, F., Herrfeldt, J. V., Peterson, D. S., and Ravetch, J. V. W. 1995. A large and diverse gene family (*var*) encodes 200-350 kD proteins implicated in the antigenic variation and cytoadherence of *Plasmodium falciparum*-infected erythrocytes. *Cell* 82:89-100.

Suerbaum, S., Maynard Smith, J., Bapumia, K., Morelli, G., Smith, N. H., Kunstmann, E., Dyrek, I., and Achtman, M. 1998. Free recombination within *Helicobacter pylori. Proceedings of the National Academy of Sciences USA* 95: 12619-12624.

Suzuki, Y., and Gojobori, T. 1999. A method for detecting positive selection at single amino acid sites. *Molecular Biology and Evolution* 16:1315-1328.

Swain, S. L. 1994. Generation and in vivo persistence of polarized Th1 and Th2 memory cells. *Immunity* 1:543-552.

Tada, Y., Hongo, S., Muraki, Y., Sugawara, K., Kitame, F., and Nakamura, K. 1997. Evolutionary analysis of influenza C virus M genes. *Virus Genes* 15:53-59.

Taddei, F., Radman, M., Maynard Smith, J., Toupance, B., Gouyon, P. H., and Godelle, B. 1997. Role of mutator alleles in adaptive evolution. *Nature* 387:700-702.

Taylor, H. P., Armstrong, S. J., and Dimmock, N. J. 1987. Quantitative relationships between an influenza virus and neutralizing antibody. *Virology* 159:288-298.

Terry, C. F., Loukaci, V., and Green, F. R. 2000. Cooperative influence of genetic polymorphisms on interleukin 6 transcriptional regulation. *Journal of Biological Chemistry* 275:18138-18144.

Thomas, D. B., Patera, A. C., Graham, C. M., and Smith, C. A. 1998. Antibody-mediated immunity. In Nicholson, K. G., Webster, R. G., and Hay, A. J., eds., *Textbook of Influenza*, pp. 267-277. Blackwell Science, Oxford.

Thursz, M., Kwiatkowski, D., Allsopp, C. E. M., Greenwood, B. M., Thomas, H. C., and Hill, A. V. S. 1995. Association of an HLA class II allele with clearance of hepatitis B virus infection in The Gambia. *New England Journal of Medicine* 332:1065-1069.

Tibayrenc, M. 1999. Toward an integrated genetic epidemiology of parasitic protozoa and other pathogens. *Annual Review of Genetics* 33:171-191.

Tibayrenc, M., and Ayala, F. J. 1988. Isozyme variability in *Trypanosoma cruzi*, the agent of Chagas' disease: genetical, taxonomical, and epidemiological significance. *Evolution* 42:277-292.

Tibayrenc, M., Kjellberg, F., Arnaud, J., Oury, B., Brenière, S., Dardé, M.-L., and Ayala, F. J. 1991. Are eukaryotic microorganisms clonal or sexual? A population genetics vantage. *Proceedings of the National Academy of Sciences USA* 88:5129-5133.

Tibayrenc, M., Kjellberg, F., and Ayala, F. J. 1990. A clonal theory of parasitic protozoa: the population genetic structure of *Entamoeba, Giardia, Leishmania* and *Trypanosomes,* and its medical and taxonomic consequences. *Proceedings of the National Academy of Sciences USA* 87:2414-2418.

Tibayrenc, M., Ward, P., Moya, A., and Ayala, F. J. 1986. Natural populations of *Trypanosoma cruzi,* the agent of Chagas' disease, have a complex multiclonal structure. *Proceedings of the National Academy of Sciences USA* 83:115-119.

Tissot, A. C., Ciatto, C., Mitti, P. R. E., Grütter, M. G., and Plückthun, A. 2000. Viral escape at the molecular level explained by quantitative T-cell receptor/peptide/MHC interactions and the crystal structure of a peptide/MHC complex. *Journal of Molecular Biology* 302:873-885.

Tortorella, D., Gewurz, B. E., Furman, M. H., Schust, D. J., and Ploegh, H. L. 2000. Viral subversion of the immune system. *Annual Review of Immunology* 18:861-926.

Turner, C. M. R. 1997. The rate of antigenic variation in fly-transmitted and syringe-passaged infections of *Trypanosoma brucei*. *FEMS Microbiology Letters* 153:227-231.

Turner, C. M. R. 1999. Antigenic variation in *Trypanosoma brucei* infections: an holistic view. *Journal of Cell Science* 112:3187-3192.

Turner, C. M. R., Aslam, N., and Angus, S. D. 1996. Inhibition of growth of *Trypanosoma brucei* parasites in chronic infections. *Parasitology Research* 82:61-66.

Turner, C. M. R., and Barry, J. D. 1989. High frequency of antigenic variation in *Trypanosoma brucei rhodesiense* infections. *Parasitology* 99:67-75.

Underwood, P. A. 1982. Mapping of antigenic changes in the haemagglutinin of Hong Kong influenza (H3N2) strains using a large panel of monoclonal antibodies. *Journal of General Virology* 62:153-160.

Underwood, P. A. 1984. An antigenic map of the haemagglutinin of the influenza Hong Kong subtype (H3N2), constructed using mouse monoclonal antibodies. *Molecular Immunology* 21:663-671.

van de Putte, P., Plasterk, R., and Kuijpers, A. 1984. A Mu gin complementing function and an invertible DNA region in *Escherichia coli* K-12 are situated on the genetic element e14. *Journal of Bacteriology* 158:517–522.

van Hattum, J., Schreuder, G. M., and Schalm, S. W. 1987. HLA antigens in patients with various courses after hepatitis B virus infection. *Hepatology* 7:11–14.

van Regenmortel, M. H. V. 1998. From absolute to exquisite specificity: reflections on the fuzzy nature of species, specificity and antigenic sites. *Journal of Immunological Methods* 216:37–48.

van Regenmortel, M. H. V., Altschuh, D., Chatellier, J., Christensen, L., Rauffer-Bruyère, N., Richalet, S., Witz, J., and Zeder-Lutz, G. 1998. Measurement of antigen-antibody interactions with biosensors. *Journal of Molecular Recognition* 11:163–167.

Vickerman, K. 1989. Trypanosome sociology and antigenic variation. *Parasitology* 99:S37–S47.

Vidal, N., Peeters, M., Mulanga-Kabeya, C., Nzilambi, N., Robertson, D., Ilunga, W., Sema, H., Tshimanga, K., Bongo, B., and Delaporte, E. 2000. Unprecedented degree of human immunodeficiency virus type 1 (HIV-1) group M genetic diversity in the Democratic Republic of Congo suggests that the HIV-1 pandemic originated in central Africa. *Journal of Virology* 74:10498–10507.

Vijayakrishnan, L., Kumar, V., Agrewala, A., Mishra, G. C., and Rao, K. V. S. 1994. Antigen-specific early primary humoral responses modulate immunodominance of B cell epitopes. *Journal of Immunology* 153:1613–1625.

Villadangos, J. A., Bryant, R. A. R., Deussing, J., Driessen, C., Lennon-Dumenil, A.-M., Riese, R. J., Roth, W., Saftig, P., Shi, G.-P., Chapman, H. A., Peters, C., and Ploegh, H. L. 1999. Proteases involved in MHC class II antigen presentation. *Immunological Reviews* 172:109–120.

Vincent, R., Louis-Plence, P., Gaillard, F., Clot, J., and Eliaou, J.-F. 1997. Qualitative and quantitative analysis of HLA-DRB gene expression. *Journal of Rheumatology* 24:225–226.

Virji, M., Evans, D., Hadfield, A., Grunert, F., Telxeira, A. M., and Watt, S. M. 1999. Critical determinants of host receptor targeting by *Neisseria meningitidis* and *Neisseria gonorrhoeae:* identification of Opa adhesiotopes on the N-domain of CD66 molecules. *Molecular Microbiology* 34:538–551.

Vogel, T., Kurth, R., and Norley, S. 1994. The majority of neutralizing Abs in HIV-1 infected patients recognize linear V3 loop sequences. *Journal of Immunology* 153:1895–1904.

Volkman, S. K., Barry, A. E., Lyons, E. J., Nielsen, K. M., Thomas, S. M., Choi, M., Thakore, S. S., Day, K. P., Wirth, D. F., and Hartl, D. L. 2001. Recent origin of *Plasmodium falciparum* from a single progenitor. *Science* 293:482–484.

Wakely, J. 1993. Substitution rate variation among sites in hypervariable region I of human mitochondrial DNA. *Journal of Molecular Evolution* 37:613–623.

Walker, G. C. 1984. Mutagenesis and inducible responses to deoxyribonucleic acid damage in *Escherichia coli. Microbiological Reviews* 48:60–93.

Wang, M.-L., Skehel, J. J., and Wiley, D. C. 1986. Comparative analyses of the specificities of anti-influenza hemagglutinin antibodies in human sera. *Journal of Virology* 57:124–128.

Watts, C., and Amigorena, S. 2000. Antigen traffic pathways in dendritic cells. *Traffic* 1:312–317.

Weaver, S. C., Brault, A. C., Kang, W., and Holland, J. J. 1999. Genetic and fitness changes accompanying adaptation of an arbovirus to vertebrate and invertebrate cells. *Journal of Virology* 73:4316–4326.

Weber, J., Fenyo, E.-M., Beddows, S., Kaleebu, P., and Bjorndal, A. 1996. Neutralization serotypes of HIV-1 field isolates are not predicted by genetic subtype. *Journal of Virology* 70:7827–7832.

Webster, R. G., Air, G. M., Metzger, D. W., Colman, P. M., Varghese, J. N., Baker, A. T., and Laver, W. G. 1987. Antigenic structure and variation in an influenza virus N9 neuraminidase. *Journal of Virology* 61:2910–2916.

Webster, R. G., and Bean, W. J. 1998. Evolution and ecology of influenza viruses: interspecies transmission. In Nicholson, K. G., Webster, R. G., and Hay, A. J., eds., *Textbook of Influenza*, pp. 109–119. Blackwell Science, Oxford.

Webster, R. G., Bean, W. J., Gorman, O. T., Chambers, T. M., and Kawaoka, Y. 1992. Evolution and ecology of influenza A viruses. *Microbiological Review* 56:152–179.

Webster, R. G., Brown, L. E., and Laver, W. G. 1984. Antigenic and biological characterization of influenza virus neuraminidase (N2) with monoclonal antibodies. *Virology* 135:30–42.

Webster, R. G., Shortridge, K. F., and Kawaoka, Y. 1997. Influenza: interspecies transmission and emergence of new pandemics. *FEMS Immunology and Medical Microbiology* 18:275–279.

Wedemayer, G. J., Patten, P. A., Wang, L. H., Schultz, P. G., and Stevens, R. C. 1997. Structural insights into the evolution of an antibody combining site. *Science* 276:1665–1669.

Weidt, G., Deppert, W., Utermöhlen, O., Heukeshoven, J., and Lehmann-Grube, F. 1995. Emergence of virus escape mutants after immunization with epitope vaccine. *Journal of Virology* 69:7147–7151.

Weidt, G., Utermöhlen, O., Heukeshoven, J., Lehmann-Grube, F., and Deppert, W. 1998. Relationship among immunodominance of single CD8$^+$ T cell epitopes, virus load, and kinetics of primary antiviral CTL response. *Journal of Immunology* 160:2923–2931.

Wettstein, P. J. 1986. Immunodominance in the T-cell response to multiple non-H-2 histocompatibility antigens. II. Observation of a hierarchy among dominant antigens. *Immunogenetics* 24:24–31.

Wetz, K., Willingmann, P., Zeichhardt, H., and Habermehl, K.-O. 1986. Neutralization of poliovirus by polyclonal antibodies requires binding of a single molecule per virion. *Archives of Virology* 91:207–220.

Whitmire, J. K., Murali-Krishna, K., Altman, J., and Ahmed, R. 2000. Antiviral

CD4 and CD8 T-cell memory: differences in the size of the response and activation requirements. *Philosophical Transactions of the Royal Society of London B* 355:373-379.

Wiley, D. C., Wilson, I. A., and Skehel, J. J. 1981. Structural identification of the antibody-binding sites of Hong Kong influenza haemagglutinin and their involvement in antigenic variation. *Nature* 289:373-378.

Willems, R., Paul, A., van der Heide, H. G. J., ter Avest, A. R., and Mooi, F. R. 1990. Fimbrial phase variation in *Bordetella pertussis:* a novel mechanism for transcriptional regulation. *EMBO Journal* 9:2803-2809.

Wilson, I. A., and Cox, N. J. 1990. Structural basis of immune recognition of influenza virus hemagglutinin. *Annual Review of Immunology* 8:737-771.

Wilson, I. A., Skehel, J. J., and Wiley, D. C. 1981. Structure of the haemagglutinin membrane glycoprotein of influenza virus at 3 Å resolution. *Nature* 289:366-373.

Wodarz, D., and Nowak, M. A. 2000. CD8 memory, immunodominance, and antigenic escape. *European Journal of Immunology* 30:2704-2712.

Wodarz, D., Nowak, M. A., and Bangham, C. R. M. 1999. The dynamics of HTLV-I and the CTL response. *Immunology Today* 20:220-227.

Wohlfart, C. 1988. Neutralization of adenoviruses: kinetics, stoichiometry and mechanisms. *Journal of Virology* 62:2321-2328.

Worobey, M. 2000. Extensive homologous recombination among widely divergent TT viruses. *Journal of Virology* 74:7666-7670.

Worobey, M., and Holmes, E. C. 1999. Evolutionary aspects of recombination in RNA viruses. *Journal of General Virology* 80:2535-2543.

Worobey, M., Rambaut, A., and Holmes, E. C. 1999. Widespread intra-serotype recombination in natural populations of dengue virus. *Proceedings of the National Academy of Sciences USA* 96:7352-7357.

Wren, B. W. 1991. A family of clostridial and streptococcal ligand-binding proteins with conserved C-terminal repeat sequences. *Molecular Microbiology* 5:797-803.

Wright, P. F., and Webster, R. G. 2001. Orthomyxoviruses. In Knipe, D. M., and Howley, P. M., eds., *Fields Virology,* 4th ed., pp. 1533-1579. Lippincott-Raven, Philadelphia.

Wright, S. 1969. *Evolution and the Genetics of Populations.* Vol. 2, *The Theory of Gene Frequencies.* University of Chicago Press, Chicago.

Wright, S. 1978. *Evolution and the Genetics of Populations.* Vol. 4, *Variability within and between Natural Populations.* University of Chicago Press, Chicago.

Wu, J., Longmate, J. A., Adamus, G., Hargrave, P. A., and Wakeland, E. K. 1996. Interval mapping of quantitative trait loci controlling humoral immunity to exogenous antigens. *Journal of Immunology* 157:2498-2505.

Xu, J., Mitchell, T. G., and Vilgalys, R. 1999. PCR-restriction fragment length polymorphism (RFLP) analyses reveal both extensive clonality and local genetic differences in *Candida albicans. Molecular Ecology* 8:59-73.

Yamaguchi-Kabata, Y., and Gojobori, T. 2000. Reevaluation of amino acid variability of the human immunodeficiency virus type 1 gp120 envelope glycoprotein and prediction of new discontinuous epitopes. *Journal of Virology* 74:4335-4350.

Yang, Z. H., and Bielawski, J. P. 2000. Statistical methods for detecting molecular adaptation. *Trends in Ecology and Evolution* 15:496-503.

Yewdell, J. W., and Bennink, J. R. 1999. Immunodominance in major histocompatibility complex class I-restricted T lymphocyte responses. *Annual Review of Immunology* 17:51-88.

Yewdell, J. W., Caton, A. J., and Gerhard, W. 1986. Selection of influenza A adsorptive mutants by growth in the presence of a mixture of monoclonal anti-haemagglutinin antibodies. *Journal of Virology* 57:623-628.

Yewdell, J. W., Webster, R. G., and Gerhard, W. U. 1979. Antigenic variation in three distinct determinants of an influenza type A haemagglutinin molecule. *Nature* 279:246-248.

York, I. A., Goldberg, A. L., Mo, X. Y., and Rock, K. L. 1999. Proteolysis and class I major histocompatibility complex antigen presentation. *Immunological Reviews* 172:49-66.

Yoshida, M. 2001. Multiple viral strategies of HTLV-1 for dysregulation of cell growth control. *Annual Review of Immunology* 19:475-496.

Young, A. C., Zhang, W., Sacchettini, J. C., and Nathenson, S. G. 1994. The three-dimensional structure of H-2Db at 2.4 Å resolution: implications for antigen-determinant selection. *Cell* 76:39-50.

Yusim, K., Peeters, M., Pybus, O. G., Bhattacharya, T., Delaporte, E., Mulanga, C., Muldoon, M., Theiler, J., and Korber, B. 2001. Using human immunodeficiency virus type 1 sequences to infer historical features of the acquired immune deficiency syndrome epidemic and human immunodeficiency virus evolution. *Philosophical Transactions of the Royal Society of London B* 356:855-866.

Zhang, J., Tang, L.-Y., Li, T., Ma, Y., and Sapp, C. M. 2000. Most retroviral recombinations occur during minus-strand DNA synthesis. *Journal of Virology* 74:2313-2322.

Zhou, J., and Spratt, B. G. 1992. Sequence diversity within the *argF, fbp* and *recA* genes of natural isolates of *Neisseria meningitidis*—interspecies recombination within the *argF* gene. *Molecular Microbiology* 6:2135-2146.

Zinkernagel, R. M., Althage, A., Cooper, S., Kreeb, G., Klein, P. A., Sefton, B., Flaherty, L., Stimpfling, J., Shreffler, D., and Klein, J. 1978. Ir-genes in H-2 regulate generation of anti-viral cytotoxic T cells. Mapping to K or D and dominance or unresponsiveness. *Journal of Experimental Medicine* 148:592-606.

Zinkernagel, R. M., Bachmann, M. F., Kündig, T. M., Oehen, S., Pirchet, H., and Hengartner, H. 1996. On immunological memory. *Annual Review of Immunology* 14:333–367.

Zolla-Pazner, S., Gorny, M. K., Nyambi, P. N., VanCott, T. C., and Nádas, A. 1999. Immunotyping of HIV-1: an approach to immunologic classification of HIV. *Journal of Virology* 73:4042–4051.

Author Index

Ishioka, G., 86, 303
Ison, C. A., 156, 283

Jack, N., 164, 276
Jackson, T., 196–99, 280, 285
Jacobson, L. P., 26, 114, 304
Jakobsen, I., 113, 306
Jameel, S., 74, 287
Jameson, S. C., 46, 86, 278, 285
Jamieson, B. D., 84, 285
Janeway, Jr., C. A., 13, 16–17, 20, 53,
    55, 74, 77, 89, 113, 115, 127, 130,
    140, 233, 286
Janitz, M., 117–18, 277
Janssens, W., 67, 183–85, 288,
    295–96
Jarra, W., 65, 298
Jaulin, C., 49, 51, 286, 291
Jeang, K.-T., 240, 303
Jenni, L., 67, 286
Jensen, L. T., 226, 286
Jetzt, A. E., 162, 286
Jiang, H., 237–38, 298
Jiménez-Clavero, M. A., 189–90,
    192–93, 304
Jing, P., 95, 235–36, 241, 270, 279
Johnston, R. E., 197–98, 272, 287
Jones, D. M., 164, 279
Jones, S. E., 132, 215, 288
Jongejan, F., 250–51, 282
Jongeneel, C. V., 51, 53, 112, 291
Jung, G., 46, 295
Jung, H. C., 119, 286
Jyssum, K., 59, 286

Kahmann, R., 64, 286
Kai, C., 162, 281
Kaiser, M., 189, 305
Kalden, J. R., 117, 299
Kaleebu, P., 183, 309
Kalish, M. L., 163, 183, 300
Kam-Morgan, L. N. W., 37, 41–42,
    288
Kamp, D., 64, 286
Kamper, S. M., 66, 271
Kampinga, G., 163, 277
Kang, W., 226, 309

Karabatsos, N., 181, 274, 288
Karlinke, U., 78, 301
Karlsson, K.-A., 216, 292
Kaslow, R., 26, 114, 304
Katlama, C., 240, 302
Katopodis, N. F., 119, 287
Katzer, F., 250–51, 282
Kaverin, N. V., 135, 217, 286, 301
Kawanishi, K., 85, 303
Kawaoka, Y., 67, 147, 159, 208,
    216–17, 219, 276, 286, 291–92,
    309
Keen, J. K., 65, 273
Keitel, T., 37, 286–87
Kennedy, K. E., 64, 285
Kepler, T. B., 117–18, 277
Kerlan-Candon, S., 117–18, 289
Keulen, W., 240, 270
Khanna, R., 85, 274
Khilko, S., 46, 275
Khurana, A., 48, 298
Kilbourne, E. D., 213, 286
Kim, A., 119, 287
Kim, C. Y., 119, 286
Kim, J. M., 119, 286
Kim, K. J., 35, 302
Kimata, J. T., 94–95, 287, 301
Kimura, H., 160, 297
Kimura, M., 149, 151, 246, 277, 287
King, A. M. Q., 196–99, 280, 285
King, G., 46, 295
Kitame, F., 160, 297, 306
Kitten, T., 63, 271
Kjellberg, F., 150, 156, 158, 307
Klarmann, G. J., 162, 286
Klein, J., 82, 170, 296, 311
Klein, P. A., 82, 311
Klenerman, P., 29, 83, 86, 88, 90–91,
    135, 224, 244, 275, 287, 295, 298
Klimstra, W. B., 197–98, 272, 287
Kloetzel, P.-M., 231–32, 272, 296
Knipe, D. M., 58, 92, 130, 287
Knossow, M., 211–13, 273, 280, 304
Knowles, B. B., 82, 278
Knowles, N. J., 196, 199, 254, 283,
    285
Kocher, T. D., 253, 283

Subject Index